Doping in Cycling

Doping in Cycling: Interdisciplinary Perspectives provides an up-to-date overview of the knowledge about doping and anti-doping in the sport that has dominated doping headlines for at least two decades. It critically addresses overarching questions related to doping and anti-doping, and topical issues being raised in the agenda of policy-makers at the global level.

The book features cross-disciplinary contributions from international leading scholars in sports sociology, history, philosophy, psychology and criminology, and even beyond human and social sciences. Split into three parts (the use and supply of doping products; threats on cycling and opportunities for anti-doping; and issues, controversies, and stakes), it covers topics such as changing patterns of drug use in professional cycling, the impact of scientific advances on doping in cycling, whether cycling teams can prevent doping, whistleblowing on doping in cycling, and how to improve the credibility of the sport.

This is a vital resource for researchers, students, policy-makers, anti-doping organisations and sports federations, and an important read for anyone involved in elite cycling.

Bertrand Fincoeur is Senior Researcher at the Institute of Sports Sciences at the University of Lausanne, Switzerland.

John Gleaves is Associate Professor of Kinesiology at the California State University, Fullerton, USA.

Fabien Ohl is Full Professor of Sociology of Sport at the University of Lausanne, Switzerland.

Ethics and Sport

Series editors

Mike McNamee
University of Wales Swansea
Jim Parry
University of Leeds

The *Ethics and Sport* series aims to encourage critical reflection on the practice of sport, and to stimulate professional evaluation and development. Each volume explores new work relating to philosophical ethics and the social and cultural study of ethical issues. Each is different in scope, appeal, focus, and treatment but a balance is sought between local and international focus, perennial and contemporary issues, level of audience, teaching and research application, and variety of practical concerns.

Recent titles include:

Body Ecology and Emersive Leisure
Edited by Bernard Andrieu, Jim Parry, Alessandro Porrovecchio and Olivier Sirost

Sport, Ethics and Philosophy
Edited by Mike McNamee

Philosophy and Nature Sports
Kevin Krein

Emotion in Sports
Philosophical Perspectives
Yunus Tuncel

Sport, Ethics, and Neurophilosophy
Jeffrey Fry and Mike McNamee

Doping in Cycling
Interdisciplinary Perspectives
Edited by Bertrand Fincoeur, John Gleaves and Fabien Ohl

For a complete series list please visit: www.routledge.com/Ethics-and-Sport/book-series/EANDS

Doping in Cycling

Interdisciplinary Perspectives

Edited by Bertrand Fincoeur,
John Gleaves and Fabien Ohl

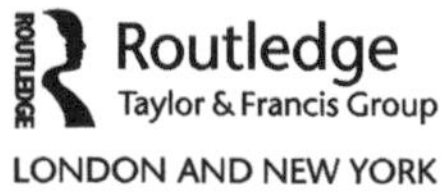

LONDON AND NEW YORK

First published 2019
by Routledge
2 Park Square, Milton Park, Abingdon, Oxon OX14 4RN

and by Routledge
52 Vanderbilt Avenue, New York, NY 10017

First issued in paperback 2020

Routledge is an imprint of the Taylor & Francis Group, an informa business

British Library Cataloguing-in-Publication Data
A catalogue record for this book is available from the British Library

Library of Congress Cataloging-in-Publication Data
A catalog record has been requested for this book

ISBN 13: 978-0-367-66385-8 (pbk)
ISBN 13: 978-1-138-47790-2 (hbk)

Typeset in Goudy
by Wearset Ltd, Boldon, Tyne and Wear

Contents

Figures

Tables

Contributors

Reid Aikin manages the Athlete Biological Passport (ABP) at the World Anti-Doping Agency. He has a BSc in Biochemistry and PhD in Surgical Research from McGill University, followed by a postdoctoral fellowship at the University of Nice. He is an avid cycling fan and has participated, albeit poorly, in regional road and MTB events for over 20 years.

Andrew Bloodworth is a Senior Lecturer in the School of Sports and Exercise Science at Swansea University. His research interests are in the field of applied ethics, related to sport policy and health. He has published research exploring athletes' attitudes toward doping, anti-doping policy, and eating disorders in elite sport. Andrew is a fellow of the higher education academy, and has taught applied ethics in healthcare, as well as in a sporting context.

Ask Vest Christiansen is an Associate Professor of sport science in the Department of Public Health at Aarhus University (AU). He is the co-director of the International Network of Doping Research (INDR). His research has followed two main branches: doping in elite sport and recreational athletes' use of drugs in fitness and strength training environments.

Luke Cox is a PhD student in the Applied Sports Technology Exercise and Medicine Research Centre within the School of Sport and Exercise Sciences at Swansea University. His current work and PhD span the realms of ethics, doping, anti-doping policy, and policy solutions.

Paul Dimeo is an Associate Professor in the Faculty of Health Sciences and Sport at the University of Stirling. His main areas of research interest and expertise relate to drug use in sport and anti-doping policy. He authored numerous publications on doping and anti-doping. Recently, he published *The Anti-Doping Crisis in Sport: Causes, Consequences, Solutions* (with Verner Møller, 2018).

Matt Englar-Carlson is a Professor of Counselling and Director and Founder of the Center for Boys and Men at California State University – Fullerton. His scholarly interest in sport focuses on how positive psychology intersects with masculinity, including the application of strength-based approaches to understanding how we view athletes, their behaviour, and how athletes themselves find positivity within their sport.

Kelsey Erickson is a Senior Research Fellow in the Institute for Sport, Physical Activity and Leisure (ISPAL) at Leeds Beckett University. Her expertise is in the psychology of drugs in sport and she is particularly interested in developing an understanding of the psychosocial factors that influence performance-enhancing drug use. Her research agenda also explores the issue of whistleblowing on doping and seeks to ascertain the determinants of the behaviour.

Raphaël Faiss is an Exercise Physiologist with specific expertise in altitude training and cycling. Former cycle messenger world champion (2003, 2004, and 2006), elite cyclist (2008–2010), and scientific advisor to the Swiss cycling national teams (track, road, and MTB) (2014–2016), he is currently research manager of the Research and Expertise in anti-Doping sciences (REDs) of the University of Lausanne.

Bertrand Fincoeur is a Senior Researcher at the Institute of Sports Sciences of the University of Lausanne. He obtained his PhD in criminology at the University of Leuven. He received the 2018 Young Researcher Award of the French-speaking International Society of Criminology (AICLF). His research focuses on controversial issues in sports (doping and anti-doping, football hooliganism).

John Gleaves is an Associate Professor of Kinesiology at the California State University, Fullerton. He currently serves as the co-director for the International Network for Doping Research and associate editor for the journal Performance Enhancement and Health. He also serves on the USA Cycling Anti-Doping Advisory Committee, the WADA Working Group on Prevalence, and as an expert witness in the US government's lawsuit against Lance Armstrong.

April Henning is a Lecturer in the Faculty of Health Sciences and Sport at the University of Stirling. Her research focuses on the intersections of health, substance use, and sport policy, with a special focus on amateur endurance athletes.

Bengt Kayser is a Full Professor at the Faculty of Biology and Medicine, and Director of the Institute of Sports Sciences, University of Lausanne. He authored numerous publications on doping and anti-doping. He also holds a PhD in Kinesiology from the University of Leuven: 'Ethical Aspects of Doping and Anti-Doping: In Search of an Alternative Policy' (2018).

Michael McNamee is a Professor of Applied Ethics at Swansea University. He is Program Chair of the Erasmus Mundus Joint Master Degree in Sport Ethics and Integrity (MAiSI). A former President of the International Association of the Philosophy of Sport, he has published widely in the ethics of sports. He is also founding editor of Sport, Ethics and Philosophy.

Fabien Ohl is a Full Professor of the Sociology of Sport at the University of Lausanne. He received mandates to study and prevent doping from organisations such as WADA, OFSP (Federal Health Office), SNSF (Swiss National Science Foundation), and UCI. He is also involved in education, analysing doping in a course at the University of Lausanne, but also thanks to a MOOC in French and in English (www.coursera.org/learn/doping/).

Letizia Paoli is a Full Professor of Criminology at the University of Leuven Faculty of Law and a life member at Clare Hall, University of Cambridge. In 2016 she was awarded the Thorsten Sellin & Sheldon and Eleanor Glueck Award by the American Society of Criminology for her 'contributions to international criminology' and the Distinguished Scholar Award of the International Association for the Study of Organized Crime.

Werner Pitsch is a Senior Researcher and Lecturer for the Department for Sociology and Economics of Sports at the Institute for Sport Sciences at Saarland University. He has conducted several studies on the prevalence of doping in elite and amateur sports as well as investigations into the quality and the unintended social consequences of the current anti-doping policy.

Flora Plassard is a PhD student in Sociology of Sport at the University of Lausanne. Her study focuses on women elite cycling. She tries to understand the link between confidence relationships and power relations in this sport.

Martial Saugy is a Biologist and Professor in Anti-Doping Sciences. Co-founder of the Swiss Laboratory for Doping Analyses in Lausanne (1990), Director of the Laboratory from 2002 to 2016, he initiated the blood test in cycling in 1997, then the athlete biological passport in 2008. He is currently director of the Research and Expertise in anti-Doping sciences (REDs) of the University of Lausanne.

Lucie Schoch is a Sports Sociologist and Senior Lecturer at the University of Lausanne. Her research focuses on the production of sports news and its content, with a specific interest for sports journalism.

Pierre-Edouard Sottas is a Senior Advisor for the Athlete Biological Passport (ABP) at the World Anti-Doping Agency (WADA). After seven years in the development of the ABP programme at the Laboratory for Doping Analyses (LAD, Lausanne), he joined WADA in 2010 to manage the implementation and use of this programme worldwide. He holds a MSc in Physics, a MSc in Biology and a PhD in Life Sciences (EPFL, Lausanne).

Marjolaine Viret, PhD, is a Swiss-qualified attorney specialising in sports and life sciences, and a researcher at the University of Neuchâtel. Her interests focus on interdisciplinary approaches to regulation in anti-doping and other science-based domains. She is the author of the book 'Evidence in Anti-Doping at the Intersection of Science & Law' (T.M.C. Asser/Springer, 2016).

Ivan Waddington is a Visiting Professor at the Norwegian School of Sport Sciences. His books include *Sport, Health and Drugs* (2000), *Pain and Injury in Sport* (with Sigmund Loland and Berit Skirstad, 2006), *An Introduction to Drugs in Sport* (with Andy Smith, 2009) and the *Routledge Handbook of Drugs and Sport* (with Verner Møller and John Hoberman, 2015).

Acknowledgements

The authors would like to warmly thank the Swiss National Science Foundation (SNSF) for the grants 'Cycling culture, organisations and doping' and 'SNSF 100017_166236 Team organization & riders' vulnerability: Their impact on doping use in elite road cycling'. These research grants have supported our research project on doping in cycling, and the subsequent workshop that resulted in this book, at the Institute of Sports Sciences of the University of Lausanne.

We are also very grateful to Mike McNamee, for his enthusiastic reaction about this book proposal, and to Rebecca Connor, at Routledge, for her amazing assistance throughout the whole publication process.

Introduction

Bertrand Fincoeur, John Gleaves, and Fabien Ohl

In September 2017, experts from various disciplines gathered in Lausanne for a two-day workshop to share and discuss their research into doping in cycling. Funded by the Swiss National Science Foundation, the collection of experts included representatives from sporting organisations as well as academics representing the social sciences, natural sciences, and the humanities. This book is one of the main outcomes of that workshop. It focuses on doping and anti-doping *in cycling*, and the reasons for that are twofold. First, there is good evidence that the history of cycling is intertwined with that of performance-enhancing drugs. Given such a history, we hypothesised that cycling could provide a benchmark allowing scholars to better measure and analyse the development of doping culture, its use and supply among athletes, and the effects of anti-doping policies in other sports. Second, the repeated doping scandals that occurred in cycling, first in the 1960s and more intensely since the late 1990s, have generated significant scholarly interest in doping within the sport. However, given the cross-disciplinary nature of doping and anti-doping, such scholarship often existed isolated from work developed in other disciplines or published in other fields. Indeed, until now, no book has systematically examined doping and anti-doping issues in cycling from various disciplines ranging from sports sociology, history, philosophy, psychology or criminology, and even beyond human and social sciences. This monograph, *Doping in Cycling: Interdisciplinary Perspectives*, provides an up-to-date overview of the knowledge about doping and anti-doping in the sport that has dominated doping headlines for at least two decades. Based on contributions from international leading scholars, this book critically addresses overarching questions related to doping and anti-doping, and very topical issues being raised in the agenda of policy-makers at the global level.

In this introduction, we briefly elaborate on two aspects that have underpinned the motives for this book: the intertwinement between doping and cycling, and the added value of interdisciplinary perspectives to analyse this relation.

The intertwined relationship between doping and cycling

Devoting a book to the doping phenomenon in cycling is not a zero-risk enterprise. Some might dismiss it as an over-studied topic with nothing new to offer. Others might point out that such attention only reinforces the feeling shared by numerous stakeholders that cycling continues to receive more than its share of negative attention for its doping past, especially from the media, public authorities, and, as matter of fact, academic researchers. Indeed, the illegal use of performance-enhancing drugs (PED) obviously extends to sports other than cycling, as evidenced repeatedly by the number of scandals pertaining to athletics, combat sports, American baseball, and weightlifting. Should one search hard enough, they could certainly find a past anti-doping rule violation in every single Olympic sport. Finally, critics might question whether such a topic, with its political and ideological baggage, can ever represent the breadth of views while treating diverging perspectives fairly.

In various respects, we can accept this criticism. In fact, they were on the forefront of our minds from the outset. We can understand that riders, sports directors, team physicians, managers, and soigneurs are fed up with requests from researchers to talk about doping. Although doping in cycling is obviously not eradicated, cycling has made significant efforts to address this issue. Cycling has also arguably conducted the most in-depth introspection into its doping past. This airing of its dirty laundry has provided ample evidence to sift through. Indeed, it is precisely because cycling was under such intense scrutiny that such a book might be worth reading, not only for those wishing to better understand doping in cycling but also those wishing to understand its lessons for other sports. With this work, scholars, students, journalists, and curious publicans draw some lessons from cycling's development of a complicated body of doping practices and the various efforts made to modify them.

So, what do we know about doping and anti-doping in cycling, and what can this book add to the existing knowledge?

Reports are known of riders using stimulants at six-day races, often in an amateurish way, as early as in the late nineteenth century (Dimeo, 2007; Gleaves, 2011). In the first part of the twentieth century, the use of PED in sport in general, and in cycling in particular, was not subject to intense policy debate (Houlihan, 2002) but it had become commonplace in the peloton, and many riders saw little problem with admitting they used enhancers (Heijmans & Mallon, 2011). Prior to World War II, professional cyclists often employed alcohol, opium, or cocaine as antidotes to the unnatural fatigue that came with their extreme efforts. For example, professional cyclists viewed doping as *faire le métier* (to 'do their job') or support for their *rendement* ('productivity' or 'output') (Thompson, 2008).

Cycling's doping culture started to change after the alleged amphetamines-related (Møller, 2005) death of the Danish rider Knud Enemark Jensen during the 1960 Olympics. Cycling found itself in a reluctant role pioneering the development of anti-doping policies in professional sport. While the UCI carried out its first anti-doping tests in 1965, its riders' reaction was strong and five riders refused to be tested at the 1966 World Championships (Christiansen, 2010). Months earlier, French legend Jacques Anquetil led riders in a protest against the drug testing at the 1966 Tour de France (Thompson, 2008). Reports that amphetamines had been found in the autopsy of British rider Tom Simpson after his death during the 1967 Tour de France (Mignon, 2003) put further pressure on sports organisations and public governing bodies to regulate doping (Hunt, 2011). The new anti-doping policies entering cycling did little to slow the sport's flourishing doping culture. New drugs including testosterone and later blood transfusions and erythropoietin proved more effective. These product's spread throughout professional cycling burst into the public's view following the 1998 Tour de France. Known as the Festina Affair, French custom officers discover a haul of doping products in a Festina cycling car, one of the most important elite teams at that time. This scandal brought various revelations following the aftermath of the 1998 season (e.g. Bassons, 2000; Menthéour, 1999; Voet, 2001) and exposed the degree that professional cycling teams had systematised their doping practices.

The Festina affair could have been a turning point in the sport's history. Yet evidence suggests that riders did not stop using illegal enhancers. The period between the 1998 Tour de France and the early 2010s witnessed repeated scandals involving various teams and riders (e.g. Blitz, 2001; Oil for Drugs, 2004; Cofidis, 2004; Puerto, 2006; Via Col Doping, 2008; Armstrong, 2012). This list is far from being exhaustive but does indicate why cycling remains the sport most closely linked to doping in the public's imagination (López, 2015). At the same time period, social scientists also started to document extensively the widespread culture of tolerance towards doping in cycling (Brissonneau, 2007; Christiansen, 2005; Hoberman, 2003; Schneider, 2006; Waddington, 2009). Alongside this research, former riders and staff created a cottage industry out of tell-all books that confirmed what everyone suspected: cycling remained seriously contaminated (e.g. Gaumont, 2005; D'Hont, 2007; Hamilton & Coyle, 2012). But are there any peculiarities of cycling?

In some regards, cycling had unique features that made doping a particularly stubborn problem. Compared to other international sports federations, the UCI has always been a rather weak organisation with limited financial means and limited power compared to race organisers and teams (Aubel & Ohl, 2015; Van Reeth & Larson, 2015). Whereas international federations for sports such as football and athletics run their own events, most of cycling's premier events are not organised by the UCI. The UCI also does control the television rights for most of their events. Additionally, UCI, teams and riders may have struggled to protect themselves against the doping allegations. In particular, they took quite paradoxical positions.

Cycling's repeated doping scandals seriously threatened the sports image and economic model throughout the 2000s. At the same time, the sport actually adopted a prominent role in the development of the current anti-doping regime. The UCI was the first international federation to conduct anti-doping tests to detect EPO (2001), and to introduce the use of the Athlete Biological Passport (ABP) back in 2008. However, not only were several teams and riders still involved in doping offences, but being an early adopter of anti-doping measures meant it drew even more attention to its doping issues. For example, during the first three years that the UCI used its ABP, 20 of the 26 riders found to be using EPO were identified through their abnormal blood profile leading to a targeted doping test and transparency. The ABP also generated unwanted headlines for cycling when two riders, Franco Pellizotti and Pietro Caucchioli, appealed their ABP cases to the Court of Arbitration for Sport. Even though the UCI won, such incidents ensured cycling garnered more attention for its doping history. And despite its efforts, critics still reminded audiences that the sport had remained complicit by hushing up its doping practices for far too long (Marty, Nicholson, & Haas, 2015).

Yet, despite various scandals in cycling's 'nonlinear' movement to clean up the sport (Dimeo, 2014; Hardie, 2011; Smith, 2017), evidence suggests numerous changes within elite cycling over the last two decades have made progress. From an institutional perspective, the Cycling Anti-Doping Foundation (CADF), an independent anti-doping entity established in 2008, provided the UCI with much needed oversight and credibility. Its development may have opened a new era for the management of the doping issue by the sports organisations. Importantly, the use of PEDs is no longer a silently accepted behaviour, and numerous riders and people active within the cycling (at least officially) increasingly condemn the practices that use to define the sport (Ohl, Fincoeur, Lentillon-Kaestner, Defrance, & Brissonneau, 2015; Smith, 2017; Waddington & Smith, 2009). Accordingly, the patterns of use and supply are not similar to those which ruled elite cycling well into the twenty-first century (Fincoeur, van de Ven, & Mulrooney, 2014). While the cycling culture is not homogeneous and there are different attitudes towards doping among cycling actors, any ongoing doping practices occur in secret, including to insiders. As a result, the existing cultural paradigm and structural theories cannot fully explain why some riders are dopers, and others are not. Indeed, while the environment has become much less conducive to doping, the interaction between the cycling teams' culture and the individual propensity to use or avoid illegal doping products could be increasingly determinant. Considering the history of doping in cycling, this is not a minor evolution. For sure, doping has been an output of the cycling culture. And just as sure, doping today occurs in a specific context that needs further investigation. Thus, scholars must devote more attention to theoretical frameworks that integrate the person–setting interaction. Such frameworks will help better understand and analyse how changes in the riders' social environment may increase their agency and impact their individual behaviour. Such a task is obviously a seminal debate in social sciences. We hope that this book, with its various contributions, provides some new insights to feed this discussion and go beyond the existing knowledge.

While studying the intertwined relationship between doping and cycling, one should, however, not look at the evolution of this relation through rose-tinted glasses. Indeed, in spite of fewer individual doping cases at the elite level, several side effects arising from the current situation deserve attention. In particular, each victory still garners some degree of suspicion. Cycling's tarnished credibility also fuels speculation about mechanical doping. At the same time, many still consider factions within amateur and masters' cycling rife with doping practices, which further challenges the precarious credibility of cycling and raises similar questions for the evolution of sport and anti-doping in general. Addressing these issues was thus also an objective of the present book.

The added value of interdisciplinary perspectives

In Gary Marx's introduction to his book about police in the US, the author wrote that 'much of the literature on controversial police topics breaks down into two categories: uncritical work by well-informed insiders and critical work by uninformed outsiders' (Marx, 1988: xiii). Can this statement be transposed to other research areas, such as doping studies? Importantly, can we find ways to perform an analysis that is both well-informed *and* critical? Doping-related research may struggle to rely on insider's shared knowledge since it concerns a sensitive topic that presents serious risks meaning that data collection about doping practices always faces social desirability bias. This presents risks that any conclusions on doping and anti-doping may not be explicitly grounded in empirical data. In contrast, researchers who have privileged access to first-hand data thanks to their relationship with certain anti-doping or sport institutions may equally run the risk of uncritically (and unintentionally?) adopting the official standpoints from the organisations regarding doping issues. This raises several important questions for (anti-)doping researchers about their collaborations with sports organisations or analyses on cultural changes. Precisely, what is the role of (social) scientists when it comes to doping practices? Are social scientists supposed to help transform sports organisations or individual behaviours? Can social scientists remain critical when their research receives funds or commissions from a sports organisation or a public governing body? How do even scholars produce well-informed knowledge on a very sensitive topic like doping? We expect that interdisciplinary perspectives help answer these questions.

Inviting authors from various scientific disciplines and institutional backgrounds to share their knowledge on the topic of this book may be considered as a means to overcome unfertile oppositions. However, beyond the existing variance between the theoretical and methodological approaches from the different scientific disciplines, we may identify two trends in doping-related research. First, many researchers do not fundamentally contest the existing grounds of anti-doping policies. Since they share most of the current objectives of anti-doping policies, they can see various reasons for which scientists can cooperate with sports organisations to better prevent doping (e.g. Aubel & Ohl, 2014; Backhouse, Patterson & McKenna, 2012; Loland, 2018; McNamee, 2012; Overbye, 2018; Petroczi, Norman, & Brueckner, 2017). These researchers may also express less scepticism about the outcomes of anti-doping policy. Second, other researchers tend to contest (part of) the existing grounds of the current global anti-doping regime. They then suggest rethinking several rules of the play while expressing doubts about the effectiveness of anti-doping policy. Much of this literature argues, in fact, that anti-doping policy has primarily been a failure since its inception, not least because it has been costly, precariously grounded in loose notions of sports ethics, and detrimental to athletes' privacy, all for poor results, which is therefore suggestive of an alternative framework to ongoing policies (e.g. Dimeo & Møller, 2018; Fincoeur, van de Ven, & Mulrooney, 2014; Hunt, Dimeo, & Jedlicka, 2012; Kayser & Tolleneer, 2017; Pitsch, 2009; Savulescu, 2015; Stewart & Smith, 2014; Waddington, Christiansen, Gleaves, Hoberman, & Møller, 2013).

Despite different appraisals of doping and anti-doping, the decision-making process may benefit from the various researchers' standpoints. Whether it concerns policy translatable research, such as new avenues or best practices of doping prevention, or critical stances encouraging organisations to rethink or reorient their current anti-doping policy, social scientists all seek to offer new insights on doping and anti-doping. Social sciences can be used as a resource to unveil the hidden structures of power and domination (e.g. Bourdieu, 1984). This is in line with a conception of social sciences based on the assumption that social sciences have liberating virtues. As a consequence, social science researchers focusing on doping and anti-doping may desire that their research helps social actors shape critical and more distant approaches to the issue. Social sciences may, however, struggle to spontaneously permeate the decision-making process from sports organisations and public governing bodies. This book, therefore, provides an opportunity to bridge the gap between academic scholars from various disciplines, and policy-makers. This raises two comments.

First, following Becker's (1998) idea to convey social actors to appropriate sociology that enables them to analyse their own culture, the assumption that social scientists are likely to provide the best solutions to problems of anti-doping actors is questionable. There is a risk here that social scientists act as 'moral entrepreneurs' (Becker, 1963), who can judge how anti-doping organisations should function. This may explain why social scientists are not always welcome in sports organisations while addressing (anti-)doping issues. In addition, the distinction between researchers and ordinary social actors is criticised by Callon (1984: 196) for whom social sciences' goal may not be to bring the truth but to 'faithfully restore the existing points of view to their places and, in addition, they rightly abstain from taking sides'. In line with the so-called 'pragmatic sociologists', researchers should then support a principle of agnosticism. It means an impartiality between actors engaged in a controversy, and a commitment for research to value all the viewpoints, which means to treat a researcher's gaze as one of the viewpoints. Such a definition of a social scientist's role (Latour, 1999) has been quite successful in the sociology of knowledge but also criticised because it pretends that 'all theories have the same credibility, but it doesn't' (Bloor, 1999: 133).

Second, anti-doping organisations and actors, often guided by beliefs in 'clean sport', may struggle to accurately grasp the limits and merits of anti-doping. Academic scholars may provide ideas to improve anti-doping and prevent doping (Aubel & Ohl, 2014; Backhouse et al., 2014), or to think out of the box to radically change it (e.g. Kayser, Mauron, & Miah, 2007; Savulescu, 2015). However, researchers' agenda is different, and that is a common mistake to believe that actors from sport and anti-doping organisations have the same conditions and tools to be reflexive and express it publicly. Many of them may not debate such sensitive issues as easily as academics because they face more constraints. Indeed, their words are scrutinised by journalists and the public, as well as their own organisation, for any deviation from the official positions. Although social scientists can provide tools and resources to critically analyse topics such as the grounds or the effectiveness of anti-doping programmes, policy-makers often face a lack of time, social sciences' knowledge and/or independence when embedded into, and confronted to, the dominant belief.

However, instead of an opposition between policy-makers and academics, we rather believe in the virtues of a dynamic process: academic scholars have much to learn from sports organisations, and anti-doping policy-makers would benefit from better integrating researchers' insights in their own reflections on policy developments. This then acknowledges the idea of 'linked ecologies' (Abbott, 2005) between the scholarly community and the public and sports organisations. The interdisciplinary perspectives presented in this book combined with the mixing of academic scholars and representatives of anti-doping organisations then rely on the idea that social scientists can give room to the diversity of the points of view, and address the various contradictions and controversies.

Structure of this book

This book comprises three parts and 17 chapters.

Part I consists of six chapters which all deal with the use and supply of doping substances and methods (hereinafter referred to as doping products). It is appropriate to start with this part because the use and supply of doping products are the core issues in doping and anti-doping research. This first part intends to answer the question: how does doping and/or anti-doping look in 2018, two decades after the Festina scandal and various changes in anti-doping policies? It addresses the changes in doping use in both elite and recreational cycling. It also concerns the issue of prevalence from both a social science and forensic science perspective. Finally, it focuses on an increasing concern for anti-doping policy-makers, which is the supply chains of doping products.

Part II comprises six chapters and addresses several threats and opportunities that are raised by the development of doping and anti-doping at a global level. It therefore answers the question: what could doping and/or anti-doping in cycling look like in the near future? In particular, this chapter addresses the (to some extent already current) threats of mechanical doping and misuse of therapeutic use exemptions. Four opportunities for anti-doping policy are then presented and critically discussed: the role of cycling teams in doping prevention, the contribution of whistleblowing in deterring doping in cycling, the use of a 'performance passport' to complement the Athlete Biological Passport approach, and the out-of-the-box proposal to rethink the anti-doping regime.

Part III comprises five chapters and concerns issues, controversies, and stakes that cross doping and anti-doping in cycling. These chapters cover important issues for the cycling culture, in particular: how the credibility of cycling is threatened, the role of the media, the focus on clean cyclists, and the ethical and juridical grounds of anti-doping, including the ways to minimise its collateral damages.

This book thus aims at documenting the changes and the challenging issues related to doping in cycling thanks to contributions of well-informed and critical scholarly researchers and policy-makers. Obviously, it by no means warrants that their various conclusions are uncontroversial. There is a large discrepancy between the methodological approaches, theoretical backgrounds, and various scientific disciplines adopted by the 17 authors of this book. Not unsurprisingly, different chapters then sometimes end up with very different conclusions about doping in general, and anti-doping policies in particular. We do not see it as a problem since this simply indicates that debate and disagreement are a normal part of sciences. We therefore invite each reader, whether he is a scholar, a policy-maker, a student, an athlete or a cycling fan, to critical reading and further discussion.

References

Abbott, A. (2005). Linked ecologies: States and universities as environments for professions. *Sociological Theory, 23*(3), 245–274.

Aubel, O. & Ohl, F. (2014). An alternative approach to the prevention of doping in cycling. *International Journal of Drug Policy, 25*(6), 1094–1102.

Aubel, O. & Ohl, F. (2015). De la précarité des coureurs cyclistes professionnels aux pratiques de dopage. *Actes de la recherche en sciences sociales, 209*, 28–41.

Backhouse, S., Collins, C., Defoort, Y., McNamee, M., Parkinson, A., Sauer, M., … Hauw, D. (2014). *Study on doping prevention: A map of legal, regulatory and prevention practice provisions in EU 28.*

Backhouse, S., Patterson, L., & McKenna, J. (2012). Achieving the Olympic ideal: Preventing doping in sport. *Performance Enhancement & Health, 1*(2), 83–85.

Bassons, C. (2000). *Positif.* Paris: Stock.

Becker, H.S. (1963). *Outsiders: Studies in the sociology of deviance.* New York: The Free Press of Glencoe.

Becker, H.S. (1998). *Tricks of the Trade: How to Think About Your Research While You're Doing it*. Chicago: University of Chicago Press.
Bloor, D. (1999). Reply to Bruno Latour. *Studies in History and Philosophy of Science*, *30*, 131–138.
Bourdieu, P. (1984). *Distinction: A Social Critique of the Judgement of Taste*. Cambridge: Harvard University Press.
Brissonneau, C. (2007). Le dopage dans le cyclisme professionnel au milieu des années 1990: une reconstruction des valeurs sportives. *Déviance et Société*, *31*(2), 129–148.
Callon, M. (1984). Some elements of a sociology of translation: domestication of the scallops and the fishermen of St Brieuc Bay. *The Sociological Review*, *32*, 196–233.
Christiansen, A.V. (2005). The Legacy of Festina: Patterns of Drug Use in European Cycling Since 1998. *Sports in History*, *25*(3), 497–514.
Christiansen, A.V. (2010). 'We are not sportsmen, we are professionals': professionalism, doping and deviance in elite sport. *International Journal of Sport Management and Marketing*, *7*(1/2), 91–103.
Dimeo, P. (2007). *A History of Drug Use in Sport, 1876–1976: Beyond Good and Evil*. London: Routledge.
Dimeo, P. (2014). Why Lance Armstrong? Historical context and key turning points in the 'Cleaning Up' of professional cycling. *The International Journal of the History of Sport*, *31*(8), 951–968.
Dimeo, P. & Møller, V. (2018). *The Anti-Doping Crisis in Sport*. London: Routledge.
Fincoeur, B., van de Ven, K., & Mulrooney, K. (2014). The symbiotic evolution of anti-doping and supply chains of doping substances: How criminal networks may benefit from anti-doping policy. *Trends in Organized Crime*, *17*, 1–22.
Gaumont, P. (2005). *Prisonnier du Dopage*. Paris: Grasset.
Gleaves, J. (2011). Doped professionals and clean amateurs: Amateurism's influence on the modern philosophy of anti-doping. *Journal of Sport History*, 38(2), 237–254.
Hamilton, T. & Coyle, D. (2012). *The Secret Race: Inside the Hidden World of the Tour de France: Doping, Cover-ups, and Winning at All Costs*. New York: Bantam.
Hardie, M. (2011). It's not about the blood! Operación Puerto and the end of modernity. In M. McNamee & V. Møller (Eds), *Doping and Anti-Doping Policy in Sport: Ethical Legal and Social Perspectives* (pp. 160–182). London: Routledge.
Heijmans, J. & Mallon, B. (2011). *Historical Dictionary of Cycling*. Plymouth: The Scarecrow Press.
Hoberman, J. (2003). 'A pharmacy on wheels': Doping and community cohesion among professional cyclists following the Tour de France scandal of 1998. In V. Møller & J. Nauright (Eds), *The Essence of Sport* (pp. 107–127). Odense: University of Southern Denmark Press.
Houlihan, B. (2002). *Dying to Win: Doping in Sport and the Development of Anti-doping Policy*. Strasbourg: Council of Europe Publishers.
Hunt, T. (2011). *Drug games: The International Olympic Committee and the Politics of Doping, 1960–2008*. Austin: University of Texas Press.
Hunt, T., Dimeo, P., & Jedlicka, S. (2012). The historical roots of today's problems: a critical appraisal of the international anti-doping movement. *Performance Enhancement & Health*, *1*, 55–60.
Kayser, B. & Tolleneer, J. (2017). Ethics of a relaxed anti-doping rule accompanied by harm-reduction measures. *Journal of Medical Ethics*, 43, 282.

Kayser, B., Mauron, A., & Miah, A. (2007). Current anti-doping policy: a critical appraisal. *BMC Medical Ethics*, *8*(1), 2.

Latour, B. (1999). For David Bloor … and beyond: A reply to David Bloor's anti-latour. *Studies in History and Philosophy of Science*, *30*, 113–130.

Loland, S. (2018). Performance-enhancing drugs, sport, and the ideal of natural athletic performance. *The American Journal of Bioethics*, *18*(6), 8–15.

Marty, D., Nicholson, D., & Haas, U. (2015). *Report to the President of the Union Cycliste Internationale*. Lausanne: Cycling Independent Reform Commission.

Marx, G. (1988). *Undercover: Police Surveillance in America*. Berkeley: University of California Press.

McNamee, M.J. (2012). The spirit of sport and the medicalisation of anti-doping: Empirical and normative ethics. *Asian Bioethics Review*, *4*(4), 374–392.

Menthéour, E. (1999). *Secret défonce. Ma vérité sur le dopage*. Paris: Lattès.

Mignon, P. (2003). The Tour de France and the doping issue. *The International Journal of the History of Sport*, *20*(2), 227–245.

Møller, V. (2005). Knud Enemark Jensen's death during the 1960 Rome Olympics: A Search for truth? *Sport in History*, *25*(3), 452–471.

Ohl, F., Fincoeur, B., Lentillon-Kaestner, V., Defrance, J., & Brissonneau, C. (2015). The socialization of young cyclists and the culture of doping. *International Review for the Sociology of Sport*, *7*, 865–882.

Overbye, M. (2018). An (un)desirable trade of harms? How elite athletes might react to medically supervised 'doping' and their considerations of side-effects in this situation. *The International Journal of Drug Policy*, *55*, 14–30.

Petroczi, A., Norman, P., & Brueckner, S. (2017). Can we better integrate the role of anti-doping in sports and society? A psychological approach to contemporary value-based prevention. *Medicine and Sport Science*, *62*, 160–176.

Pitsch, W. (2009). The 'science of doping' revisited: Fallacies of the current anti-doping regime. *European Journal of Sport Science*, *9*(2), 87–95.

Savulescu, J. (2015). Why we should legalise performance-enhancing drugs in sport. In I. Waddington, V. Møller, & J. Hoberman (Eds), *Routledge Handbook of Drugs and Sport* (pp. 350–362). London: Routledge.

Schneider, A. (2006). Cultural nuances: doping, cycling and the Tour de France. *Sport in Society*, *9*, 212–226.

Smith, C. (2017). Tour du dopage: Confessions of doping professional cyclists in a modern work environment. *International Review for the Sociology of Sport*, *52*(1), 97–111.

Stewart, B. & Smith, A. (2014). *Rethinking Drug Use in Sport: Why the War Will Never be Won*. London: Routledge.

Thompson, C. (2008). *The Tour de France: A Cultural History*. Berkeley: University of California Press.

Van Reeth, D. & Larson, D.J. (2015). *The Economics of Professional Road Cycling*. New York: Springer.

Voet, W. (2001). *Breaking the Chain: Drugs and Cycling – The True Story*. New York: Yellow Jersey Press.

Waddington, I., Christiansen, A.V., Gleaves, J., Hoberman, J., & Møller, V. (2013). Recreational drug use and sport: Time for a WADA rethink? *Performance Enhancement & Health*, *2*(2), 41–47.

Waddington, I. & Smith, A. (2009). *An Introduction to Drugs in Sport: Addicted to Winning?* London: Routledge.

Part I

The use and supply of doping products

Chapter 1

Assessing and explaining the doping prevalence in cycling

Werner Pitsch

In recent years, a line of empirical studies succeeded in validly estimating the doping prevalence in elite sport as a whole and specifically in cycling. In each study, variations of the randomised response technique (RRT) were used, but they nevertheless ended up with more or less comparable results. Empirical social research thus provides a reliable description of the extent of doping in different contexts, while the development of theories explaining doping lacks the quality to provide coherent explanations of quantitative phenomena. This discrepancy was mentioned by Pitsch and Emrich (2012), but despite this desideratum, theoretical reasoning and empirical research did not succeed in closing this gap.

The following chapter will begin with a brief explanation of indirect questioning techniques to enable the reader to assess both the reliability and limitations of results from these methods. After an overview of empirical results on doping prevalence in elite sport, and especially in elite and amateur cycling, theories of doping will be contrasted using research questions arising from these results. Based on an astonishingly consistent pattern of results across different settings, we will demonstrate how social scientific theory can be linked explicitly to empirical data. The potential of this methodology in terms of clarifying essential and abundant elements of the description of the empirical field, as well as pointing at research desiderata and to new hypotheses, will be highlighted in the end.

Indirect questioning techniques

Indirect questioning techniques allow respondents in surveys on embarrassing or threatening topics to answer honestly without compromising themselves. The randomised response technique was the first of these techniques, developed more than 50 years ago (Warner, 1965). Since then there have been many methodological studies investigating advantages and risks of different variants of this technique (for an overview, see the meta-analysis by Lensvelt-Mulders, Hox, van der Heijden, & Maas (2005) and the recent review by Wolter (2012)). The rationale of these techniques is to use some randomisation like flipping a coin or rolling a dice in the process of answering an embarrassing question. This randomisation is implemented in a way that is clearly understood by the respondent. Thus, respondents understand that an embarrassing answer can be the result of the randomising process or of answering the embarrassing question truthfully. There is much evidence that indirect questioning techniques effectively reduce the social desirability bias for sensitive issues (Lensvelt-Mulders et al., 2005). As the researcher knows the characteristics of the randomising device, he or she can calculate the proportion of honest yes- and no-answers to the embarrassing question, while the respondent recognises that there is no way to infer his/her property or behaviour from his/her individual answer.

Although respondents are more prone to answer the sensitive questions honestly, there remains a bias due to either inappropriately handling the randomising device or to deliberately cheating when answering. In order to control for this effect, Clarke and Desharnais (1998) developed the first cheater-detection technique, typically used for no-cheating when the embarrassing answer is 'yes' (see Figure 1.1). Feth, Frenger, Pitsch, & Schmelzeisen (2017) expanded this technique to a total cheater detection, which can be used to detect no- as well as yes-cheaters.

RRT has been used for doping in sport repeatedly on different populations by performance (elite athletes: Elbe & Pitsch 2018; de Hon, Kuipers, & van Bottenburg, 2015; Pitsch & Emrich, 2012; Pitsch, Emrich, & Klein, 2007; amateur athletes: Frenger, Pitsch, & Emrich, 2016) and from different disciplines (track-and-field athletes: Ulrich et al., 2017; triathletes: Dietz et al., 2013; Schröter et al., 2016). In particular, concerning doping in cycling, there have been studies

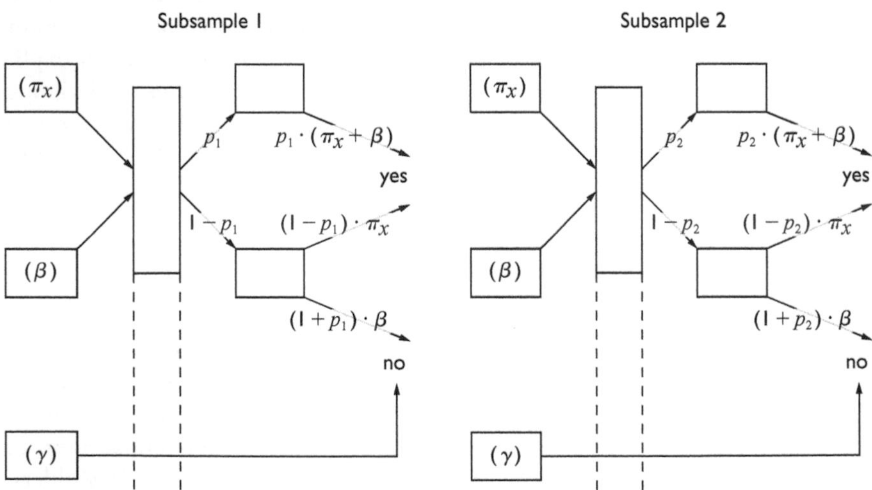

Figure 1.1 RRT with no-cheater detection.

on elite Flemish cyclists (Fincoeur, Frenger, & Pitsch, 2014; Fincoeur & Pitsch, 2017) as well as among amateur cyclists licenced by USACycling (see below). For this chapter, the results from two studies among cyclists are considered. A population of Flemish cyclists was studied in May and July 2013 (Fincoeur, Frenger, & Pitsch, 2014). Among other questions, there was an RRT question on doping during the last season:

> Have you used forbidden substances or methods in order to enhance your cycling performance during the last season? (TUE excluded)

An invitation to participate in this study was sent to 2776 Flemish cyclists by e-mail. After three reminders, there were 767 responses. Due to the cheater-detection method used, one cannot calculate for a point estimate of the rate of dopers in a population. Rather, an interval indicating the span between the rate of honest yes-responders – which equals the lowest possible level of dopers in the population – and the rate of honest yes responders plus the rate of cheaters, which reflects the upper limit of the interval. In contrast to the suspicion that cycling is a debauched sport with professional cyclists all being doping sinners, the results for the prevalence estimates for this study indicated the overwhelming majority of respondents is likely a non-doper. The rate of honest yes-responders for last season doping was estimated at 0.4%, with 26.3% cheaters and 73.3% honest no-responses. The important issue when interpreting these results is that the rate of honest no-responses is surely an unbiased estimation of the no-doping prevalence, as the rate of no-cheaters (presumably due to social desirability) is explicitly estimated with this technique. Besides this, the rate of honest yes-responders is also very likely to be a valid lowest threshold estimate, as the probability that this rate is inflated by yes-cheaters can, especially among elite athletes, be plausibly assumed to be extremely low. Accordingly, both the rate of honest yes- and of honest no-responses are the lowest assumable figures for dopers and non-dopers in the population.

The same questions were used in a survey among amateur cyclists who were licenced by USACycling in 2014. As USACycling did not share their list of contact data with the researchers, the communication with the respondents could not perfectly be controlled. Concerning the response rate, this was not seen a priori as a massive disadvantage as the large population count (51,782 licence holders in 2014) left enough room to end up with a sufficiently large record set even at low response rates. A total of 39,000 members of USACycling who had opted for e-mail communication were invited via a newsletter to participate in the survey. The reminder was sent to 44,133 members of USACycling. The discrepancy in the number of addressees between the two communications remained unclear to the researchers. The survey started on 04 September 2014 and was finished on 27 October 2014.

The response added up to 3756 records from respondents who had at least started to answer the questionnaire and 2949 complete records. Due to question- and/or item non-response, this figure is higher than the number of exploitable results for single items and especially higher for calculations referring to more than one item (e.g. estimating the doping prevalence by licence level).

Although USACycling provided in-depth information on the distribution of the population by age, discipline, sex, and performance class, the return could not be tested for being representative. The 'doping' focus of the study made only cyclists who actively participated in competitions relevant for the research. This was attained by a question in the beginning of the questionnaire asking if the respondent participated at least in one competition during the last two years. Respondents answering 'no' were immediately directed to a webpage thanking them for their interest in the research and explaining that they did not belong to the relevant subpopulation. The main objective of this technique was to avoid an artificial underestimation of doping prevalence as a result of cyclists with other motivations than being successful in competitions (e.g. saving money for accident insurance) entering the sample. As a side effect of targeting this subpopulation, the researchers were unable to test if the sample represents the subpopulation of actively competing amateur cyclists, as this subpopulation is not recorded by USACycling.

Analysis resulted in a best estimate of 3.15% for the prevalence of last year doping, which did not differ significantly from zero. The estimated rate of honest 'no'-responders is 74.88%. The true score of the last year prevalence thus ranges between at least 3.15% and 25.12%. Compared to other studies in amateur sport (Frenger, Pitsch, & Emrich, 2016), this rate is not astonishing and there is no hint that doping in amateur cycling was more prevalent than in any amateur sport in general. What was especially interesting is the pattern of doping prevalence when differentiating by performance category. To conduct these analyses, cyclists were grouped according to their USACycling amateur performance category. These categories range from 1 (topmost performers) to 5 (lowest performance category). Due to the low number of records among category 1 cyclists, we grouped categories 1 and 2 together and conducted no-cheater detection analyses. The reasons for omitting the yes-cheater detection are as follows: (1) the overall estimate of this proportion yielded a value of 0 (see above) and (2) the no-cheater detection already provides stable results for sample sizes that are too low to perform a total cheater detection (Feth et al., 2017). The results for the last year prevalence (Table 1.1) strongly support the findings from elite sport, discussed above. As can be seen in the following table, the rate of honest 'yes'-responders was calculated to be zero for categories 1 and 2 as well as for category 5, while the estimates for categories 3 and 4 were above this level. The significant differences support the pattern showing doping is less prevalent at the highest levels of competition. Additionally, doping is less prevalent where performance and success are the least important (category 5).

Similar results were repeatedly reported in elite sport, as internationally competitive athletes showed a lower doping prevalence than the category of

Table 1.1 Comparison of doping prevalence at different licence categories

Last year prevalence	*Honest 'yes'*	*Cheater 'no'*	*Honest 'no'*
cat. 1 + 2	0.0000	0.1799	0.8201
cat. 3	0.0226	0.2505	0.7269
cat. 4	0.0849	0.2672	0.6479
cat. 5	0.0000	0.1758	0.8242
Significant differences for honest responses			
	cat. 1 + 2	*cat. 3*	*cat. 4*
cat. 3, honest 'yes'	–	–	–
cat. 3, honest 'no'	–	–	–
cat. 4, honest 'yes'	–0.0849	–0.0623	–
cat. 4, honest 'no'	0.1723	–	–
cat. 5, honest 'yes'	–	–	0.0849
cat. 5, honest 'no'	–	–0.0973	–0.1764

nationally competitive ones (Pitsch & Emrich, 2012; Pitsch, Emrich, & Klein, 2007). As a result of this research, we find nearly equal overall levels of doping prevalence among elite and amateur cyclists, while the pattern of reduced doping prevalence among the top performers compared to athletes at lower performance levels persists at both levels.

Initial ad hoc explanations (Pitsch, Emrich, & Klein, 2007) for this prevalence pattern in elite sports were built on the assumption of athletes rationally making doping decisions based on balanced utilities from doped and non-doped sports, and the probabilities of success, detection, and sanctioning. With this rationale, the lower prevalence among the top performers was thought to originate from the higher risk of detection as well as the higher loss in utility after being detected and sanctioned. Therefore, present anti-doping policies that concentrate doping tests at higher levels of performance were thought to reduce the amount of doping at these levels, but also to increase doping prevalence at lower levels of competition. Nevertheless, this rationale does not hold for amateur sport as (1) there are no massive gains to win from being successful in competition and (2) doping tests are scarce at every level and therefore the probability of detection at the top level nearly equals the probability at lower levels.

The aim of the following considerations is to find a coherent explanation that works on both levels of performance. To end up with different explanations for similar patterns in elite and in amateur sport would also require explanation of how these areas differ qualitatively and how this difference yields similar results when it comes to decisions for deviant behaviour. In this context, the difference between amateur sport and professional sport is only a qualitative one from the perspective of sport organisations. Differences at the athlete level are mostly quantitative in terms of performance, but also in terms of loss such as time spent on training, money spent on equipment and travel, as well as in terms of utility like prize money and public attention. At least between high-level amateur sport and low-level professional sport, this is a very blurred line.

The explanation developed in the following chapter also accounts for results from studies on the relationship between the level of prize money and the doping prevalence in different sports. Frenger, Pitsch, & Emrich (2012) had studied the relationship between prize money and prize money gradation in Olympic disciplines and the estimated doping risk in these disciplines. The doping risk was estimated by experts, forming the group of independent observers at the 24th Olympic Games in Beijing (WADA, 2009). The results showed that the level of the mean prize money in different sport disciplines was positively correlated with the estimated doping risk. However, within each discipline there was no correlation between the possible relative gain by performing higher and the doping risk estimate. Therefore, economic incentive-theories (like e.g. used by Maennig, 2002) may well explain different levels of doping between sports but cannot explain doping decisions of athletes at different levels of performance within one sport.

Problems of theory development in the doping field

Social scientific theories used to explain doping so far cover both domains of sport but ignore empirical evidence showing different doping prevalence in different disciplines and at different levels of competition (e.g. psychological explanations, building on moral (dis-) engagement, Melzer, Elbe, & Brand, 2010, or on social-cognitive theory, Lucidi et al., 2008, Lazuras, Barkoukis, Rodafinos, & Haralambos, 2010, Petróczi & Aidman, 2008, or sociological theories of deviant behaviour, based on subculture theories). Theories, developed for elite sport often (implicitly or explicitly) model doping as a rational behaviour, assuming that the subjectively expected utility from doping (*ud*) equals the probability of success (*ps*) times the costs to be successful (*cs*) minus the probability of detection (*pd*) times the costs due to being detected and sanctioned as a doper (*cd*) – in short: $ud = ps * cs - pd * cd$. By limiting the scope of the explanation, these approaches typically ignore empirical evidence that doping prevalence in amateur and in elite sport show similar quantitative patterns, presented above. Patterns for this shortcoming can be found in simplifying game theoretical explanations following Breivik (1992), like e.g. Eber & Thépot (1999), but also more sophisticated n-person games like Buechel, Emrich & Pohlkamp, (2014). Other theories, especially those developed for elite sport, ignore that their assumptions concerning utility from doping fail when tested empirically (e.g. Houlihan, 2008). Few papers have discussed doping in amateur and in elite athletes together, but the focus was mostly on the differences between these two domains and the widely qualitative approach did not allow for calculating the doping prevalence (Henning & Dimeo, 2015).

As a result, sport science has so far found explanations that work on both levels but fail to explain the differences within competitive levels, or explanations that work on one level but fail on the other. It is questionable whether the artificial – and mostly normative – differentiation between elite and amateur level sport, which is first and foremost an organisational one made by sport associations, is helpful when trying to explain human behaviour in this context. Therefore, the starting point for the following discussion was very much inspired by the argument of parsimony in theory development (for the context of theoretical language see 'Occam's Razor'; for the context of empirical content of hypotheses see Popperian philosophy of science). Nevertheless, omitting the assumption that amateur and elite sport differ by principle calls for a coherent explanation that (1) can explain the differences in the overall level of doping between these domains and (2) can also explain the differences between performance levels within these domains. This is done through the concept of 'consumption capital'.

Consumption capital

The term 'consumption capital' was created by Stigler and Becker (1977) as the pivotal element of their theory of 'rational addiction'. Stigler and Becker used 'getting used to good music' as an example for their concept of 'rational addiction'. This as well as the title of their first publication on this theory 'de gustibus non est disputandum' (there is no accounting for taste) points to the fact, that this theory was not only developed to rationally explain addictions, which are often thought to be harmful but also to explain the development of passion and commitment. The concept builds on the idea that humans get addicted to goods which, when consumed, lead to an increased stock of human capital to consume the good in the future. These goods were called 'consumption capital goods'. Accordingly, the proficiency to consume these goods was called 'consumption capital'. The utility of this concept in the context of sport is immediately understood from the following examples:

- For a beginner, every tennis lesson increases his/her capability, to consume 'tennis' in the future in multiple ways. It increases his/her ability to play tennis, but also the understanding of what is happening in the court when watching broadcasted tennis matches, and his/her ability to discuss tennis-related issues;
- For a top-level athlete in athletic gymnastics, every training session increases his/her capability to consume 'gymnastics' in the future, as not training would reduce the chances of winning in competition, and learning new athletic skills as well as automatising already learned skills increases the chances of competing successfully.

This means that the utility from consumption is not only defined by present consumption but also a function of consumption in the past. If we understand 'competing' as 'consumption' in this model, the utility from consuming is defined by the years spent exercising and training, as well as the economic resources spent on equipment and on travel costs. This utility is only realised if the athlete is successful, in whatever way, he/she defines 'success'.

This idea is very different from the idea of 'utility' used in sociological and economic rational choice models of doping behaviour. As in these models, utility was only seen as influenced by the outcome of the single competition under study. With this idea, utility from doping (doped) sport is embedded in the sporting biography of the individual and, therefore, biographical marginal conditions like their age as well as the age at the beginning of their sporting career become important in the context of this explanation. Nevertheless, the idea that the utility accrues only with the probability of success persists with this model.

Up to now, these assumptions only are ex-ante formulated ideas that might explain the pattern of data, resulting from the empirical studies. This means that although derivations from these assumptions match the pattern of empirical data, they are not (yet) empirically tested. This would afford a similar study to be conducted as the USACycling study and data to be gathered on relevant biographical attributes such as age, age at the beginning of the career, etc. Additionally, data acquisition would also have to cover plausible confounding variables such as sporting careers in similar disciplines (e.g. triathlon), if the sporting career was interrupted (e.g. by injuries), and so on. In the light of the limited chances to approach amateur athletes to conduct doping studies, the methodological effort to conduct indirect questioning surveys, the limitations of statistical analyses due to indirect questioning, and the huge sample sizes which are needed, the hypotheses which one tries to test should be scrutinised in advance. This can be reached by formalising these assumptions in a mathematical model and predicting the effect these assumptions will yield if effective in a population. Comparing the results of such a model to already available empirical evidence then allows testing to see if the posteriori 'explanation' is at least plausible. Additionally, formalising such a model and predicting from it requires explicitly modelling any marginal condition that may influence the results. Therefore, this technique also draws one's attention to necessary preconditions that were not included in the provisional explanation because they were not perceived as crucial issues.

For the issue under study, a numerical model was written in R (R Core Team, 2017). For numerical simulation, the model massively used parallel computing (Microsoft Corporation & Weston, 2017). Graphical illustrations used the ggplot2 package (Wickham, 2009). Basic ideas of the formalised model were taken from Pitsch (2003, 2005a).

Pivotal elements in the formalisation were athletes, who were represented by a record containing an athlete ID, talent, age at the beginning of the athletic career, and athlete's current age. The present model is not an agent-based model in the sense of Ferber (1999) or Woolridge (2002) although it could easily be expanded accordingly. Nevertheless, the basic elements in the formalisation are called 'agents' in order to differentiate these model elements from athletes who are the elements of the original population. To generate meaningful predictions from such models to compare to real-world populations, it is important to select starting values for the agent population as close as possible to the original. Information for some variables like age can be drawn from information from the sport association (here, USACycling) or from empirical studies. Other information may not be easily available (e.g. the typical age of cyclists at the beginning of athletic career) or may not be accessible in principle (e.g. talent distribution in a cycling population). For these variables the only way to start is with plausible guesses.

We used the following:

- A lognormally distributed random variable for age at beginning the cycling career that fits a distribution for a comparable population (elite athletes) from Germany. The lognormal shape accounts for the fact that more athletes begin at lower ages than at higher ages;
- A normally distributed random variable for age with mean and standard deviation derived from the study presented above;
- The right half of a standard normal distribution for talent (see Figure 1.2). The rationale to use only the right half of the distribution was that those whose talent is lower than the mean in a population are unlikely to compete in a sport.

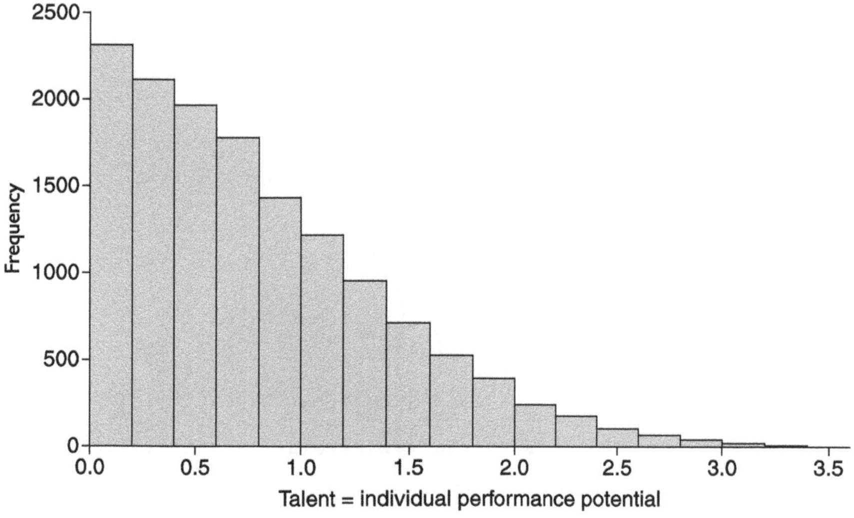

Figure 1.2 Distribution of the variable 'talent', indicating the individual performance potential at the age of maximum performance (26 years).

Up to that point, the model implementation only refers to known or assumed properties of the individuals within this population. In this first step, called instantiation, the population is built by assigning random values to individuals under the assumption that the modelled properties are independent. In the following step, further parameters are derived from these initial values. We calculated the performance of the athletes whose age exceeded the age at the beginning. For these athletes, their performance was calculated as a reverse u-shaped function of the agent's age and his maximum performance age, which was normatively defined at 26 years. This means that every agent in the population reaches his/her maximum performance potential, defined by the variable 'talent', at this age. Further influences on the agents' performance were not modelled. The influence of training on athletic performance was omitted because all agents were assumed to train and the influence of different levels of training was found to be negligible in previous models (Pitsch, 2005b). The common effect of randomly distributed talent and the reverse u-shaped function resulted in the distribution of agents by performance (see Figure 1.3).

Besides the performance of the athletes, we also calculated the utility of training in the discipline. We assumed that the utility of training is at its highest in the beginning of a career and diminished with every subsequent year. The cumulative utility from training has the form of an inclining curve with permanently receding positive slope (see Figure 1.4), thus asymptotically increasing up to the limit 1.

The probability of doping to increase performance was calculated for each individual as a function of the performance difference between this individual and both the next better one and the next worse. This follows the rationale that

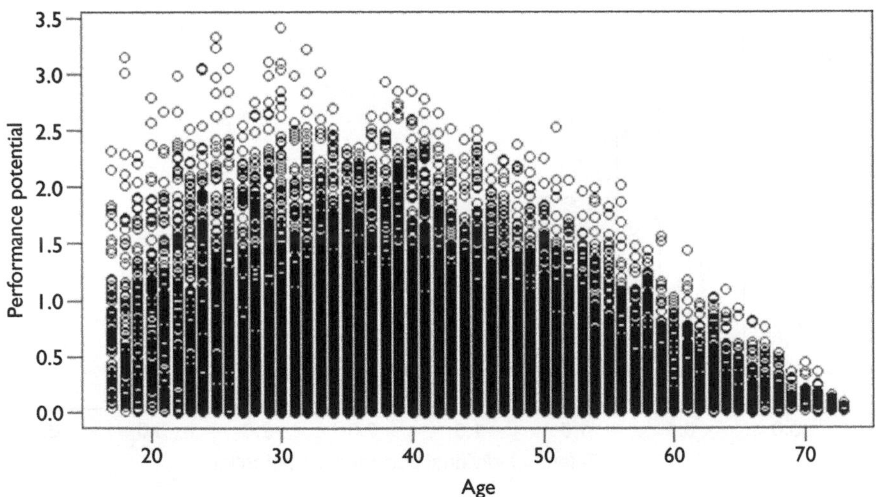

Figure 1.3 Levels of performance potential in the population by age.

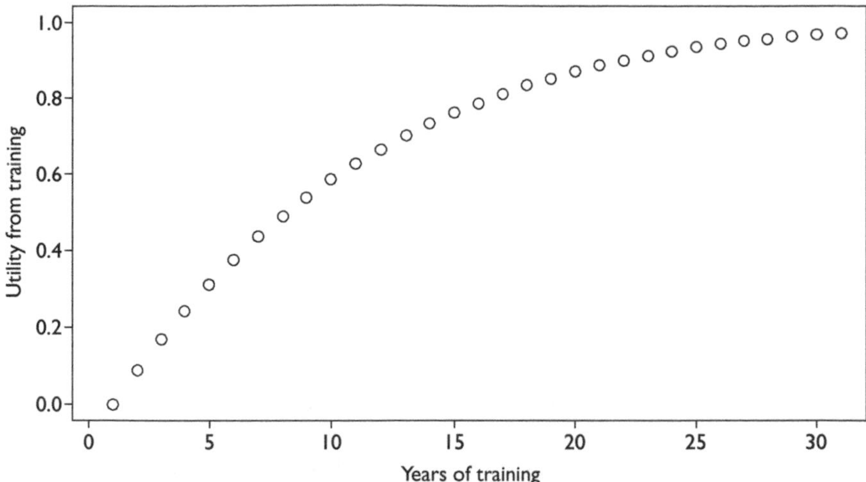

Figure 1.4 Cumulative utility from training.

the utility from competition can only be gained if the individual is successful. The temptation to illegally increase performance in order to rank higher by surpassing an opponent who is supposed to compete better than the individual increases with a decreasing difference in performance. If this difference is low, the probability of gaining a higher ranking by using illegal techniques is high. With large differences, the probability to gain a higher ranking by doping diminishes. The same holds for the idea of avoiding being surpassed by a weaker opponent. By and large, the mean doping temptation is a function of the performance density in a performance class, but for individuals this temptation may vary widely due to their individual position in the performance ranking.

In order to keep the model as simple as possible, we did not calculate for individual doping decisions based on the modelled utility multiplied by the probability of using doping substances. Instead we used the outcome of this multiplication as an indicator for higher or lower doping propensity in different classes. Adding a decision rule at the individual level would have made it necessary to explicitly model this decision and required implementing more assumptions into the model that are, at best, only weakly empirically substantiated. Additionally, this more complicated model would not have led to any advantage if the decision is made based only on the probability of being successful with doping and the utility from competing successfully. The so-modelled doping prevalence would have only been a linear function of the mean doping propensity.

First results and refining the model

First simulations with this model revealed an important property was missing from the model. Up to now, agents were only stratified into performance classes and the competition at every level was a total one. This led to the effect that with decreasing performance classes, the mean individual probability to use doping substances increased massively due to the much higher performance density at lower levels. Therefore, it became apparent that since lower level athletic competitions in the real world are stratified by age classes, and often also into regional classes, is an important influence reducing the doping propensity in mass sport.

To model the stratification of competition by age classes, the limits for these classes were taken from the USACycling website and applied accordingly. The refined model contained one additional agent property named 'location', which was then used to assign athletes at lower performance levels to different regional classes. This variable was instantiated as a uniformly distributed random variable. Regional classes were assigned as follows: the top performance class was kept as one group, the second performance class was divided into two, the third class into four, the fourth class into six, etc. This was built on plausibility as there was no information available from the USACycling's website concerning this issue. However, because the model would end up with incorrect predictions if all competitions at different levels were total competitions, some kind of random stratification was needed. In the real world original, this is typically accomplished through the spatial distribution of athletes in a discipline, either explicitly by local, regional, and nation-wide competitions for different levels of performance, or implicitly by the assumed differing willingness of athletes to travel long distances to participate in competitions. Therefore, we called the stratification pattern we used 'regional classification' although there was no explicitly spatial character in the model.

Results from the final model

The simulated doping propensity inclines with inclining performance class but declines again from the second highest to the highest class (see Figure 1.5). For the tier of only young adult high performers (age ranging from 18 to 35 and performance above the ninety-ninth percentile), doping propensity is shown in Figure 1.6. It is clear that the decline between the second and the top tier is even larger than in the 'amateur' case in Figure 1.5, but that this pattern persists on both levels. Additionally, comparing Figure 1.5 to Figure 1.6 reveals that the doping propensity at the elite level is lower than at the amateur level, which also concurs with the empirical results presented above. Both aspects that were to be explained are provided in this simulation. Nevertheless, as the difference between amateur and elite in one sport had only been shown once and the empirical difference is far from significant, the amateur–elite difference should not be over-interpreted.

The results indicate that the model provides the explanation the research sought. But a direct comparison to the empirical results (see Figure 1.7) reveals that this effect is only qualitative and mostly fits to the first-second-tier

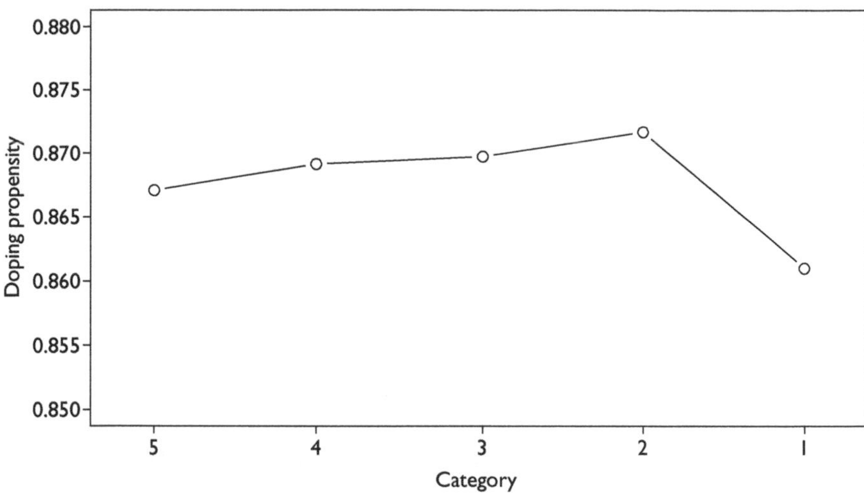

Figure 1.5 Simulated doping propensity by performance class at the amateur level.

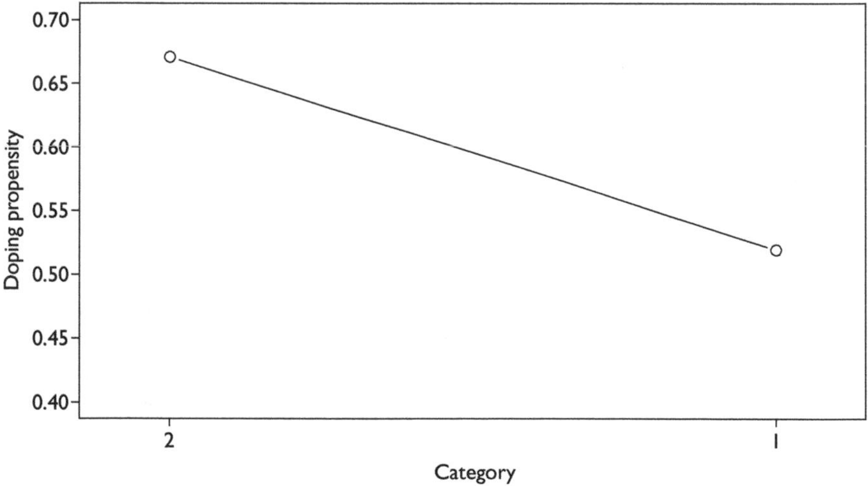

Figure 1.6 Simulated doping propensity for two tiers at the elite level (young adult high-performers).

difference, while the conditions at the other levels are not met equally well. The explanation in itself may provide a sufficient qualitative explanation, but either the explanation or the numerical specificities of the realised model fail to render numerically correct results.

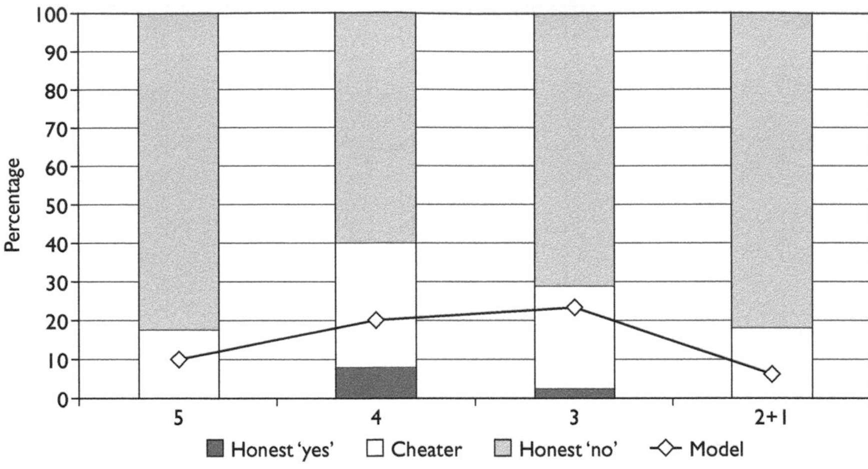

Figure 1.7 Comparison of simulated results and empirical data.

Final remarks and discussion of further potential

The assumption of sport as consumption capital led to the following:

1 A coherent explanation without the need to a priori or ad hoc assume substantial differences between the processes leading to doping in elite and in amateur sport;
2 Predictions that are qualitatively coherent with the presented empirical evidence.

The quantitative fit might still be improved, but this would come either by implementing further assumptions into the model, or by artificially changing model parameters in order to end up with a better fit without changing the model itself, though this would not add value to the explanation. While the latter technique merely presents the model builder's proficiency in mathematics, the first one is always at risk of providing over-complicated models that do not improve the explanation and offer only more numerically exact predictions. At this point, there is an explicit trade-off between the requirements according to Occam's razor argument and the objective to end up with numerically exact predictions. This is the reason there is, in principle, no 'correct' or 'false' model, only appropriate models for pre-defined objectives.

For the sociology of sport, the essence of this explanation is that there is no need to assume a mythical 'point of no return' or similar qualitative differences between the elite and the amateur domains in sport to explain patterns of doping prevalence by performance classes. This characteristic concurs with descriptions of athletes' biographies that often depict the way into professional sports from the individual perspective as a successive sliding into a new career phase that are retrospectively categorised as 'amateur' and 'elite' (Bette, 2002).

Formally modelling this explanation provides the often-missing link between explanations at an individual level and empirical evidence at the population or subgroup level. In this model, we assume that doping decisions at the individual level are influenced by

- one's individual consumption capital, accumulated by doing sport; and
- one's estimated probability of gaining a higher ranking, or at least securing an expected ranking; independently of the performance domain, to the collective empirical phenomenon of maximum prevalence within the second tier, in elite as well as in amateur sport.

The idea that the (a posteriori assumed) concept of sport as consumption capital at the individual level provides a coherent explanation for the collective phenomenon cannot be taken for granted. This is well illustrated by the first simulations without the spatial and age classification, which led to non-fitting results. The fact that athletic competitions are stratified competitions at lower performance levels is an important part of this explanation that would have remained hidden without explicitly modelling and simulating.

The development of this model must not be finished at that point. The most straightforward way to further develop the model is to calibrate it in order to better meet the conditions in the original (e.g. the distribution of agents by the age of beginning the sport). Additionally, further information on the original can be included (e.g. drop-out rate at different levels of age and performance) and the model can be further calibrated to produce similar conditions as the original (e.g. age distribution of top-level performers). All this may lead to an increased fit between the predictions and empirical evidence.

The model can also be used to generate new hypotheses (e.g. prevalence by age classes), which in turn can be tested using existing datasets. In this sense, it can provide insight on the limitations of the present explanation (e.g. the observation that stratification of competition influences doping propensity at the amateur level). This can be the basis for further hypothesis testing because doping prevalence within one sport, in different countries, and with different stratifications of competition should differ accordingly.

The formalisation of social scientific models leads to a high level of intersubjectivity and enables a high level of constructive criticism. The explanation provided by the model cannot only be criticised, but suggested changes to the model can be tested for their effect on the outcome. Additionally, this technique allows testing if hypothesised explanations miss crucial elements (as in the present case), if social scientific theories are free from contradictions and if they can be tested empirically. Furthermore, it allows comparing existing explanations to new ones. By and large, this technique renders the process of theory development by indicating essential and dispensable elements of theories and by pointing towards research desiderata. Nevertheless, one shortcoming is that the development of formalised models is extremely time consuming and laborious, and currently there is no common template for how to present the steps of model development, including the assumptions made and the marginal conditions selected. These may be the reasons why developing formalised models of social interaction remains a marginal phenomenon in social sciences in spite of its obvious advantages.

References

Bette, K.H. (2002). *Biographische Dynamiken im Leistungssport*. Köln: Strauss.

Breivik, G. (1992). Doping games. A game theoretical exploration of doping. *International Review for the Sociology of Sport, 27*(3), 235–255.

Buechel, B., Emrich, E., & Pohlkamp, S. (2014). Nobody's innocent: The role of customers in the doping dilemma. *Journal of Sports Economics, 17*(8), 767–789.

Clark, S.J. & Desharnais, R.A. (1998). Honest answers to embarrassing questions: Detecting cheating in the randomized response model. *Psychological Methods, 3*, 160–168.

de Hon, O., Kuipers, H., & van Bottenburg, M. (2015). Prevalence of doping use in elite sports: A review of numbers and methods. *Sports Medicine, 45*(1), 57–69.

Dietz, P., Ulrich, R., Dalaker, R., Striegel, H., Franke, A.G., Lieb, K., & Simon, P. (2013). Associations between physical and cognitive doping – a cross-sectional study in 2.997 triathletes. *PLOS One*, 8(11), e78702.

Eber, N. & Thépot, J. (1999). Doping in sport and competition design. *Recherches Économiques de Louvain – Louvain Economic Review, 65*(4), 435–446.

Elbe, A.-M. & Pitsch, W. (2018). Doping prevalence among Danish elite athletes. *Performance Enhancement & Health*, 6(1), 28–32.

Ferber, J. (1999). *Multi-Agent System: An Introduction to Distributed Artificial Intelligence*. Harlow: Addison Wesley Longman.

Feth, S., Frenger, M., Pitsch, W., & Schmelzeisen, P. (2017). *Cheater Detection for Randomized Response-Techniques: Derivation, Analyses and Application* (Schriften des Europäischen Insituts für Sozioökonomie e.V., 12). Saarbrücken: universaar. Online available under http://universaar.uni-saarland.de/monographien/volltexte/2018/161/pdf/europ_inst_band_12_engl_komplett.pdf

Fincoeur, B., Frenger, M., & Pitsch, W. (2014). Does one play with the athletes' health in the name of ethics? *Performance Enhancement & Health, 2*, 182–193.

Fincoeur, B. & Pitsch, W. (2017). Omgaan met sociale wenselijkheid: Inschatting van de dopingprevalentie aan de hand van de Randomized Response Technique. *Panopticon, 38*(5), 376–386.

Frenger, M., Pitsch, W., & Emrich, E. (2012). Erfolg(+)reich und verdorben? Eine empirische Überprüfung verbreiteter Vorurteile zur Kommerzialisierung im Sport // Erfolg(+)reich und verdorben? *Sportwissenschaft, 42*(3), 188–201.

Frenger, M., Pitsch, W., & Emrich, E. (2016). Sport-induced substance use – an empirical study to the extent within a German sports association. *PLOS ONE, 11*(10), e0165103.

Henning, A. & Dimeo, P. (2015). Questions of fairness and anti-doping in US cycling: The contrasting experiences of professionals and amateurs. *Drugs: Education, Prevention, and Policy*, 1–10.

Houlihan, B. (2008). *Sport and society. A student introduction* (second ed.). Los Angeles: Sage.

Lazuras, L., Barkoukis, V., Rodafinos, A., & Haralambos, T. (2010). Predictors of doping intentions in elite-level athletes: a social cognition approach. *Journal of Sport and Exercise Psychology*, *32*, 694–710.

Lensvelt-Mulders, G.J.L.M., Hox, J.J., van der Heijden, P.G.M., & Maas, C.J.M. (2005). Meta-analysis of randomized response research. Thirty-five years of validation. *Sociological Methods and Research*, *33*, 315–348.

Lucidi, F., Zelli, A., Mallia, L., Grano, C., Russo, P.M., & Violani, C. (2008). The social-cognitive mechanisms regulating adolescents' use of doping substances. *Journal of Sports Sciences*, *26*(5), 447–456.

Maennig, W. (2002). On the economics of doping and corruption in international sports. *Journal of Sport Economics*, *3*, 61–89.

Melzer, M., Elbe, A.-M., & Brand, R. (2010). Moral and ethical decision-making: A chance for doping prevention in sports? *Nordic Journal of Applied Ethics*, *4*(1), 69–85.

Microsoft Corporation & Weston, St. (2017). *doParallel: Foreach Parallel Adaptor for the 'parallel' Package*. R package version 1.0.11. https://CRAN.R-project.org/package=doParallel.

Petróczi, A. & Aidman, E.V. (2008). Psychological drivers in doping: The life-cycle model of performance enhancement. *Substance Abuse Treatment Prevention and Policy*, 3. doi:10.1186/1747-597x-3-7.

Pitsch, W. (2003). Social-scientific modelling supporting theory development: A model of socioepidemiology of success in top-level sport. *International Journal for Computer Science in Sport*, Special edition 01/2003.

Pitsch, W. (2005a). Ein Modell zur Simulation von Spitzensportlerlaufbahnen: Methodologische Grundlagen und Struktur des Modells. In E. Emrich, A. Güllich, M.P. Büch (Eds), *Nachwuchsleistungssport – Theoretische Reflexionen und empirische Analysen* (pp. 285–319). Schorndorf: Hofmann.

Pitsch, W. (2005b). Ein Modell zur Simulation von Spitzensportlerlaufbahnen: Parametrisierung und Ergebnisse einer ersten Simulation. In E. Emrich, A. Güllich, M.P. Büch (Eds), *Nachwuchsleistungssport – Theoretische Reflexionen und empirische Analysen* (pp. 321–346). Schorndorf: Hofmann.

Pitsch, W., Emrich, E., & Klein, M. (2007). Doping in elite sports in Germany: results of a www survey. *European Journal of Sport and Society*, *4*(2), 89–102.

Pitsch, W. & Emrich, E. (2012). The frequency of doping in elite sport – results of a replication study. *International Review for the Sociology of Sport*, *47*, 559–580.

R Core Team (2017). *R: A language and environment for statistical computing*. R Foundation for Statistical Computing, Vienna, Austria. URL www.R-project.org/.

Schröter, H., Studzinski, B., Dietz, P., Ulrich, R., Striegel, H., Simon, P., & Barkley, J. (2016). A comparison of the cheater detection and the unrelated question models: A randomized response survey on physical and cognitive doping in recreational triathletes. *PLOS ONE*, *11*(5), e0155765.

Stigler, G. & Becker, G.S. (1977). De Gustibus Non Est Disputandum. *American Economic Review*, *67*, 76–90.

Ulrich, R., Pope, H.G., Cléret, L., Petróczi, A., Nepusz, T., Schaffer, J., Kanayama, G., Comstock, R.D., & Simon, P. (2017). Doping in two elite athletics competitions assessed by randomized-response surveys. *Sports Medicine*, *45*, 57.

WADA (2009). *Report of the Independent Observers, XXIX Olympic Games, Beijing 2008.* Vancouver: WADA.

Warner, S.L. (1965). Randomized-response. A survey technique for eliminating evasive answer bias. *Journal of the American Statistical Association*, 60, 63–69.

Wickham, H. (2009). *ggplot2: Elegant Graphics for Data Analysis*. New York: Springer.

Wolter, F. (2012). *Heikle Fragen in Interviews*. Wiesbaden: VS Verlag für Sozialwissenschaften.

Woolridge, J.M. (2002). *Econometric Analysis of Cross Section and Panel Data*. Cambridge: MIT Press.

Chapter 2

Changing patterns of drug use in professional cycling

Implications for anti-doping policy

Ivan Waddington

In an important recent paper, Christophe Brissonneau (2015) draws upon the Marxist concept of the mode of production to analyse changing patterns of drug use in modern cycling. Brissonneau identifies what he calls two modes of production of the cycling performance, the first of which characterised professional cycling in the period from about 1970 to the 1980s, while the second developed from the mid-1980s. Each mode of production is characterised by a particular pattern of relationships between those involved in producing the cycling performance and, suggests Brissonneau, each mode of production is associated with a distinctive pattern of drug use.

The first mode of production Brissonneau describes as artisanal. Teams were small in size, composed of about 20 people and staff consisted of family members and former riders. All shared a personal history in cycling. There was a simple division of labour with relatively little specialisation. The *directeur sportif* was a former cyclist and had many functions including those of manager and trainer. He also liaised with sponsors, recruited the team members, arranged the racing schedule, and hired mechanics and *soigneurs* (also former cyclists) who helped riders with everyday jobs like washing clothes and cleaning bikes. The team was paid to represent the sponsor and for this reason cyclists rode many races, perhaps two or three a week in the season.

Training was based on empiricism and reflected an emphasis on quantity rather than quality, with riders typically riding long distances in training day after day; there was no question of carefully honing one's fitness according to a carefully worked out plan. Subject to deep fatigue because of the physical effort involved in training, racing, and travel, drug use was common. Amphetamines were used to relieve tiredness in racing and in travelling between races, while steroids were also used to relieve tiredness and to allow heavier training loads, though their use was unsystematic. Consistent with the empiricist approach to training, this period was, suggests Brissonneau, characterised by dabbling in drugs, rather than the systematic scientific use of drugs to enhance performance (Brissonneau, 2015: 184–185).

This mode of production of the cycling performance – small scale, artisanal and based on small budgets and family support – gave way from the early 1980s to a better financed and more highly rationalised system based on an increasingly scientific approach to training. This change was linked with an economic boom in cycling associated with growing internationalisation and spectacularisation and by a reorganisation of cycle racing by the sport's governing bodies. These changes generated higher levels of sponsorship from large international companies and a change in the management of teams, with a move away from family management towards an enterprise model of management. With greater funds available, staffing levels increased with a significant increase in role specialisation. The team director no longer did everything but specialised in finding sponsors and hiring and supervising staff. Within teams, riders became more specialised (sprinters, climbers, lead-out riders) while other specialists, outsiders to the cycling family, were also recruited. Of particular significance in this regard were doctors and specialists in exercise physiology, imposed by sponsors and team directors in order to look after the riders' health and to improve the cycling performance. Team doctors now mediated between riders and biological knowledge so that riders who had previously just dabbled in drugs such as amphetamines and steroids were now introduced to newer and more powerful drugs and were able to plan the systematic and scientific use of drugs and training schedules under the direction of team physicians. If the artisanal or family-based mode of production was based on empiricism, the key process in the second phase, the enterprise model, was the medicalisation of elite cycling (Brissonneau, 2015: 186–187).

Since the 1970s there has developed a substantial literature on the process of medicalisation of society (Zola, 1972; Waitzkin & Waterman, 1974; Illich, 1975; Clarke, Shim, Mamo, Fosket, & Fishman 2003; Conrad, 2005) and, more recently, on the medicalisation of sport and the relationship between medicalisation and drug use in sport (Waddington, 1996, 2000, 2004, 2005; Waddington & Murphy, 1992; Malcolm, 2017). Brissonneau's analysis, and particularly his analysis of the second stage – the enterprise model of management in cycling – is entirely consistent with this approach. It might be noted that some medical sociologists have recently pointed to a new phase, which has been termed biomedicalisation, in the relationship between medicine and other aspects of society. According to Clarke et al. (2003) there are five new and key dimensions involved in the shift from medicalisation to biomedicalisation: (i) an integration of business and medicine; (ii) a focus emphasising health status, risk, and surveillance; (iii) a 'technoscientisation' of medical practice; (iv) transformations of biomedical knowledge production including especially informatics and medicine's 'evidence-base'; and (v) biomedical intervention to transform bodies, including an increased focus on optimisation and enhancement. In a recent analysis of British professional football and cycling, Faulkner et al. (2017) argued that these dimensions of biomedicalisation can be observed

> in the academic disciplines of sports science and sports medicine, in the increasing corporatisation and globalisation of sport, in the availability of

> elite 'evidence-based' medical practitioners in sport, in the high levels of monitoring of sports performance through informatics, in the continual search for science-based higher levels of performance and the implications of this for the professional and personal identities of sports performers and their organisations.
>
> (p. 137)

It may, then, be appropriate to consider the process of biomedicalisation as a third mode of production of the sporting performance to be added to Brissonneau's two earlier stages.

Some years before Brissonneau's paper, Benjamin Brewer (2002) and Ask Vest Christiansen (2005) offered a broadly similar analysis in which they identified three major periods in the development of modern professional cycling and, as in the case of Brissonneau's analysis, each period was associated with a different pattern of social relationships and each pattern of relationships generated a distinctive pattern of drug use.

Drug use as a social process

What is the significance of the work of Brissoneau, Brewer, and Christiansen? And what are the implications for anti-doping policy? In order to understand this, it may be useful to draw upon Howard Becker's (1963) classic sociological analysis of the process of becoming a drug user. Although Becker's analysis focused on drug use outside of the sports context – Becker focused specifically on the process of becoming a marihuana user – the principles of his approach are no less relevant for understanding key aspects of drug use in sport. Becker noted that attempts to understand drug use are mainly concerned with the question: why do they do it? He noted that attempts to account for the use of marihuana 'lean heavily on the premise that the presence of any particular kind of behavior in an individual can best be explained as a result of some trait which predisposes or motivates him (sic) to engage in that behavior'. He notes that this trait is usually identified as psychological but he adds: 'I do not think such theories can adequately account for marihuana use' (Becker, 1963: 41–42).

The bulk of Becker's analysis is devoted to showing that the process of becoming a drug user is *necessarily* – that is it cannot be other than – a *social* process and that any attempt to understand the drug user as an isolated, self-contained individual is necessarily misleading and unhelpful. Thus, any drug user – inside or outside of sport – needs to get information from others about the kinds of drugs that are available and their effects, they need to learn how to use those drugs and how to recognise the effects of the drugs. And since illicit drug use both inside and outside of sport is generally held to be a deviant or immoral – perhaps even illegal – activity, drug users need to develop a relationship with a reliable 'connection', that is a dealer in illicit drugs, and also to establish their own credibility as a person who can be trusted to buy and use drugs without endangering anyone else. In addition, and since drug use is illicit and/or illegal, they are also required, first, to understand, and to accept, the importance of maintaining secrecy concerning the use of drugs not just by themselves but also by others and, second, they are constrained to reject conventional definitions of drug use as immoral and to develop a rationalisation for their own use of drugs (Becker, 1963: 41–78).

As in the case of Becker's analysis, the great strength of the work of Brissonneau, Brewer, and Christiansen is that it seeks to understand drug use not in terms of isolated acts of individual deviance but as a social process, that is, in terms of patterns of social relationships. For example, Christiansen emphasises that 'doping requires the cooperation of others' and, in a passage which is very reminiscent of Becker's classical analysis, he adds:

> There is a need for contact with people who can help with storage and delivery, for example, but especially with expertise and relevant knowledge. Without people who know which drugs to take, when to take them, and how they work, access to drugs is useless.

And like Becker, he emphasises the need to build up networks, which:

> have to be established gradually through friends and colleagues who can help the rider gain contact with 'the right people'. And again like Becker, he emphasises that 'the doping networks … are largely built on trust, which requires time to establish.'
>
> (Christiansen, 2005: 505–506)

Of course, Brewer, Christiansen, and Brissonneau are not the only, nor were they the first, social scientists to make this point; indeed, a similar point has been made by many sociologists of sport in recent decades. In 2000, for example, I drew attention to what I called 'the doping network' and wrote that 'it is clear that at the elite level it is simply unrealistic to see the individual drug-using athlete as working alone, without the assistance and support of others' (Waddington, 2000: 159). My own work over the last 25 years has focused in particular on the process of medicalisation of sport and the centrality of the relationship between athletes and sports physicians and other sports scientists (Waddington, 1996, 2000, 2001, 2004, 2005, 2007, 2015, 2016; Waddington & Murphy, 1992; Waddington & Smith, 2009) a theme which has also figured strongly in the work of John Hoberman (1992, 2002, 2012, 2013). Among many other themes which have been examined by social scientists one might mention the development of a culture of tolerance of doping in some sports, including cycling (Waddington, 2000; Waddington & Smith 2009); drug culture and community cohesion in cycling (Hoberman, 2003); cyclists' and other athletes' understanding of, and rationales for, their own use of drugs (Brewer, 2002; Monaghan, 2001) and drug use and athletic career structures (Bette, 2004). The key distinguishing characteristic of all these social science perspectives on drug use in sport is:

> they seek to understand the behaviour of drug-using athletes not by focusing on the athlete as an individual, but by locating athletes within the network of relationships in which they are involved within sport. This typically involves a focus not just on the athletes' relationships with others in what Nixon (1992) has called the 'sportsnet', that is the web of interaction with other athletes, coaches, managers, team physicians and others, but also on broader social changes such as the increasing competitiveness and commercialization of sport.
>
> (Waddington, 2016: 22)

But how has this research been received by anti-doping organisations and what impact has it had on anti-doping policy? For the most part it would seem that those with the responsibility for developing anti-doping policy have been largely unaware of, or perhaps simply uninterested in, social scientific research and that it has had little impact on anti-doping policy. In their recent work, *Detecting Doping in Sport*, Moston and Engelberg (2017: 134) have noted: 'One of the most frustrating problems in research is seeing how findings are abused, or (sometimes worse) simply ignored by the people the research was aimed at informing'.

If anti-doping policy-makers have largely ignored social science research, the reasons for this are not difficult to see. Ever since anti-doping policy began to develop from the 1960s, anti-doping organisations have implicitly – and therefore uncritically – accepted as a basis for policy the individualism which is such a marked feature of modern western societies. Thus, anti-doping policy has been based on a highly individualised conception of the elite athlete, who is presented as an asocial, isolated individual who is able to make more or less free and unconstrained choices. But such a conceptualisation is fundamentally flawed. It reflects what Norbert Elias called a 'Homo clausus' conceptualisation of the elite athlete (significantly conceptualised in the singular) as a 'closed person', rather than a more adequate conceptualisation of athletes (in the plural) as 'Homines aperti', that is 'open people', bonded together with other people in various ways and whose actions and choices are constrained, to varying degrees, by those bonds with others (Elias, 1970).

This individualistic bias underpins many aspects of anti-doping policy. It fits very well, for example, with the persistent – though frankly incredible – claim which has been made by anti-doping organisations over many years, that the fact that only 1–2% of tests on athletes are positive indicates not the limited effectiveness of testing, but rather that we are dealing with only a few isolated and deviant individuals, the occasional 'bad apple' in an otherwise good barrel of fruit. But more significantly, these individualistic assumptions can be seen in the two central aspects of anti-doping policy: the emphasis on detecting and punishing the individual drug-using athlete and, second, the emphasis on biological testing as a means of doing this.

And let there be no doubt that biological testing has always been, and remains, the very heart of anti-doping policy. In recent years, the number of samples analysed by WADA-accredited laboratories increased every year from 2011 through to 2015, with a 7.1% increase from 2014 to 2015, when no fewer than 303,369 samples were analysed (WADA, 2016: 4), with a small decrease of 0.9% from 2015 to 2016, to 300,546) (WADA, 2017: 1). The introduction of the athletes' biological passport scheme has, of course, served to further emphasise the reliance on biological testing; in 2009, 6082 samples were analysed for the scheme and this figure has regularly increased – in some years by over 60% – and in 2016 the number of samples analysed stood at 28,173, more than a fourfold increase in seven years (WADA, 2017: 1).

As a means of illustrating the individualism which underpins this approach, as well as the obvious limitations of this approach, consider the landmark positive drug test of Ben Johnson at the Seoul Olympics. That test told us that Johnson had used the steroid stanozolol but it told us almost nothing else of value. It told us nothing about Dr Jamie Astaphan, the physician who supplied the drugs to Johnson and who monitored his drug use. It told us nothing about the fact that Dr Astaphan had become an expert in the use of performance-enhancing drugs, or that he had an international clientele of elite athletes from many countries in North America, Europe, and Africa. It told us nothing about the network of doctors in North America who were prepared to supply performance-enhancing drugs to athletes. It told us nothing about relationships between athletes, nothing about the culture of drug-using athletes and, in particular, the 'brotherhood of the needle', which bound drug-using athletes together in a code of silence. And it told us nothing about the competitive and other pressures on elite athletes to use performance-enhancing drugs. In effect, it told us nothing about the 'doping network'. Put simply, Johnson's positive test told us nothing about what was going on outside, as opposed to inside, his body. The mass of detailed information, indicated above, about the doping network in Canadian sport was generated only by the decision of the Canadian government to establish the *Commission of Inquiry into the Use of Drugs and Banned Practices Intended to Increase Athletic Performance* (Dubin, 1990); had the matter been left to the anti-doping organisations, we would probably have found out nothing other than that Johnson, the 'bad apple' of Canadian athletics, had used stanozolol.

The limits of biological testing

Of course, many researchers have expressed doubts, on a variety of grounds, about the effectiveness of biological testing as a means of detecting and controlling drug use and, indeed, WADA has itself recognised the lack of effectiveness of its testing programmes. A working group established by WADA to examine the effectiveness of testing programmes accepted that there is '(n)o research-based evidence that OOC (out-of-competition) testing as conducted is effective' (WADA, 2013, Appendix 'A': 11) and that 'drug testing programs have been generally unsuccessful in detecting dopers/cheaters' (WADA, 2013: 2). In what can only be regarded as a serious indictment of its own programmes, WADA noted that over the last 20 years – and despite increased testing, increasingly sophisticated tests, more out-of-competition testing, more targeted testing, and greatly increased intrusion into the private lives of athletes through the whereabouts programme – still only around 1% of tests produce adverse analytical findings; as WADA has itself noted, there has not been any statistical improvement since about 1985 (WADA, 2013: Appendix 'A': 1). In other words, WADA's testing system appears to be no more successful at identifying drug-using athletes than the widely discredited and corrupt system previously operated by the IOC.

More recently, Moston and Engelberg (2017) have noted that micro-dosing of drugs is difficult to detect, the reliability of the tests themselves often fails to meet normal scientific standards, tamper detection features on sample bottles can be overcome relatively easily, while athletes may adopt any of a variety of evasive manoeuvres to avoid testing. This has led them to suggest that 'the detection of doping through a primary strategy of biological analysis is fatally flawed'; indeed, they argue that 'the detection of doping has hitherto been conducted in ways that effectively ensure that doping will *not* be detected' (Moston & Engelberg, 2017: vii, emphasis added).

I do not wish to comment on the technical problems with testing on which Moston and Engelberg focus; their argument is very different from that being presented here. My central argument is not that the tests are technically imperfect, thus allowing them to be defeated by smart athletes and their advisers. My argument about the limitations of any policy based on biological testing is more fundamental and it is this: no matter how technically sophisticated and effective the analysis of urine and blood samples may become, and no matter how sophisticated the process of biological profiling may become – and also assuming that major problems involving corruption and lack of commitment to anti-doping among some anti-doping and federation officials (WADA, 2013) can also be overcome – such techniques will, by their very nature, *remain inherently incapable of telling us anything at all about the social processes which constrain and encourage and facilitate and conceal drug use in sport.* As we noted earlier, such tests can tell us nothing about the culture of doping, or about relationships between drug-using athletes, doctors, managers, coaches, drug suppliers, and others in the doping network. In other words, the results of such tests – even where they are successful in identify individual drug-using athletes – can tell us nothing about those processes an understanding of which is essential for an understanding of drug use in sport. And without a proper understanding, the possibilities of effective control are minimal.

It is important to recognise that there is an inherently close relationship between the ineffectiveness of anti-doping programmes and their overwhelming dependence on biological testing. If it is accepted that drug-using athletes rarely work alone, unaided by others – and the evidence is overwhelming – then it is clearly important to identify and to sanction not only the athletes who use drugs but also those who supply the drugs, the doctors who administer them, and the coaches, team managers, and others who collude with or conceal their use. But a positive urine or blood sample can only provide evidence of an anti-doping violation on the part of the individual athlete who supplied that sample; it can tell us nothing about who supplied or administered a banned substance and, of course, it cannot be used as evidence against anyone other than the athlete. Put simply, biological testing does nothing – *and can do nothing* – to identify the other people involved in the 'doping network'.

Whither anti-doping policy?

Moston and Engelberg (2017) have noted that there has been a lack of research on the detection of doping in sport and they comment that:

> Coming from a background in forensic interviewing, specifically the questioning of suspects by police officers, we couldn't understand why anti-doping authorities seemed to think that doping could best be detected through biological testing. This would be similar to the police detecting criminals based on a strategy of only collecting fingerprint evidence (suspects would quickly learn that the simple expedient of wearing gloves would render them virtually uncatchable).
>
> (Moston & Engelberg, 2017: vi)

They note that 'It is a popular fallacy, known as the CSI effect … that most criminal investigations are solved through the use of scientifically verifiable evidence (such as fingerprints or DNA)' (p. 65). In fact, however,

> most police investigations centre on talking to people, both witnesses and suspects. Scientific evidence, like DNA matching, is important and sometimes crucial to a case, but by and large most cases are solved by the simple expedient of talking to people.
>
> (p. vi)

Moston and Engelberg's (2017: 63) central argument is that biological testing is, in comparison with forensic interviewing, both an ineffective and a very expensive way of detecting drug-using athletes. In this they are almost certainly correct. Paoli and Donati (2014: 10) have noted that it has been suggested that an elite athlete who is doping may undergo 150 tests before testing positive, suggesting that each positive test costs approximately $300,000. Although Paoli and Donati note that this is a 'back of the envelope calculation', it is clear that biological testing is a remarkably cost-ineffective way of identifying drug-using athletes.

However, the significance of forensic interviewing in anti-doping goes much further than Moston and Engelberg's contention that it is a more effective and more efficient – because more cost-effective – way of identifying drug-using athletes. In this regard, even Moston and Engelberg seem unaware of the full implications of the shift in policy for which they argue. This is because, like the anti-doping organisations they criticise, Moston and Engelberg themselves appear locked into the ideology of individualism and their primary focus therefore remains on identifying the drug-using athlete. However, what they call the 'simple expedient of talking to people' is not simply a more effective way of identifying the individual drug-using athlete; much more importantly, it is the *only* way of identifying, and securing evidence against, other members of the doping network. The key strengths of forensic interviewing – not just identifying the individual drug-using athlete but uncovering the wider structure of the doping network and those involved in it – as well as the importance of non-analytical (i.e. non-biological) data in this process, can be clearly illustrated by reference to one of the most infamous cases of doping not just in cycling, but in any sport: the case of Lance Armstrong.

Learning the lessons of the Armstrong case

It is important to note that the case against Armstrong was not initiated as a result of a positive drug test. Rather, it had its origins in another case which the United States Anti-Doping Agency (USADA) was investigating, against another American cyclist, Kayle Leogrande, which was also based on non-analytical data. Leogrande received a two-year suspension for the use of erythropoietin (EPO) but, in the course of the investigation, witnesses provided USADA with information about people who may have supplied Leogrande and other cyclists with drugs and also information about an alleged doping programme on the United States Postal Service (USPS) team. It was this which led to the USADA investigation which uncovered what USADA (2012: 5) described as 'a massive team doping scheme, more extensive than any previously revealed in professional sports history'.

The USADA investigation did not focus on Armstrong as an isolated individual but on the social organisation of the doping network within the USPS/Discovery Channel teams. As the USADA report documented, 'Armstrong did not act alone. He acted with the help of a small army of enablers, including doping doctors, drug smugglers, and others within and outside the sport and in his team' (USADA, 2012: 6). The report documented in great detail the relationships between those within the doping network, even down to the role of 'Motoman', a motorcycle enthusiast and sometime personal assistant to Armstrong, who used his motorcycle to follow the Tour de France and deliver EPO to riders before mountain stages. And it documented the variety of prohibited substances and methods used by Armstrong and his teammates, not just EPO but also blood transfusions, testosterone, corticosteroids, and masking agents.

As the USADA report (2012: 4) made clear, 'the most critical evidence' came from Armstrong's former teammates and former employees of his cycling teams, that is from what Moston and Engelberg call 'the simple expedient of talking to people'. More specifically, USADA interviewed and took sworn statements from more than two dozen witnesses, including 15 professional cyclists and 12 members of Armstrong's cycling teams. In addition, they also used other non-analytical evidence of the kind frequently used in criminal investigations: banking and accounting records which showed that Armstrong had paid Dr Ferrari, the doctor at the heart of the doping network, more than a million dollars, and e-mails between Ferrari and Armstrong.

It is also important to stress that forensic interviewing not only proved an effective means of successfully bringing a case against someone against whom it was not possible to bring a case based on analytical evidence – at the time there was no publicly available evidence that Armstrong had ever failed a doping test – but, more importantly, by focusing on the social network of doping, USADA was able to generate 'more than enough evidence to proceed with charges' not just against Armstrong but also against former USPS and Discovery Channel team director Johan Bruyneel, former USPS and/or Discovery Channel doctors Pedro Celaya, Luis Garcia del Moral, and Michele Ferrari, and team trainer Jose 'Pepe' Marti (USADA, 2012: 4).

It is sobering to compare how little we have learnt from positive drug tests of individual athletes with how much we have learned from enquiries which, like the USADA inquiry, have focused not on the individual athlete but on building up a picture of doping networks; other significant examples of the latter, all of which have provided very detailed pictures of such networks, include the Dubin Commission in Canada (Dubin, 1990), the investigation and subsequent prosecutions by French police after the 1998 Tour de France (Waddington, 2000), and the report into drug use in American baseball by the former US Senator George Mitchell (Mitchell, 2007). In this regard, it is instructive to engage in a Weberian 'what if', or counterfactual, 'thought experiment' – Weber (1949: 173) himself referred to the production of 'imaginative constructs' – in relation to the Armstrong case.

The USADA investigation revealed that, contrary to Armstrong's frequent public claims that he had never tested positive, he had in fact tested positive for EPO at the 2001 Tour of Switzerland. However, the Union Cycliste Internationale did not make the test result public and no action was taken against Armstrong after he and his team director, Johan Bruyneel, visited the UCI headquarters and Armstrong made a donation of at least $100,000 'to help the development of cycling' (USADA, 2012: 51–52). But consider the following 'what if' scenario: 'what if', instead of the detailed investigation by USADA, the UCI had initiated action against Armstrong on the basis of that positive biological test? What would have been the likely consequences of that?

Of course, we cannot be sure about what would have happened in this situation – as Weber noted, such thought experiments cannot generate certainty – but it is probable that Armstrong would simply have served a sanction of up to two years and that he would then have resumed his cycling career (and probably continued doping). But the critical question is this: had the UCI followed the WADA Code and initiated a case based on the analysis of a biological sample, would this have opened up the Armstrong case for wider analysis of the kind provided by the USADA enquiry or would it, on the contrary, have represented the end point of the process, the conclusion of the case and, far from opening the case up, closed it down to further investigation?

The overwhelming probability is that action against Armstrong based on his positive test would have resulted in Armstrong's suspension and the closure of the case. We would not have discovered anything about the detailed organisation of doping within the USPS and Discovery Channel teams or the central involvement of other people both inside and outside the teams. And, of course, action against Armstrong on the basis of his positive drug test would not have provided any evidence to proceed with charges against anyone other than Armstrong himself.

Despite the significance of investigations of this kind in going beyond the individual drug-using athlete and opening up the wider doping network for examination, such investigations have rarely been initiated by anti-doping organisations, although USADA should perhaps be noted as an exception. In addition to the Armstrong case, USADA was also involved in a highly successful joint investigation from 2003 with the San Mateo County narcotics task force into the Bay Area Laboratory Co-operative (BALCO). It might be noted that investigations of this type have not only generated much more – and more useful – information about doping than could ever be obtained from biological testing of individual athletes, but they have also been instrumental in identifying athletes, like Armstrong, who despite a long history of regular and systematic drug use, had not been detected by biological testing. For example, while not a single cyclist failed a drug test carried out by the race organisers within the 1998 Tour de France – a truly astonishing fact on which neither the UCI nor any anti-doping organisation appears ever to have commented – the French police operation identified a considerable number of cyclists who were using drugs and led to suspensions of riders and prosecutions of other team members. The BALCO investigation also implicated a number of world-class athletes in drug use, including Dwain Chambers, Kelli White and, perhaps most significantly, Marion Jones, a world-class athlete who, like Armstrong, had previously escaped detection despite being tested on innumerable occasions.

Can WADA kick its addiction?

There are signs that WADA is finally – albeit very belatedly – beginning to recognise the significance of investigations of this kind and their potential to reveal the wider structure of doping networks. In 2015, the WADA President, Sir Craig Reedie, announced that 'WADA is increasingly of the belief that athletes do not dope alone, and that often there is a member of their entourage encouraging them to cheat' (WADA, 2015a). This recognition of a basic aspect of drug use is welcome, though those who have argued for evidence-based anti-doping policy will be disappointed that WADA has only just discovered what social scientists have been saying for over half a century.

Reedie's comment was made in relation to a new 'prohibited association' rule in the 2015 WADA Code (WADA, 2015b, article 2.10), which prohibits athletes and other persons from working with athlete support personnel who are currently sanctioned or who have been sanctioned in the previous six years for an anti-doping violation. Perhaps of greater significance, however, is another change in the 2015 Code which gives WADA power to 'initiate its own investigations of anti-doping rule violations and other activities that may facilitate doping' (WADA, 2015b, article 20.7.10). It was this rule which was used to establish the McLaren Independent Investigation which revealed widespread state-sponsored doping of Russian athletes involving more than 1000 athletes and more than 30 sports – and which thereby pointed up once again the ineffectiveness of biological testing of individual athletes as a means of detecting doping. The 2016 WADA Annual Report recognised that such investigations 'helped prove that non-analytical evidence is of tremendous value to anti-doping and that WADA's investigations and intelligence-gathering capacity need to be enhanced' (WADA, 2017: 8). Few social scientists would disagree with this statement, though some may express doubts about whether WADA and other anti-doping organisations can really kick their own addiction to biological testing.

References

Becker, H. (1963). *Outsiders*. New York: Free Press.

Bette, K.-H. (2004). Biographical risks and doping. In J. Hoberman, V. Møller (Eds) *Doping and Public Policy* (pp. 101–111). Odense: University of Southern Denmark.

Brewer, B. (2002). Commercialization in professional cycling 1950–2001: institutional transformations and the rationalization of doping. *Sociology of Sport Journal, 19*, 276–301.

Brissonneau, C. (2015). The 1998 Tour de France: Festina, from scandal to an affair in cycling. In V. Møller, I. Waddington, J. Hoberman (Eds), *Routledge Handbook of Drugs and Sport* (pp. 181–192). London: Routledge.

Christiansen, A.V. (2005). The legacy of Festina: patterns of drug use in European cycling since 1998. *Sport in History, 25*(3), 497–514.

Clarke, A.E., Mamo, L., Fishman, J.R., Shim, J.K., & Fosket, J.R. (2003). Biomedicalization: Technoscientific transformations of health, illness and U.S. medicine. *American Sociological Review*, 68(2), 161–194.

Conrad, P. (2005). The shifting engines of medicalization. *Journal of Health and Social Behaviour*, 45, 3–14.

Dubin, Honourable C.L. (1990). *Commission of Inquiry into the Use of Drugs and Banned Practices Intended to Increase Athletic Performance*. Ottawa: Canadian Government Publishing Centre.

Elias, N. (1970). *What is Sociology?* London: Hutchinson.

Faulkner, A., McNamee, M., Coveney, C., & Gabe, J. (2017). Where biomedicalization and magic meet: Therapeutic innovations of elite sports injury in British professional football and cycling. *Social Science and Medicine, 178*, 136–143.

Hoberman, J. (1992). *Mortal Engines: The Science of Performance and the Dehumanization of Sport*. New York: Free Press.

Hoberman, J. (2002). Sports physicians and the doping crisis in elite sport. *Clinical Journal of Sport Medicine, 12*, 203–208.

Hoberman, J. (2003). 'A pharmacy on wheels': doping and community cohesion among professional cyclists following the Tour de France scandal of 1998. In V. Møller, J. Nauright (Eds), *The Essence of Sport* (pp. 107–127). Odense: University Press of Southern Denmark.

Hoberman, J. (2012). Sports physicians and doping: medical ethics and elite performance. In D. Malcolm, P. Safai (Eds), *The Social Organization of Sports Medicine* (pp. 237–264). New York: Routledge.

Hoberman, J. (2013). Sports physicians, human nature, and the limits of medical enhancement. In J. Tolleneer, S. Sterckx, P. Bonte (Eds), *Athletic Enhancement, Human Nature and Ethics* (pp. 255–270). Dordrecht: Springer.

Illich, I. (1975). *Medical Nemesis*. London: Calder and Boyars.

Malcolm, D. (2017). *Sport, Medicine and Health: The Medicalization of Sport?* London: Routledge.

Mitchell, G.J. (2007). *Report to the Commissioner of Baseball of an Independent Investigation into the Illegal Use of Steroids and other Performance Enhancing Substances by Players in Major League Baseball*. New York: Office of the Commissioner of Baseball.

Monaghan, L. (2001). *Bodybuilding, Drugs and Risk*. London: Routledge.

Moston, S. & Engelberg, T. (2017). *Detecting Doping in Sport*. London: Routledge.

Nixon, H.L. II (1992). A social network analysis of influences on athletes to play with pain and injuries. *Journal of Sport and Social Issues, 16*(2), 127–135.

Paoli, L. & Donati, A. (2014). *The Sports Doping Market*. New York: Springer.

USADA (2012), *Report on Proceedings Under the World Anti-Doping Code and the USADA Protocol: Reasoned Decision of the United States Anti-Doping Agency on Disqualification and Ineligibility*. Colorado Springs: USADA.

WADA Working Group (2013), *Report to WADA Executive Committee on Lack of Effectiveness of Testing Programs*. www.wada-ama.org/en/resources/world-anti-doping-program/lack-of-effectiveness-of-testing-program, accessed 27 November 2017

WADA (2015a). WADA publishes global list of suspended athlete support personnel, 14 September, www.wada-ama.org/en/media/news/2015-09/wada-publishes-global-list-of-suspended-athlete-support-personnel, accessed 30 October 2017.

WADA (2015b). *World Anti-Doping Code*. Montreal: WADA.

WADA (2016). *2015 Anti-Doping Testing Figures*, by laboratory. Montreal: WADA.

WADA (2017). *2016 Anti-Doping Testing Figures*, Executive summary. Montreal: WADA.

WADA (2017). Annual Report 2016. Montreal: WADA.

Waddington, I. (1996). The development of sports medicine. *Sociology of Sport Journal, 13*(2), 176–196.

Waddington, I. (2000). *Sport, Health and Drugs*. London: E & FN Spon.

Waddington, I. (2001). Doping in sport: a medical sociological perspective. In *Research on Doping in Sport* (pp. 11–21). Oslo: Norwegian University of Sport and Physical Education.

Waddington, I. (2004). Doping in sport: some issues for medical practitioners. In J. Hoberman, V. Møller (Eds), *Doping and Public Policy* (pp. 31–44). Odense: University Press of Southern Denmark.

Waddington, I. (2005). Le dopage sportif: la responsibilité des praticiens médicaux/ Doping in sport: the responsibilities of medical practitioners. *Revue internationale des sciences du sport et de l'education physique/International Journal of Sport Science and Physical Education*, 26, 9–23.

Waddington, I. (2007). Doping in de sport – Naar een sociologische verklaring. In J. Van Gestel (Eds), *Figuraties in de Sport* (pp. 185–211). Gent: Academia Press.

Waddington, I. (2015). Towards an understanding of drug use in sport: a medical sociological perspective. In V. Møller, I. Waddington, J. Hoberman (Eds), *Routledge Handbook of Drugs and Sport* (pp. 405–417). London: Routledge.

Waddington, I. (2016). Social and behavioural perspectives on drug use in sport. In N. Ahmadi, A. Ljungqvist, & G. Svedsäter (Eds), *Doping and Public Health* (pp. 22–37). London: Routledge.

Waddington, I. & Murphy, P. (1992). Drugs, sport and ideologies. In E. Dunning & C. Rojek (Eds), *Sport and Leisure in the Civilizing Process: Critique and Counter-Critique* (pp. 36–64). London: Palgrave Macmillan.

Waddington, I. & Smith, A. (2009). *An Introduction to Drugs in Sport*. London: Routledge.

Waitzkin, H. & Waterman, B. (1974). *The Exploitation of Illness in Capitalist Society*. New York: Bobbs-Merrill.

Weber, M. (1949). *The Methodology of the Social Sciences*. New York. Free Press.

Zola, I. (1972). Medicine as an institution of social control. *Sociological Review*, 20, 487–504.

Chapter 3

Substance use, anti-doping, and health in amateur cycling

April Henning

Cycling is no stranger to issues and scandals around doping with performance enhancing substances (PES). In particular, cycling's relationship with doping was a driver of many anti-doping developments that now have a global and cross-sport reach through the World Anti-Doping Agency (WADA). Founded on the twin principles of health and fairness, anti-doping has focused mainly on the elite levels of sport though its rules to extend to govern non-elites in member sports. However, research on non-elite cycling has begun to emerge both from academics and from sport-authorised commissions that increasingly shows amateur cyclists also engage in doping (CIRC Report, 2015). Among these non-elite athletes are those at the very top of the amateur divisions who may later become professionals, as well as those who compete at lower levels or in masters divisions and who are unlikely to win competitions, turn professional, or even identify as more than a recreational cyclist (Henning & Dimeo, 2015). With an increased awareness of doping among amateur cyclists, sport governing bodies have begun to respond. USA Cycling increased its attention and resource allocation for testing amateurs under its RaceClean programme for the 2016 competitive year, resulting in an increased number of tests conducted and positive samples returned (Whiteman, 2017).

While it is not unreasonable for WADA or a sport to limit or prohibit the use of demonstrably dangerous substances in the name of athlete health, it is often taken for granted that the current policies are fair, effective, and pro-health. While these views of the risks of all doping substances and the effectiveness of anti-doping policy is not the view shared by some sport scholars (e.g. Alexander, 2014; López, 2013; 2014; Smith & Stewart, 2015; Waddington, Christiansen, Gleaves, Hoberman, & Møller, 2013), anti-doping policies have continued to take the same detect-and-punish approach to athletes across the competitive spectrum. This has come, seemingly, without much regard for how athlete health may be negatively impacted by the current approach to anti-doping. Negative health effects of anti-doping policies may be less of a concern among elites with resources and expertise to draw on for planning training and monitoring health. However, amateurs differ in significant ways from elites and expecting cyclists competing in weekend Gravel Grinders to have the same lifestyles, resources, and needs as the pros in the Grand Tours ignores these distinctions. Simply expanding anti-doping programmes designed for elite athletes to include amateurs carries several risks that can undercut the effectiveness of the programme, but that also may negatively impact athlete health and overall wellbeing.

The result of such a move for amateur cycling is that in some cases anti-doping is at odds with athlete health. There are various reasons for this, several of which are especially relevant to amateur cyclists. Below I will identify three health-related themes that illustrate problem areas for the wholesale application of current anti-doping to amateur cycling. Drawing on cases from cycling, including the results from the 2016 RaceClean programme, I will show where policy rethinks, adjustments, and overhauls may be necessary. I argue that amateur cyclists require an approach focused on health needs and harm reduction, rather than on detection and punishment.

Background and literature

WADA was established in 1999 to set global standards for anti-doping regulations and ensure that these are consistently applied across signatory countries and sports. Under its Code, WADA defines the rules around doping – including what is considered a violation of these rules – and provides a framework for their enforcement (WADA, 2015). As part of these policies, WADA also manages the annually updated List of Prohibited Substances and Methods (WADA, 2016). Together, these two documents form the basis for anti-doping efforts. Though all participants in sports governed by Code signatories are subject to the Code, most anti-doping efforts have focused on elite-level athletes, especially in Olympic sport.

WADA relies on health as one rationale for rendering a substance prohibited, along with fairness and the 'spirit of sport'. Health, or the risk a substance potentially presents to health, is one of three criteria used to determine which substances are banned. The other two criteria are the potential for enhancing performance and whether a substance is contra the 'spirit of sport'.[1] A substance meeting two of these three criteria may be banned from use. It is important to highlight that section 4.3.1.2 of the WADA Code specifies that substances or methods need only to present a *potential* health risk, not necessarily an *actual* risk, to meet the health criteria; section 4.3.1.1 gives a similar specification for a substances' potential to enhance performance (WADA, 2015: 30). The unclear decision-making process obscures the basis for inclusions to the list and can raise questions and confusion about why some substances are included (McNamee, 2012).

The extent to which doping occurs is an ongoing question at all levels of competition. While testing returns an annual 1–2% rate of positives across all samples, this is widely thought to be significantly lower than actual prevalence rates (Dimeo & Taylor, 2013; Pitsch, Emrich, & Klein, 2007). Statistical modelling has put the single season prevalence of banned substance use among elite athletes closer to 48% (Dimeo & Taylor, 2013). A study of elite athletes using a combination of modelling plus athlete questionnaires estimated prevalence between 14% and 39% (de Hon, Kuipers, & van Bottenburg, 2015). A recently published study of elite track and field athletes surveyed using the randomised response technique (RRT) found that past year doping at two events was estimated at 43.6% and 57.1% (Ulrich et al., 2017). At non-elite sport levels, studies have begun to show that lower level competitors use banned substances. A study of recreational sports populations in Germany using an indirect questioning method, randomised response technique, found the prevalence for lifetime use of doping substances fell between 3.35% and 10.55% (Frenger, Pitsch & Emrich, 2016). Similar use rates have been found in studies of fitness centre users, with 8.2% in Dutch gyms (Stubbe, Chorus, Frank, Hon, & Heijden, 2014) and 12.5% in a German sample (Simon, Striegel, Aust, Dietz, & Ulrich, 2006). Each of these studies use different methods and focus on differing populations and comparisons should be considered with a critical eye. However, the clear trend is that each puts the likely prevalence rate well above the rate of returned positives. As anti-doping testing and educational resources tend to be concentrated at the elite levels of sport, findings of high prevalence among lower competitive groups raises questions about the effectiveness and ability of the anti-doping system to achieve its stated goals.

Though only a few studies have looked at amateur cycling directly, there is evidence of doping behaviours at lower competitive levels of the sport. In a study of doping cases in cycling, amateur use patterns sometimes differed from elites (Henning & Dimeo, 2015). A study of Australian elite amateur cyclists found those cyclists saw a close relationship between doping and being a professional cyclist, with some drawing parallels between legal supplement use for enhancing purposes and using banned substances (Outram & Stewart, 2015). Results of an online survey of Spanish adult amateur cyclists showed 'amateur cyclists in general and amateur cyclists with experience in competition in particular as groups at risk for PED use' (Zabala, Morente-Sánchez, Mateo-March, Sanabria, 2016: 73). Cyclists may also have more tolerant attitudes towards doping than other sports, as a survey of Spanish female competitive cyclists and triathletes found (Morente-Sánchez, Leruite, Mateo-March, & Zabala, 2013). However, health may be overlooked in discussions of anti-doping in cycling in favour of the drive to retain sponsors responsible for the financial survival of cycling (Waddington & Smith, 2009). Rather, the focus on morality, detection, and punishment may come at the expense of athlete health.

Amateur cycling: anti-doping vs. health?

Anti-doping and health likely were not intended to be at odds with one another. On its face it would seem logical that prohibiting the use of potentially harmful substances would be in the interests of both health and fairness. The realities of these policies highlight where they collide with health, the former potentially undermining the latter. I have identified three key health related obstacles for implementing anti-doping in amateur cycling. Of course, these themes overlap and are related to one another. For clarity, I have broken them down across these three themes: deterrence, motivation/intent, and inadvertent consumption/knowledge.

Deterrence

The focus on testing athletes has often been rationalised in terms of deterrence. The logic is that athletes will weigh the cost of being caught using banned substances against the potential rewards of doping. More testing means a greater likelihood of detection, altering the cost calculation in ways that deter use (Donovan, Egger, Kapernick, & Mendoza, 2002; Strelan & Boeckmann, 2006). Testing may act as a deterrent at the elite level, where cyclists are tested frequently and have livelihoods at stake. However, expanding anti-doping testing to include amateur cyclists may catch a few cyclists who are intentionally doping, but it will likely catch more cyclists who are unknowingly using banned substances or using them for reasons not related to enhancement (see M. Viret's paper in this book). One illustrative case is the results from USA Cycling's 2016 RaceClean programme, targeted at amateur athletes. The programme was responsible for a total of 185 tests during 2016 (Whiteman, 2017) conducted on a membership of more than 60,000 (USA Cycling, 2016). While the number of tests was a large increase over previous years, there was a very low likelihood that any given amateur would be tested under the programme. Because of the cost of anti-doping testing it is improbable that the vast majority of USA Cycling's amateur members will ever be tested. When there is no real threat of being tested, and therefore having any banned substance use detected, the existence of a testing programme is unlikely to have a real deterrence effect.

Seeking to deter amateur cyclists also does little in the way of promoting health when use of a banned substance is medically necessary. Cyclists using a banned substance under medical advice may find their health is negatively impacted by stopping use to remain within sport rules or by ending their participation in cycling and potentially losing the social and health benefits of participation. An athlete may also remain within cycling rules but endanger health by using or overusing potentially risky substances that are allowed in sport, such as some pain killers during endurance events (Küster, Renner, Oppel, Niederweis, & Brune, 2013). It is here that the question of what motivates a cyclist to use a prohibited substance becomes important to consider.

Motivation and intent

Amateur cyclists, including competitive amateurs, are often differently motivated to either knowingly or unknowingly use banned substances than elites (Henning & Dimeo, 2015; Outram & Stewart, 2015). Amateurs' motivations for using banned substances can vary widely beyond seeking to directly enhance performance. Additional motivations may include the desire to improve health, overcome training fatigue or injury, controlling weight, body image reasons, or for recreation and relaxation (Henning & Dimeo, 2014). However, intent to use a prohibited substance does not need to be shown in order for an athlete to receive a sanction under the principle of strict liability (Koh, Edwards, Freeman, & Zaslawski, 2012). For cyclists unknowingly using prohibited substances, or who are using a medication containing one under the care of a medical doctor, they are held responsible in the same way as an athlete intentionally using a substance for performance enhancement.

The effect an amateur cyclist is seeking will also influence the substance he or she chooses. One growing challenge is the increasing legality of cannabis as it remains banned under WADA rules. According to available United States Anti-Doping Agency (USADA) records, eight cyclists have been banned for positive anti-doping tests showing Tetrahydrocannabinol or THC, the psychoactive component of cannabis (USADA, 2017). In every case, the cyclists were given reduced bans from the maximum available penalty. While this allowed cyclists to return to competition more quickly than those who receive the maximum ban, it did nothing to prevent them being labelled a doper. This, along with the lack of evidence for performance enhancing benefits and any major health risk potential, has led to debate over its inclusion on the Prohibited List (Henne, Koh, & McDermott, 2013; Waddington et al., 2013). Given its status as a primarily recreational drug makes it unlikely that these athletes were seeking a direct performance benefit from their use, though there is evidence cannabis can be useful medicinally (Hill, 2015). The recent wave of cannabis decriminalisation in several countries or localities has left cannabis-using cyclists in a tricky spot. In terms of local law, they are within the bounds of acceptability. However, they remain in violation of WADA rules prohibiting cannabis use.

Amateur athletes may also face a choice between anti-doping rules and medical advice. As I have argued elsewhere (Henning, 2017) it should be expected that amateur athletes would follow the advice of their personal medical professionals when treating illness or injury. Even when an athlete uses a prescription medication containing a banned substance under a doctor's supervision and advice they still face a sanction if tested for anti-doping purposes. The system for issuing exemptions for medically necessary use of banned substances, called therapeutic use exemptions or TUEs, is intended to prevent such situations by allowing athletes to apply for and receive a waiver for using a banned substance. Applying for a TUE does not ensure one will be granted.

In 2016, masters cyclist Mary Verrando-Higgins applied for a TUE after receiving a prescription for a medication containing an anabolic agent (USADA, 2016). Verrando-Higgins was denied a TUE, but chose to compete while taking her medication. She tested positive for an anabolic agent in May 2016, but was given a reduced one-year competition ban 'due to the nature and extent of the medical records provided, USADA accepted Verrando-Higgins' explanation that she used the substance with a prescription under the care of a licenced physician for therapeutic purposes and without the intent to enhance her athletic performance' (USADA, 2016). Despite denying her request for a TUE, USADA saw fit to reduce Verrando-Higgins' sanction on the grounds that it was for medical purposes and not an unfair enhancement. Other amateur and masters cyclists may now face similar dilemmas under USA Cycling's Race-Clean programme.

Inadvertent consumption and knowledge

The question of motivation is complicated by amateur cyclists' knowledge of places where banned substances might be found. Even well-intentioned cyclists are vulnerable to the unexpected presence of banned substances in products they purchase legally and are widely available. This is underscored by the fact that cyclists may inadvertently ingest a banned substance, including those found in over-the-counter (OTC) medications, prescription medications, and nutritional supplements (Cox, 2014; Pluim, 2008). Research into doping cases has shown that up to 40% of all positive tests may be due to inadvertent consumption of banned substances, likely through nutritional supplements and OTC medications (de Hon, 2016).

Inadvertent consumption has real consequences for cyclists at all competitive levels. As just one example, US cyclist Logan Loader was banned for eight months in 2014 for using a supplement containing a banned stimulant (USADA, 2014). Though Loader was racing with a professional team at the time of his test and could expect to be tested for anti-doping, he was unable to avoid a product containing a prohibited substance. Amateurs with less knowledge of anti-doping and of the risks posed by unverified supplements could easily find themselves in a similar situation. Though Loader's shortened ban reflects the acceptance that his use was likely unintentional, Loader is still considered a 'doper' despite his positive test resulting from using a legal supplement. The social stigma associated with doping in sport (Coomber, 2013) may have harsher consequences for amateurs than the formal competition ban outside of sport. For example, a future employer searching an athlete's name could see a press release announcing the suspension among the top search returns. The association with doping is likely to come up in Internet searches for the person's name even years after an athlete has served their ban.

Compounding the problem of the knowledge gap is the scale of the global supplement industry and the lack of regulations on supplements in many countries where these products are manufactured or sold. Contamination of supplements and the presence of ingredients not listed on product labels, as well as manufacturers that intentionally add unlisted ingredients, are each issues that leave cyclists at risk for inadvertent consumption (Maughan, 2005; Rocha, Amaral, & Oliveira, 2016). Inadvertent consumption might be curtailed through better education on the risks around supplements, along with strategies for improving the chances of using unadulterated products. However, given the vast number of amateur cyclists in the US and globally, educating cyclists at all levels is a challenge. In the absence of such education amateur athletes are often left to self-educate about doping and anti-doping, relying on a variety of sources (Erickson, McKenna, & Backhouse, 2015). Taking the wrong advice can result not only in a positive test, but might also result in a negative health outcome for the user. Allergic reactions and accidental overdoses are just two risks of products with incomplete or unclear labels.

Conclusion: focus on health

Simply expanding current anti-doping policies to amateurs are likely to be ineffective at either reducing the number of dopers caught or better promoting athlete health. The outcomes of such moves are particularly relevant for cycling and cyclists as pushes to increasingly test amateurs continue. Given the resource-intensive nature of conducting testing and the comparatively low levels of resources available, amateurs are unlikely to see testing as a strong enough threat to deter intentional use. Athletes inadvertently using banned substances through other means (i.e. supplements, medications) are also unlikely to be deterred unless testing is accompanied by comprehensive anti-doping education and resources for identifying risky products. Anti-doping will also need to better address cannabis, as its shifting legal status can leave athletes caught between legality and sport prohibition. This is similar to the position of athletes using prohibited substances under medical supervision, forcing a choice between medical advice for health and anti-doping policies.

A solution to the health conundrum of anti-doping, at least for amateurs, is to take a different approach altogether. Several scholars have called for harm reduction or harm minimisation approaches to anti-doping (Henning & Dimeo, 2017; Kayser & Broers, 2012; Kirkwood, 2009; Stewart & Smith, 2010; Waddington & Smith, 2009). Though the approaches differ in their details, each takes health as its central focus. Often borrowing from the body of research on successful harm reduction approaches for recreational drug use (i.e. Des Jarlais & Friedman, 1998; Ritter & Cameron, 2006), harm reduction accepts that substance use is occurring and then seeks to reduce the risks of such use. In cycling, this could mean empowering athletes to critically evaluate their own use through educational outreach, resource provision, and access to trustworthy experts who can inform them of the risks and rewards of substances. At the amateur level, harm reduction would likely better serve athlete health than the current approach that is focused on detecting and punishing athletes for any use, including medical, recreational, and inadvertent.

However, it seems unlikely that any such shifts are on the horizon. At the conclusion of the two-day workshop on doping in cycling that preceded this volume, I was struck by the seeming acceptance among the gathered experts from research, sport, and anti-doping that anti-doping policies overlook the unintended health risks. No fewer than three presentations – those by Bertrand Fincoeur and Ivan Waddington, as well as my own – directly noted that anti-doping policy misses opportunities to create a more nuanced approach to athlete health in various ways. Rather than discussing or questioning these assertions, discussion bypassed health in favour of other topics. Of course, it is possible that the gathered experts viewed these other topics as more pressing, urgent, or interesting. However, the silence around health was and is emblematic of the way that many have come to accept some of the negative consequences of the current anti-doping approach. It seems that if health – one of the underpinning rationales for anti-doping – is to be taken seriously, stakeholders must engage with the negative effects of anti-doping policies.

Whether anti-doping organisations and sports governing bodies are unaware of the issues around athlete health or have accepted that anti-doping policies fall short of promoting health in some ways, the implications are becoming more pressing for amateur cyclists. The WADA Code may not be well suited for the realities of amateur competition in its current form. Cyclists participating for recreation, personal drive, or health reasons may weigh their chances of actually being tested and decide to simply continue on in defiance – or ignorance – of the rules. However, others may choose to leave the organised aspects of the sport rather than bother with medical exemptions or chance being labelled a doper. Those in cycling often view its doping past as a black mark on the sport, with credibility that can only be saved by rigorous and harsh anti-doping. But racking up 'collateral damage' (Cox, 2014) among amateur cyclists caught up in strict liability while simultaneously unable to prevent intentional doping does not seem to warrant new confidence in old methods.

Note

1 WADA defines the spirit of sport as a set of sporting values: 'ethics, fair play and honesty; health; excellence in performance; character and education; fun and joy; teamwork; dedication and commitment; respect for rules and laws; respect for self and other participants; courage; community and solidarity' (WADA, 2015: 14).

References

Alexander, B.R. (2014). War on drugs redux: Welcome to the war on doping in sports. *Substance Use & Misuse*, 49(9), 1190–1193.

Cox, T.W. (2014). International war against doping: Limiting the collateral damage from strict liability. *The Vanderbilt Journal of Transnational Law*, 47, 295.

de Hon, O.M. (2016). *Striking the right balance: Effectiveness of anti-doping policies*. Doctoral dissertation. Utrecht University.

de Hon, O., Kuipers, H., & van Bottenburg, M. (2015). Prevalence of doping use in elite sports: a review of numbers and methods. *Sports Medicine*, 45(1), 57–69.

Des Jarlais, D.C. & Friedman, S.R. (1998). Fifteen years of research on preventing HIV infection among injecting drug users: what we have learned, what we have not learned, what we have done, what we have not done. *Public Health Reports*, *113*(Suppl. 1), 182–188.

Dimeo, P. & Taylor, J. (2013). Monitoring drug use in sport: The contrast between official statistics and other evidence. *Drugs: Education, Prevention and Policy*, *20*(1), 40–47.

Donovan, R.J., Egger, G., Kapernick, V., & Mendoza, J. (2002). A conceptual framework for achieving performance enhancing drug compliance in sport. *Sports Medicine*, *32*(4), 269–284.

Erickson, K., McKenna, J., & Backhouse, S.H. (2015). A qualitative analysis of the factors that protect athletes against doping in sport. *Psychology of Sport and Exercise*, *16*, 149–155.

Frenger, M., Pitsch, W., & Emrich, E. (2016). Sport-induced substance use – an empirical study to the extent within a German sports association. *PloS one*, *11*(10), e0165103.

Henne, K., Koh, B., & McDermott, V. (2013). Coherence of drug policy in sports: Illicit inclusions and illegal inconsistencies. *Performance Enhancement & Health*, *2*, 48–55.

Henning, A. (2017). Challenges to promoting health for amateur athletes through anti-doping policy. *Drugs: Education, Prevention and Policy*, *24*(3), 306–313.

Henning, A. & Dimeo, P. (2014). The complexities of anti-doping violations: A case study of sanctioned cases in all performance levels of USA cycling. *Performance Enhancement & Health*, *3*(3), 159–166.

Henning, A. & Dimeo, P. (2015). Questions of fairness and anti-doping in US cycling: The contrasting experiences of professionals and amateurs. *Drugs: Education, Prevention and Policy*, *22*(5), 400–409.

Hill, K.P. (2015). Medical marijuana for treatment of chronic pain and other medical and psychiatric problems: a clinical review. *JAMA*, *313*(24), 2474–2483.

Kayser, B. & Broers, B. (2012). The Olympics and harm reduction? *Harm Reduction Journal*, *9*(1), 33.

Kirkwood, K. (2009). Considering harm reduction as the future of doping control policy in international sport. *Quest*, *61*(2), 180–190.

Koh, B., Edwards, J., Freeman, L., & Zaslawski, C. (2012). Doping knowledge in sports: Actus reus versus mens rea. *Journal of Science and Medicine in Sport*, *15*, S52–S53.

Küster, M., Renner, B., Oppel, P., Niederweis, U., & Brune, K. (2013). Consumption of analgesics before a marathon and the incidence of cardiovascular, gastrointestinal and renal problems: A cohort study. *BMJ Open*, *3*, e002090.

López, B. (2013). Creating fear: The social construction of human Growth Hormone as a dangerous doping drug. *International Review for the Sociology of Sport*, *48*(2), 220–237.

López, B. (2014). Creating fear: the 'doping deaths', risk communication and the anti-doping campaign. *International Journal of Sport Policy and Politics*, *6*(2), 213–225.

Maughan, R.J. (2005). Contamination of dietary supplements and positive drug tests in sport. *Journal of Sports Sciences*, *23*(9), 883–889.

McNamee, M.J. (2012). The spirit of sport and the medicalisation of anti-doping: empirical and normative ethics. *Asian Bioethics Review*, *4*(4), 374–392.

Morente-Sánchez, J., Leruite, M., Mateo-March, M., & Zabala, M. (2013). Attitudes towards doping in Spanish competitive female cyclists vs. triathletes. *Journal of Science and Cycling*, *2*(2), 40–48.

Outram, S.M. & Stewart, B. (2015). Condemning and condoning: Elite amateur cyclists' perspectives on drug use and professional cycling. *International Journal of Drug Policy*, *26*(7), 682–687.

Pitsch, W., Emrich, E., & Klein, M. (2007). Doping in elite sports in Germany: Results of a www survey. *European Journal for Sport and Society*, *4*(2), 89–102.

Pluim, B. (2008). A doping sinner is not always a cheat. *British Journal of Sports Medicine*, *42*, 549–550.

Ritter, A. & Cameron, J. (2006). A review of the efficacy and effectiveness of harm reduction strategies for alcohol, tobacco and illicit drugs. *Drug and Alcohol Review*, *25*(6), 611–624.

Rocha, T., Amaral, J.S., & Oliveira, M.B.P. (2016). Adulteration of dietary supplements by the illegal addition of synthetic drugs: a review. *Comprehensive Reviews in Food Science and Food Safety*, *15*(1), 43–62.

Simon, P., Striegel, H., Aust, F., Dietz, K., & Ulrich, R. (2006). Doping in fitness sports: estimated number of unreported cases and individual probability of doping. *Addiction*, *101*(11), 1640–1644.

Smith, A.C. & Stewart, B. (2015). Why the war on drugs in sport will never be won. *Harm Reduction Journal*, *12*(1), 53.

Strelan, P. & Boeckmann, R.J. (2006). Why drug testing in elite sport does not work: Perceptual deterrence theory and the role of personal moral beliefs. *Journal of Applied Social Psychology*, *36*(12), 2909–2934.

Stubbe, J.H., Chorus, A.M., Frank, L.E., de Hon, O., & van der Heijden, P.G. (2014). Prevalence of use of performance enhancing drugs by fitness centre members. *Drug Testing and Analysis*, 6(5), 434–438.

Ulrich, R., Pope, H.G., Cléret, L., Petróczi, A., Nepusz, T., Schaffer, J., ... & Simon, P. (2017). Doping in two elite athletics competitions assessed by randomized-response surveys. *Sports Medicine*, 1–9.

USA Cycling (2016). 2015 Annual Report. Retrieved from https://s3.amazonaws.com/USACWeb/forms/2015%20Annual%20Report.pdf

USADA (2014). US Cycling Athlete, Loader, Accepts Sanction for Anti-Doping Rule Violation. Retrieved from www.usada.org/us-cycling-athlete-loader-accepts-sanction-anti-doping-rule-violation/ (16 July).

USADA (2016). U.S. Cycling Athlete, Verrando-Higgins, Accepts Sanction for Anti-Doping Rule Violation. Retrieved from www.usada.org/mary-verrando-higgins-accepts-doping-sanction/ (15 August).

WADA (2015). World Anti-Doping Code. Retrieved from www.wada-ama.org/en/resources/the-code/world-anti-doping-code.

WADA (2016). List of Prohibited Substances and Methods. Retrieved from www.wada-ama.org/en/resources/science-medicine/prohibited-list-documents

Waddington, I., Christiansen, A.V., Gleaves, J., Hoberman, J., & Møller, V. (2013). Recreational drug use and sport: Time for a WADA rethink? *Performance Enhancement & Health*, *2*, 41–47.

Waddington, I. & Smith, A. (2009). *An introduction to drugs in sport: Addicted to winning?* London: Routledge.

Whiteman, J. (2017). 2017 Q1 update. Retrieved from https://s3.amazonaws.com/USACWeb/forms/anti-doping/Q1-RC-Update.pdf

Zabala, M., Morente-Sánchez, J., Mateo-March, M., & Sanabria, D. (2016). Relationship between self-reported doping behavior and psychosocial factors in adult amateur cyclists. *The Sport Psychologist*, *30*(1), 68–75.

Chapter 4

The impact of scientific advances on doping in cycling

Reid Aikin and Pierre-Edouard Sottas

Under the World Anti-Doping Code – the document harmonising anti-doping rules and regulations in all sports and countries – the fundamental target of anti-doping is '*to protect the Athletes' fundamental right to participate in doping-free sport and thus promote health, fairness and equality for Athletes worldwide*'. The ability of a clean athlete to compete fairly relates to (1) the prevalence of doping and (2) the effect size of doping regimes on performance, where the prevalence of doping is independent of the effectiveness of the doping regimes used. While considerable emphasis has been placed on the reduction of the prevalence of doping as the key measure of success of anti-doping programmes, the reduction of the effectiveness of anti-doping regimes should be considered of equal, or arguably greater, importance. For example, a high prevalence of doping with substances that have little or no benefit on performance will provide a higher likelihood of a clean athlete competing fairly than a situation of a relatively low prevalence of doping with substances with high effect sizes. Thus, an effective anti-doping programme should seek to reduce not only the prevalence but also the effectiveness of doping by simultaneously deterring athletes from doping and by limiting their available options to dope in terms of substances, doses, and timing of doping regimes.

Here we review several key advances in anti-doping over the past decade that have significantly reduced doping in cycling. These include the development of direct tests for erythropoiesis-stimulating agents (ESAs), the creation of a whereabouts system for out-of-competition testing, and the Athlete Biological Passport (ABP).

ESA detection

The transport of oxygen to muscles is a major limiting factor in endurance performance (Bassett & Howley, 2000). Therefore, strategies to increase oxygen delivery to muscles can increase endurance performance. In particular, increasing the total amount of the oxygen carrying protein haemoglobin (HGB) can increase the amount of oxygen that can be delivered to working muscles. Increases in haemoglobin can be triggered naturally through endurance training over a long period and more rapidly through an exposure to hypoxia (e.g. altitude), but also, and potentially with a significantly larger effect size on performance, artificially through the use of ESAs or blood transfusion (Ekblom, Goldbarg, & Gullbring, 1972; Ekblom & Berglund, 1991; Birkeland et al., 2000; Russell, Gore, Ashenden, Parisotto, & Hahn 2002; Thomsen et al., 2007; Durussel et al., 2013; Clark et al., 2017).

Erythropoietin (EPO) is a protein produced by the kidney under conditions of reduced oxygen levels (e.g. a stay at altitude) which favours the differentiation, survival and proliferation of young erythroid cells, resulting in a faster release of immature red blood cells from the bone marrow into the circulation (Hattangadi, Wong, Zhang, Flygare, & Lodish, 2011). The administration of recombinant EPO (rEPO) was shown to increase HGB levels in patients with anemia (Eschbach, Egrie, Downing, Browne, & Adamson, 1987), and was subsequently approved for medical use in 1989. Shortly after its introduction in the clinics, rEPO made its way into the professional peloton and, according to numerous rider testimonials, its use was rampant during the 1990s, including by top riders (Cycling Independent Reform Commission (CIRC) report).

The first-generation rEPO test was launched in the summer of 2001 (Lasne & de Ceaurriz, 2000). However, unscrupulous athletes learned quickly that rEPO was excreted rapidly from the body (within a few days) with the effects on performance remaining over a significantly longer period (a few weeks). In summer 2001, only three months after the introduction of the test, blood profiles characterised by a high erythropoietic simulating index, known as the OFF-score (Gore et al., 2003), appeared in the elite peloton, demonstrating that doping athletes changed their behaviour to dope outside of competitions and escape the tests that were, until that time, mostly carried out during competitions.

Out-of-competition testing, new ESAs, and blood transfusion

Testing athletes outside of competitions was problematic for the simple reason that it was difficult to locate the athletes. To address this issue, the so-called 'whereabouts' system was developed and launched in 2005. This system requires athletes to provide specific location for a one-hour time slot every day, so they can be tested. Many riders testified that the introduction of out-of-competition testing had a significant impact to both deter and alter doping practices (CIRC report).

The number of ESAs that became available in the 2000s exploded, including modified forms of EPO such as Dynepo, MIRCERA and Peginesatide (formerly Hematide), multiple EPO biosimilars and small molecules that act to stabilise hypoxia inducible factor (HIF-stabilisers), which stimulates endogenous EPO production in the kidney. Of particular concern is that HIF-stabilisers are cheaper and easier to produce than rEPO, easier to store, and are taken orally.

Anti-doping labs responded quickly by developing sensitive methods capable of detecting all these novel ESAs.

While ESAs aim to produce more red blood cells, an unmediated means to increase red cell mass is blood transfusion (Giraud, Sottas, Robinson, & Saugy, 2010), would it be using blood from a matched donor (homologous) or from the athlete himself (autologous). Homologous blood transfusion can be detected by flow cytometry (Nelson, Ashenden, Langshaw, & Popp, 2002) with a time detection window that may be the longest of all anti-doping tests – up to several months. For example, the rider Tyler Hamilton tested positive in September 2004 for a blood transfusion carried out in Spring 2004. The detection of autologous blood doping is more of a challenge because the blood that is reinjected is not exogenous in the sense that it originates from inside the own athlete's body. Another approach was necessary to overcome this challenge.

The Athlete Biological Passport

A shortcoming of the rEPO test is that it is resource-demanding and costly to perform and thus cannot be performed on all anti-doping samples. The rEPO test must therefore be targeted to specific samples based on suspicion of doping. Blood testing in the 1990s and early 2000s raised the suspicion that particular athletes were doping, and could be used to target rEPO testing. Another shortcoming of the rEPO test is that at the end of the 2000s recombinant DNA technology succeeded to produce a 'designer' rEPO that is completely similar in mass and glycosylation pattern as endogenous EPO. The availability of substances identical to those produced by the human body, as well as the undetectable autologous transfusion, necessitated a new testing paradigm in sports based on the use of biomarkers of doping (Sottas et al., 2011). While a drug test aims to detect an exogenous substance in a biological fluid, a biomarker of doping is an indicator of the effect of doping. Doping leaves a characteristic fingerprint on the biology of the athlete and biomarkers of doping as formalised in the Athlete Biological Passport (ABP) programme are used to detect that fingerprint. The haematological module of the ABP was developed in the middle of the 2000s to fight against any form of doping that aims to increase red cell mass, including both EPO use and homologous and autologous forms of blood transfusions.

In response to the trend already present in the mid-2000s towards decreasing doses of ESAs, the ABP was directly developed to detect low dose ESA use. In particular, the sensitivity and specificity of the ABP was evaluated on one of the first 'rEPO micro-dosing' studies (Robinson, Saugy, Buclin, Gremion, & Mangin 2002; Robinson, Sottas, Mangin, & Saugy, 2007). These studies demonstrated that the ABP was able to detect micro-dosing and that the sensitivity was not only associated to the amount of rEPO injected but also on the response of the body to the doping regimen: athletes who had a higher response had a higher chance to return a positive result than athletes for which the drug had a negligible effect. This study also demonstrated that some individuals do not respond to rEPO treatment.

The sensitivity of the haematological module of the ABP to rEPO micro-dosing and other sophisticated transfusion doping regimes was further confirmed in other studies (Sottas, Robinson, & Saugy, 2010). Several of these studies also showed that the timing of the test was crucial (Pottgiesser et al., 2011), something unfortunately not properly integrated in the design of other studies that were focusing on testing at a high frequency.

Outcomes for cycling

Effective anti-doping programmes rely on a combination of complementary tools. For the detection of blood doping, the combination of the whereabouts system to locate athletes, the ABP to identify suspicious changes in blood values, and finally an arsenal of sensitive ESA tests offers a powerful toolset to identify doping athletes.

As soon as the haematological module of the ABP was introduced in cycling at the end of 2007, the number of riders caught for blood doping increased drastically. The statistics of the World Anti-Doping Agency show an increase of more than 300% in the number of athletes sanctioned annually for blood doping upon implementation of the ABP in 2008. This includes a significant and immediate increase in the number of rEPO positives based on improved targeting using the ABP (Figure 4.1), and starting in 2010, anti-doping rule violations

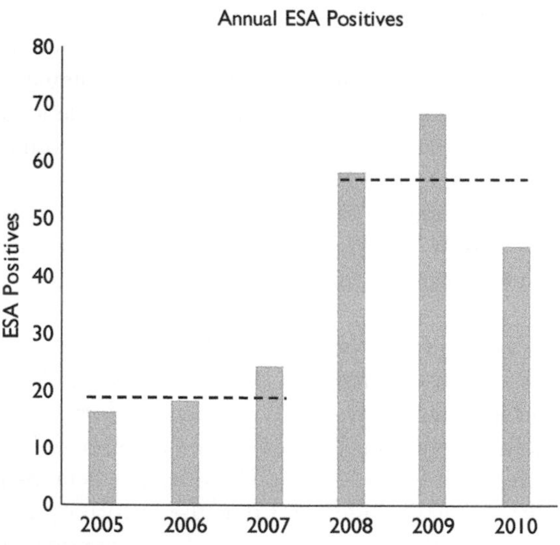

Figure 4.1 Annual ESA positives for three years before and after the implementation of the ABP.

proved by the ABP, including cases of autologous blood transfusions. Many see the years 2008–2009 as the years when blood doping moved from a rampant problem in elite cycling capable of changing unscrupulous dopers into winners of major competitions to an issue still present sporadically and often based on dosing regimes too low to produce any significant effect on performance.

With the ABP, the amount of rEPO that can be taken without generating an Atypical Passport Finding is now reduced to the point that its effects are similar to what can be achieved through training at a high altitude (a gain similar to the injection of doses as low as 5–10 U/kg taken intravenously). This has two important implications for sport. First is that the ABP has greatly improved the ability of endurance athletes to win clean, something that was much more difficult in some endurance sports a decade ago. Second, as reduced doses result in reduced benefit, the risk/reward ratio has now shifted to a point where EPO use is not considered a viable option for many dopers.

Importantly, it is not even clear that the low doses used by athletes are even effective. By definition of a biomarker of doping, there is a direct relation between the effect of the doping regimen and the ability of the ABP to detect it. In other words, the haematological module of the ABP only detects blood doping regimes that are effective. Ineffective doping, with no effect on erythropoiesis, will therefore not be detected by the ABP despite the fact that a prohibited substance was being used. Regardless of the relationship between dose and effect, once the dose is reduced to a point where its effect size is within the range of normal physiological variation then the likelihood for a clean athlete to win is significantly increased. Ongoing studies suggest that we may have reached the point where doses of EPO are so small that they have become ineffective in terms of having an effect on blood parameters.

WADA statistics show that more than 600 athletes have been sanctioned worldwide for blood doping since the launch of the ABP, with the vast majority of cases being athletes target tested for rEPO analysis because of an atypical passport and athletes sanctioned solely on their blood passport. At the end of 2007, the Union Cycliste Internationale (UCI), through the Cycling Anti-Doping Foundation (CADF), was the first International Federation to implement the haematological module of the ABP and the number of rEPO cases strongly increased in 2008–2009 in cycling. This increase in cycling contributed significantly to the threefold increase in global ESA positives seen across all sports at this time (Figure 4.1). Other sports followed in turn by implementing the blood module of the ABP.

The introduction of the ABP was seen as a major paradigm shift for anti-doping in cycling. Rider testimonies made to the Cycling Independent Reform Commission (CIRC) attested to the fact that the introduction of the ABP significantly changed doping practices in cycling, dramatically reducing the effect size of available blood doping regimes. The implications of the ABP on blood doping was also seen in other endurance sports, such as on doping regimes in athletics documented during the Pound Independent Commission investigation in

2015. Recordings from discussion from top Russian officials show the difficulties the ABP posed on their doping plans (WADA Independent Commission Report I, chapter 11).

In terms of reducing the effectiveness of doping, another significant change in behaviour has been to change the timing of blood doping regime altogether. An 'optimal' doping regime aims to provide an athlete with improved performance for a given competition period. With this in mind, anti-doping testing is often carried out in the weeks leading up to an important competition for an athlete. Knowing that the risk of being tested increases in the lead up to a competition, some athletes now dope far from competitions. While the return to normal HGB mass following blood doping can take up to several weeks, it is hypothesised that blood doping far from competition may allow improved training that will then translate into improved performance over a period longer than any performance gain directly caused by the increase in HGB mass. Evidence that such a doping regime remains performance-enhancing is lacking, however the direct benefits of an increased muscle oxygenation for a competition are suppressed and this represents another means by which the effect size of doping has diminished.

Extreme blood values seen in the late 1990s and early 2000s are no longer observed in the professional peloton. These extreme blood values are attributed to the use of high dose EPO and/or transfusion of large volumes of blood, both of which can induce a significant performance advantage. The majority of atypical blood passports are no longer characteristic of rEPO doping. The passport data suggest a shift away from rEPO in the professional peloton. In addition, the prevalence of blood doping (rEPO doping and transfusion) as calculated from all blood profiles (Sottas et al., 2011) coming from the ABP blood tests has significantly decreased in several sports, including cycling (unpublished observation).

The necessity of doping strategies to stay within the limits of the ABP to avoid detection also has implications for the use of novel ESAs aiming to increase red cell mass. Even with the emergence of new doping substances, dopers must ensure that the effect is not strong enough to be detectable by the passport. Indeed, there is no hiding the cells that are needed for oxygen transport within the body, and the effects of blood doping are long lived in the body. The duration of effect on the haematopoetic system is one of the strengths of the haematological module of the ABP. In order to carry out their function, red blood cells are present in the blood and are therefore easily accessible for measurement. Any doping substance – past, present, or future – aimed at increasing the oxygen carrying capacity of blood, if effective, will therefore affect these blood cells in some way that will be detectable by the ABP. So we will likely never see a 'heyday' for a new blood doping method equivalent to the EPO era, with unprecedented effects on physiology and blood variables, due simply to the fact that moving forward any such changes will be detected by the ABP. Whereas in the 2000s anti-doping was often viewed to be one step behind the cheaters in a never-ending pharmaceutical race, the ABP is a game changer in anti-doping because the blood module of the ABP is able to detect any substances that will be developed in the future to increase red cell mass.

Overcoming shortcomings of the current system

Blood doping is the doping method of choice in endurance sports but its effect size has significantly decreased over the past decade thanks to several improvements in the anti-doping fight. There are however two main shortcomings of current system: the first associated to the resources required, the second is the use of substances that are not detectable by the current modules of the ABP.

First, athletes must be tested, or be at risk of being tested, in order to influence their risk/reward ratio. Out-of-competition testing is resource demanding because a doping control officer has to travel to the athlete's location and then transport samples to a WADA-accredited laboratory. As a result, significant resources must be invested in order to ensure an adequate, year-round test distribution plan for a given athlete. While this may be the case for athletes in the professional ranks, many continental teams are tested far less, and so the opportunities to dope are higher. Atypical passports, EPO positives and estimates of the prevalence of doping all point out to a higher use of blood doping in second-tier teams. The athletes also fall under the jurisdiction of national anti-doping organisations, who must ensure adequate resources are allocated to testing national and junior level riders as they progress up the ranks. For example, some riders are living or training in locations that do not have heavily resourced anti-doping organisations to carry out testing. Other athletes are not part of the registered testing pool of athletes who must provide whereabouts information, and so they have a lower risk of being targeted out of competition. In addition to testing, education programmes are critical in curbing doping in young athletes and ensuring the next generation of riders is less likely to dope in the first place. In practice, for the case of blood doping only, there has been a shift from a higher prevalence in elite riders to a higher prevalence in second-tier riders.

Second, there are substances that are not detectable by the current modules of the ABP. Although these substances – that we will not mention here for obvious reasons – have a significantly lower effect size than ESAs and other blood doping methods, their effect size remains non-negligible. These substances should be the main target of anti-doping research including new direct tests and new biomarkers to be included in novel modules of the ABP. The effect size of these substances appears not to be significantly higher than nutritional products that are known to be performance-enhancing when properly titrated, such as caffeine, ketones, creatine, beta-alanine, bicarbonate, nitrate, and phosphate (Burke & Peeling, 2018), so that the risk/reward ratio of doping with a prohibited substance is significantly higher today than it was in the 2000s. In summary, when the effect size is taken into the equation of doping versus performance, some riders may continue to dope today but the current system in place improves the ability of clean athletes to win competitions. A comparison of performance data between the 1990s and the 2010s supports this viewpoint (Perneger, 2010; El Helou, 2010; Kruse, Carter, Rosedahl, & Joyner, 2014).

The future of anti-doping in cycling

Anti-doping tools continue to improve and evolve due primarily to basic research in anti-doping. Research into new biomarkers for the ABP will continue to improve the sensitivity, specificity, and coverage of the ABP. Efforts to improve the integration of ABP data with other anti-doping data will also significantly improve the effectiveness of anti-doping programmes. The use of intelligence to drive test planning has been successful in uncovering doping in cycling, such as seen at the 2017 Vuelta a Colombia and the 2017 Vuelta a Costa Rica. The monitoring of changes in athlete performance is also actively being explored as a means to uncover abnormalities that may be due to doping (Hopker et al., 2018). The ability of information system to integrate such datasets has a tremendous potential to improve anti-doping practices.

The past decade has seen a significant effect of anti-doping efforts on doping practices in cycling. This has been due to both scientific advances and the significant investment of the UCI/CADF in order to put these advances into practice. Global anti-doping programmes must continue to grow in order to ensure broad application of anti-doping methods. National anti-doping organisations are in a particularly important phase of worldwide growth, and every year new programmes come online. Investment in both basic research and anti-doping programmes must be a global effort in order to ensure a future where all clean athletes can compete with a fair chance to win across all sports.

References

Bassett, D.R. Jr & Howley, E.T. (2000). Limiting factors for maximum oxygen uptake and determinants of endurance performance. *Med. Sci. Sports Exerc.*, *32*(1), 70–84.

Birkeland, K.I., Stray-Gundersen, J., Hemmersbach, P., Hallen, J., Haug, E., & Bahr, R. (2000). Effect of rhEPO administration on serum levels of sTfR and cycling performance. *Med. Sci. Sports Exerc.*, *32*, 1238.

Burke, L.M. & Peeling, P. (2018). Methodologies for investigating performance changes with supplement use, *Int. J. Sport Nutr. Exerc. Metab.*, *28*(2), 159–169.

Clark, B., Woolford, S.M., Eastwood, A., Sharpe, K., Barnes, P.G., & Gore, C.J. (2017), Temporal changes in physiology and haematology in response to high- and microdoses of recombinant human erythropoietin. *Drug Test Anal.*, 9(10), 1561–1571.

Durussel, J., Daskalaki, E., Anderson, M., Chatterji, T., Wondimu, D.H., Padmanabhan, N., Patel, R.K., McClure, J.D., & Pitsiladis, Y.P. (2013). Haemoglobin mass and running time trial performance after recombinant human erythropoietin administration in trained men. *PLoS One*, 8, e56151.

Ekblom, B. & Berglund, B. (1991). Effect of erythropoietin administration on mammal aerobic power. *Scand. J. Med. Sci. Sports*, *1*, 88.

Ekblom, B., Goldbarg, A.N., & Gullbring, B. (1972). Response to exercise after blood loss and reinfusion. *J. Appl. Physiol.*, *33*(2), 175–180.

El Helou, N., Berthelot, G., Thibault, V., Tafflet, M., Nassif, H., Campion, F., Hermine, O., & Toussaint, J.F. (2010) Tour de France, Giro, Vuelta, and classic European races show a unique progression of road cycling speed in the last 20 years. *J. Sports Sci.* *28*(7), 789–796.

Eschbach, J.W., Egrie, J.C., Downing, M.R., Browne, J.K., & Adamson, J.W. (1987). Correction of the anemia of end-stage renal disease with recombinant human erythropoietin. Results of a combined phase I and II clinical trial. *The New England Journal of Medicine*, *316*(2), 73–78.

Giraud, S., Sottas, P.E., Robinson, N., & Saugy, M. (2010). Blood transfusion in sports. *Handb. Exp. Pharmacol*, *19*, 295–304.

Gore, C.J., Parisotto, R., Ashenden, M.J., Stray-Gundersen, J., Sharpe, K., Hopkins, W., Emslie, K.R., Howe, C., Trout, G.J., Kazlauskas, R., & Hahn, A.G. (2003). Second-generation blood tests to detect erythropoietin abuse by athletes. *Haematologica*, 88(3), 333–344.

Hattangadi, S.M., Wong, P., Zhang, L., Flygare, J., & Lodish, H.F. (2011). From stem cell to red cell: regulation of erythropoiesis at multiple levels by multiple proteins, RNAs, and chromatin modifications. *Blood*, *118*(24), 6258–6268.

Hopker, J., Schumacher, Y.O., Fedoruk, M., Mørkeberg, J., Bermon, S., Iljukov, S., Aikin, R., & Sottas, P.E. (2018). Athlete performance monitoring in anti-doping. *Front Physiol.*, 9, 232.

Kruse, T.N., Carter, R.E., Rosedahl, J.K., & Joyner, M.J. (2014) Speed trends in male distance running. *PLoS One*. 9(11), e112978.

Lasne, F. & de Ceaurriz, J. (2000). Recombinant erythropoietin in urine. *Nature*, *405*(6787), 635.

Nelson, M., Ashenden, M., Langshaw, M., & Popp, H. (2002). Detection of homologous blood transfusion by flow cytometry: a deterrent against blood doping. *Haematologica*, *87*(8), 881–882.

Perneger, T.V. (2010) Speed trends of major cycling races: does slower mean cleaner? *Int. J. Sports Med.* *31*(4), 261–264.

Pottgiesser, T., Sottas, P.E., Echteler, T., Robinson, N., Umhau, M., & Schumacher, Y.O. (2011). Detection of autologous blood doping with adaptively evaluated biomarkers of doping: a longitudinal blinded study. *Transfusion*. *51*(8), 1707–1715.

Robinson, N., Saugy, M., Buclin, T., Gremion, G., & Mangin, P. (2002). The interpretation of secondary blood markers can get hazardous in case of a discontinuous rhEPO treatment. *Haematologica*, *87*(6), ELT28.

Robinson, N., Sottas, P.E., Mangin, P., & Saugy, M. (2007). Bayesian detection of abnormal hematological values to introduce a no-start rule for heterogeneous populations of athletes. *Haematologica*, *92*(8), 1143–1144.

Russell, G., Gore, C.J., Ashenden, M.J., Parisotto, R., & Hahn, A.G. (2002). Effects of prolonged low doses of recombinant human erythropoietin during submaximal and maximal exercise. *Eur. J. Appl. Physiol.*, 86, 442.

Sottas, P.E., Robinson, N., & Saugy, M. (2010). The athlete's biological passport and indirect markers of blood doping. *Handb. Exp. Pharmacol.*, *195*, 305–326.

Sottas, P.E., Robinson, N., Fischetto, G., Dollé, G., Alonso, J.M., & Saugy, M. (2011). Prevalence of blood doping in samples collected from elite track and field athletes. *Clin. Chem.*, *57*(5), 762–769.

Sottas, P.E., Robinson, N., Rabin, O., & Saugy, M. (2011). The athlete biological passport. *Clin. Chem.*, *57*(7), 969–976.

Thomsen, J.J., Rentsch, R.L., Robach, P., Calbet, J.A., Boushel, R., Rasmussen, P., Juel, C., & Lundby, C. (2007). Prolonged administration of recombinant human erythropoietin increases submaximal performance more than maximal aerobic capacity. *Eur. J. Appl. Physiol.*, *101*, 481.

Chapter 5

Kicked out

How experts are being deterred from playing on the doping market

Bertrand Fincoeur

For athletes in elite cycling using banned performance-enhancing substances and methods (hereinafter referred to as doping products), evidence shows that several important changes over the last two decades have changed this process (Christiansen, 2005; Dimeo, 2014; see also Ohl's and Waddington's chapters in this book). Yet until recently, limited systematic research has examined the peculiarities of the supplying networks of doping products in a sports context (Athey & Bouchard, 2013; Fincoeur & Paoli, 2014; Paoli & Donati, 2014; van de Ven, 2016). In this chapter, I will thus address the recent changes in the supply-side of the doping market in elite cycling. Then I will elaborate on several research and policy implications. This chapter draws upon aggregated results from my previous research about the doping market in Belgium and France (Fincoeur, 2016), and an ongoing project on performance-enhancement in international elite cycling, funded by the Swiss National Science Foundation. Both projects rely primarily on qualitative data, i.e. semi-structured interviews (respectively, 77 and 47) with elite riders, sports directors, trainers, team physicians, team managers, and other stakeholders (sports agents, anti-doping policy-makers).

The embeddedness of cycling- and medicine-related experts within the doping supply

In order to correctly understand the functioning and the evolution of the supply chains in elite cycling, I need to briefly outline, and refer to, the demand-side of the doping market. Indeed, the doping market is a semi-illegal market (Paoli, 2016) and semi-illegal markets are, for structural reasons, especially driven by demand (Beckert & Dewey, 2017). The demand- and supply-side of the doping market are therefore intertwined and presented jointly in this chapter.

The use of performance-enhancing drugs in cycling dates back as early as in the late nineteenth century. It then took various and amateurish forms which differed from one country to another (Dimeo, 2007). A few decades later, in 1924, the French journalist Albert Londres reported about the use of enhancers by the 'slaves of the road', that is the Pélissier brothers, for whom the Tour de

France was 'an ordeal' that made it necessary to use cocaine for the eyes, chloroform for the gums, and horse liniment to keep the knees warm (Mignon, 2003). However, we know almost nothing about how riders were provided with products at that time and until the first half of the twentieth century. The patterns of drug supply were at most supposed to mirror the seemingly amateurish way that characterised the patterns of drug use.

The knowledge on the supply-side perspective is somewhat more developed for the post-WWII period since Waddington (1996), then Brissonneau and Montez de Oca (2018), addressed the increasing development of sports medicine from the 1950s onwards, which led several sports doctors to play an active part in the use of (illegal) performance-enhancing drugs among elite athletes. The report published by the investigation commission set up after the Ben Johnson scandal at the 1988 Seoul Olympics (Dubin, 1990) then provided some evidence about the involvement of health professionals in the doping supply to athletes, including the information that the 1984 Olympic US cycling team had been supplied with blood transfusions (Voy, 1991: 70). The disclosure of the 1998 Festina doping scandal provided further evidence about the particular situation within elite cycling. In his book published in the aftermath of the 1998 scandal, the former soigneur Willy Voet (2002) detailed the hidden drug-related practices of the cycling world (see especially chapters 5 and 6; see also Fignon, 2010). Importantly, such accounts illustrate the then-existing flourishing culture of tolerance towards doping that had developed within elite cycling: doping was best understood as a 'deviant overconformity' (Coakley, 2015). Consequently, people involved in the supplying networks of doping products belonged to the 'cycling family'. At least until the mid-1980s, riders, trainers, and masseurs 'were behind the distribution of the drugs, and the dosages were determined according to other riders' experiences, through "trial and error"'. The use of drugs then 'reflected the social organisation of training and preparation which was common at the time: unsophisticated and bound by tradition' (Christiansen, 2005: 500). Yet, by focusing on the importance of performance and winning, sport provided favourable conditions for its scientisation and medicalisation (Waddington & Smith, 2009). As a result, EPO turned out to be endemic in the mid-1990s after that a biomedical research team from the Italian University of Ferrara, headed by Professor Francesco Conconi with his assistants Luigi Cecchini and Michele Ferrari, ensured the appropriate use of EPO among elite riders (Donati, 2012; see also Gleaves' and Paoli's chapters in this book).

Due to the widespread acceptance of doping among elite cycling actors, a doped rider could purchase various products in pharmacies thanks to a prescription from his team doctor, or he was supplied by a teammate who then acted as a user–dealer. In the late 1990s, Italian rider Rodolfo Massi's nickname was 'the little chemist' because he allegedly supplied many riders by smuggling illegal medicine across the border from Italy to France.[1] His case is nevertheless far from being isolated. The French rider Philippe Gaumont, who was investigated in the 2004 Cofidis scandal, published an autobiography which is overflowing with anecdotes and details about the doping culture, and the role of riders and team physicians in supplying illegal enhancers (Gaumont, 2005). As illustrated below, I also collected numerous research data about that period.

> We had the yellow jersey before the last stage at the Tour of (...). The guys were concerned about losing it on the last day. In the evening, the riders asked me a little extra for the last stage. They had made a lot of efforts during the previous race days, and they were particularly tired. I did call my secretary, asking him to bring a suitcase with everything necessary for our riders. He arrived just after the dinner and we did injections for the whole team.
>
> (Mark,[2] team physician)

In the late 1990s, several teams then directly provided doping products to their riders. The richest and most supportive teams even allocated part of their annual budget to purchasing doping products. During the Festina trial, the team manager and the team physician of the Festina cycling team justified such organised practices because this strategy was intended to reduce the health risks associated with unmonitored doping practices (Roussel, 2001). The team-sponsored doping practices did, however, not exclude additional individual behaviours.

> I was team physician of a second league team but I also followed some additional riders in other teams. In particular, O. was my patient (a top rider in the late 1980s/early 1990s). I assisted him for several major races. Although I did care only of him, I could stay at the hotel with his team during the races. The team physician injected, for example, insulin to each rider of the team but I did some extras for O. In fact, the team was extremely professional and I very much appreciated this professionalism.
>
> (James, team physician)

There is thus some evidence of the (past) embeddedness of cycling- and medicine-related experts within the doping supply chains at least until the late 1990s and probably the early 2000s. Until then, the doping supply was a real insider's business. These insiders who could supply, assist, or advise the riders were experts *by experience*. They shared either cultural values or experiences with the riders. Numerous soigneurs–suppliers were former elite or semi-pro riders, as is the case of Jef D'Hont, the former Belgian soigneur of the German cycling team Telekom, whose riders Bjarne Riis and Jan Ulrich won the 1996 and 1997 Tour de France (D'Hont, 2007).

The embeddedness of actors belonging to the 'cycling family' did not fit a strategy of maximising profits since the doping networks consisted of a limited amount of people and relied on low prices (see similar conclusions regarding other sports environments: Coomber et al., 2015; Kraska, Bussard, & Brent,

2010). The experts by experience can then be considered as 'minimally commercial suppliers' (Coomber & Moyle, 2014). The then team physicians' attitudes towards doping may illustrate this minimally commercial standpoint. Although doping products were also supplied for their performance-enhancing properties and we cannot exclude that several doctors have been primarily motivated by financial incentives, health considerations were not absent from team doctors' discourse. In his book written in jail, the former team physician Georges Mouton pointed out:

> There is clear evidence that, among elite cyclists and high-level amateur cyclists, some injectable products that can be administered in the evening after a competition to help recover and contribute to a better general condition in the long term. Of course, one can argue that they also enhance the next day's performance. It does not correspond to my definition of doping which could otherwise be applied to the training and to a good sleep! Something enhancing both the performance and the health should not be considered as doping. Only thinkers completely disconnected from real world may defend such hare-brained ideas. The philosophy of anti-doping consists in avoiding everything harmful for the health but it may not attack what helps the athletes to be healthy – even if those products or methods are performance-enhancing.
>
> (Mouton, 2001: 128)

Finally, it is also unclear whether such practices could be defined as a 'market' since there was no real competition at both the demand and supply level (Beckert & Wehinger, 2013). The increasing efforts to tackle doping over the last two decades have, however, partly modified the patterns of doping supply in cycling.

The partial experts' shift

Claiming that there is a world of difference between the doping practices in elite cycling 20 years ago and these practices anno 2018 may always be risky because the period between the 1998 Tour de France and the mid-2010s was affected by repeated scandals involving various teams and/or riders (e.g. Blitz, Mantova doping investigation, Oil for Drugs case, Puerto affair, Rabobank, Lance Armstrong/US Postal, etc.). However, the aftermath of the repeated scandals, in particular the (threat of) sponsors' withdrawal, and the increased individual risks of having his contract voided after testing positive have likely had an impact on the doping prevalence and the riders' and teams' attitudes towards doping (Ohl, Fincoeur, Lentillon-Kaestner, Defrance, & Brissonneau, 2015; see also Aikin & Sottas', and Waddington's chapters). Consequently, due to both internal and external pressures, the use of (illegal) performance-enhancing drugs is today no longer overwhelmingly accepted by the riders, and the teams officially promote a zero-tolerance anti-doping stance. Roughly said, the harsher anti-doping regime and the need for a sustainable business model have fostered the cycling family to be increasingly committed with clean sport. Not unsurprisingly, these changes did not only affect the patterns of drug use. They have also had an impact on the organisation of the supply-side of the doping market. In fact, the patterns of supply simply followed what could be observed about the patterns of use. Since the doping use had lost its perceived legitimacy, the traditional suppliers became much less inclined to take risks in openly providing doping products to riders (Fincoeur, van de Ven, & Mulrooney, 2014).

> I did dope many riders in my career but today I wouldn't dare to supply an illegal stuff to any of our riders. I know what are the risks for the team vis-à-vis our sponsor, and I don't want to be responsible for making 60 guys unemployed.
>
> (Bob, team physician)

Yet, irrespective of its prevalence, each demand needs to be supplied. This then opened the doors to another category of suppliers: the experts *by expertise.*

Unlike the expert by experience, who can share his experience as an insider, the expert by expertise counts on his technical or scientific knowledge about drugs. He is, however, not necessarily familiar with elite cycling since his clients may consist of athletes from sports other than cycling or from beyond sport. Obviously, the physicians (sports doctors and other doctors, such as nutritional doctors and general practitioners) are the principal experts by expertise. This category of experts also includes the team physicians, who have a cross-sectional position between insiders and outsiders. Pharmacists, vets, physiotherapists, and trainers may also be considered as experts by expertise since they hold some (para-medical) knowledge about the products and their expected (side-)effects. Since the early 2000s, the history of cycling-related doping scandals is riddled with such experts' profiles, as illustrated by the prominent role of the veterinarian José Landuyt[3] in the doping scandal involving several Belgian top riders including the one-day races and world champion Johan Museeuw, or the pharmacist Guido Nigrelli in the Mantova doping investigation (Paoli & Donati, 2014: 69). Over-the-counter drugs, forged prescriptions, and/or thefts in hospital pharmacies by nurses have also been reported (Fincoeur, 2016). Importantly, several doctors and other health professionals unrelated to a particular elite team began to play an increasing role in prescribing, monitoring, administering, and/or providing riders with illegal enhancers. The various publicly released cases of the Italian Dr. Michele Ferrari, the Spanish Dr. Eufemiano Fuentes, the French naturopath Bernard Sainz, and the sports medicine department of the German University of Freiburg-im-Breisgau (about the latter, see Paoli's chapter) came out to illustrate this shift towards experts by expertise. Of course, I do not support the claim that these team-unrelated physicians have *appeared* on the doping market in the early 2000s, but they began to play an *increased* role because of the changes that occurred in elite cycling at that time. In fact, several team-unrelated doctors, such as Francesco Conconi and Luigi Cecchini in Italy (Paoli & Donati, 2014), Patrick Nédélec in France (Gaumont, 2005), Luis Garcia del Moral in Spain,[4] already supplied the riders before 1998. Similarly, the team-sponsored doping model did not completely fade away in the 2000s, as evidenced by numerous doping scandals pertaining to various teams such as Cofidis, Rabobank, Saunier-Duval, US Postal, etc. Despite having been investigated or reported for doping activities, several doctors have also continued their activity of team physician across the years in different teams: Massimo Besnati,[5] Pedro Celaya,[6] José Ibarguren,[7] Thomas Klimaschka,[8] Geert Leinders,[9] Andrei Mikhailov,[10] Manuel Rodriguez Alonso,[11] Yvan Van Mol,[12] etc. However, just as riders and sports directors have likely changed their attitudes towards doping, there is no reason not to acknowledge that similar changes may equally happen with team doctors. Moreover, most elite teams are now committed to a new approach of anti-doping (see Ohl's chapter), and a new generation of team doctors progressively replaces the older generation that worked through the team-sponsored doping era.

With the increasing efforts made to tackle doping, not least the development of the Athlete Biological Passport (see Aikin & Sottas' chapter), the access to the role of doping supplier seemingly more than ever relies on the capacity to appropriately monitor the use of performance-enhancing drugs. In fact, an elite rider willing to dope will unlikely do it on his own, with the notable exception of Italian elite rider Riccardo Ricco, who was admitted in February 2011 to a hospital in critical condition due to a blood transfusion he performed on himself with 25-day-old blood.[13] As illustrated by the BALCO case (Athey & Bouchard, 2013), elite athletes almost consistently need the security offered by the experts' intervention. However, insiders, such as teammates or former elite riders, can still play an important role by helping the rider gain contact with 'the right people', then acting as a broker, that is someone 'positioned between disconnected others within a network' (Morselli, 2009: 16). The reliability of the team-unrelated supplying networks will then be strengthened by the fact that the illegality entails risks for each member of the network. Becoming a partner in illegal transactions presupposes credible signals of trustworthiness on the side of the trust-taker and intensive monitoring on the side of the trust-giver (Beckert & Wehinger, 2013: 24). At a time when doping was undoubtedly widespread and culturally accepted, team doctors and soigneurs, in their quality of insiders, made this trust process probably easier. Nevertheless, the doping market within elite cycling has always been primarily a matter of experts. It therefore mainly consists of embedded actors into legitimate professions, roles, and institutional settings which are suggestive of corporate or occupational crime, defined respectively as the offences committed by corporate officials for their corporations and the offences of the corporation itself, and the violation of the criminal law in the course of activities of a legitimate occupation (Clinard

& Quinney, 1973). Due to the above-mentioned shift, the experts by expertise seem to better fit the concept of occupational criminals because the corporation – here, the teams – no longer supports doping practices. It should, however, be stressed that not all professional activities of those who administer/provide/etc. doping products are illegal, and that occupational criminals actually benefit from the legal status of their main activities to cover illegal practices. Legal and illegal activities are thus largely intertwined.

However, should these practices also be considered as part of organised criminal activities? Although the many different actors and practices that have been subsumed under this label make it a vague umbrella concept, and despite the fact that organised crime 'is nowadays simply equated with illegal enterprises or even networks of loose partnerships and individuals trading in illicit products' (Paoli & Donati, 2014: 127), it should also be stressed that the various criminal networks do not necessarily rest on a criminal organisation (Morselli, 2009). In fact, while the supply of doping products may evoke several patterns of mafia-like organisations (e.g. *omerta*), it causes little to no physical violence, although violence usually forms a main feature of illegal markets (Arlacchi, 1998). The harmful properties of the supply chains that have up to now ruled the doping market in cycling should therefore not be taken for granted. Even further, one could argue that as far as the supply-side of the doping market was in hands of experts, it has likely circumscribed the health risks associated with the use of drugs. Despite the existing evidence about the widespread doping use among elite cyclists over decades, a significant lower mortality in participants in the Tour de France, compared with the general male population, has been established (Marijon et al., 2013). Several scholars then defend that the claims concerning alleged health risks of doping may contribute to a 'discourse of fear' which can be used to legitimate the war on doping (Coomber, 2013; López, 2013). Yet, since anti-doping policies increasingly tackle the suppliers of doping products, there is a risk that experts will be replaced by, or complemented with, non-experts.

How anti-doping policy could kick out the experts

The idea of tackling the suppliers of doping products is not something really new. As early as in 1965, Belgium and France each adopted an anti-doping law establishing criminal provisions against the trafficking networks of doping products. However, these legislations were barely applied. Moreover, there was – and still is – considerable variance between the different national doping-related criminal laws, although today there is even a debate about the opportunity to criminalise not only the suppliers but also the doping users (Kayser & Kornbeck, 2018). As a result, several international initiatives were undertaken to foster the empowerment of, and the cooperation between, law enforcement agencies in the fight against doping at the global level (Kornbeck, 2013). In 2008, the World Anti-Doping Agency signed a cooperation agreement with Interpol, which led to exchange liaison officers. Significantly, the latest version of the World Anti-Doping Code (2015) has introduced a new doping offence (article 2.10), that is the 'prohibited association', which forbids athletes from associating with a coach, a doctor, or any support personnel who has committed an anti-doping rule violation. In July 2018, the prohibited association list consisted of 168 blacklisted people. In addition, various countries endorse sanctions against suppliers, including health professionals, who assist athletes in doping practices. As a consequence, after the sidestep of the experts by experience, several experts by expertise are increasingly being deterred from playing on the doping market.

> I know Greg (= an independent sports physician) for years. I can even say he is my friend. Five years ago, if you wanted a blood-transfusion or IGF-1, you could easily get it. He agreed to do everything for me. Not necessarily for making money. I think primarily for the vanity to have an elite athlete as a patient. Well, he also prescribed cortisone to young riders. But today, it's all in the past. I think he has understood that such attitudes may affect the credibility of cycling. In addition, he fears for being investigated. Let's imagine the impact on his career. He does not want to lose all what he has built.
>
> (Daniel, elite rider)

> I don't want to get fines and go to prison because of my job. I see how things are turning out. Today, I did stop with athletes. I focus on nutrition issues, other type of patients, and that's it. (...) Quite frankly, from an intellectual point of view, the job of team physician has become much less interesting than it used to be. Increasingly, it equates to a task of policeman who is expected to verify that his riders are compliant with anti-doping rules. Basically, my motivation to do this job got lost.
>
> (James, team physician)

> I am not crazy. My career is important to me. I may sometimes disagree with the WADA-list but if I was asked to prescribe or provide anything illegal, I would simply decline and say to my patient: just visit someone else.
>
> (Alan, independent sports physician)

> I have seen important changes over the past ten years. Elite riders are today much cleaner but I now received amateurs and young riders with their parents asking how I can help their child to be more performant. I prefer not to know where they will go to be provided with their bullshit stuff.
>
> (Philip, independent sports physician)

In the same vein, results from a Belgian survey among competitive riders have shown that the 'non-experts' form the category of suppliers that Belgian riders would consider in the first place if they wanted to use an illegal enhancer (Fincoeur, Frenger, & Pitsch, 2014). There are thus some indications that athletes could (slowly) turn to the 'black market' to obtain products. The sharpening of the anti-doping policy over the last two decades and, more particularly, the targeting of the riders' entourage could suggest a future reorganisation of the supply networks. What would then be the implications of such reorganisation, should the experts be deterred from operating on the doping market because of their fear of economic, symbolic, and/or criminal sanctions?

I would not want to be a bird of ill omen. There is so far no empirical evidence of massive involvement of criminal or mafia-like organisations in the supply chains within elite cycling. Even further, in a sport like bodybuilding, which is supposed to be deeply contaminated by doping practices, and which could thus be very attractive for criminal networks, there are no indications of organised crime, nor that economic incentives are the primary motivator for dealing, even at the wholesale level (van de Ven, 2017). In cycling, social supply – defined as the non-commercial or non-profitmaking distribution of drugs to non-strangers (Hough et al., 2003), or as the activity of those who may make some profit but are driven by other factors (prestige, social status) and would continue to supply even if no financial gain was made (Potter, 2009) – has so far characterised the organisation of the doping market. However, regarding the peculiar case of cycling, this analysis in terms of minimally commercial suppliers (Coomber & Moyle, 2014) may confuse causes and effects. Indeed, do suppliers in cycling limit themselves because they are principally insiders–dealers, or do they struggle to go beyond the glass ceiling as a result of the differential opportunity theory (Cloward & Ohlin, 1960)? In other words, are social suppliers not simply what they are because of the lack of resources and opportunities to further extend their illegal activities?

Yet, there is evidence that some cultural proximity between users and suppliers remains necessary (Kraska, Bussard, & Brent, 2010). The analysis of the doping market in cycling shows that the operators are mainly male, white, and educated people. This is a major difference with several traditional drug markets, such as those of heroin and cocaine (Paoli & Reuter, 2008). Moreover, the doping networks often rely on little scale organisations (see similar conclusion on drug markets: Desroches, 2007) that are primarily made up of people from a similar territorial origin, with the notable exception of the Puerto affair (Soulé & Lestrelin, 2011). In addition, alongside their status of corporate or occupational criminals, the doping suppliers rarely have a criminal background prior to committing doping support activities (Fincoeur, 2016; Paoli & Donati, 2014). Consequently, and given the changing policy context, could other avenues to obtain products be an option for athletes who increasingly struggle to find lenient experts? Finally, and although the aim is not to figure out a short-term threat, what could be academic researchers' and policy-makers' contribution to prevent the situation from turning into a self-fulfilling prophecy?

Concluding remarks: policy and research implications

Since the doping market has so far relied on proximity networks, either for cultural reasons or because riders needed the quality and security offered by reliable experts, it has not really developed within a globalised economy. However, due to the increased efforts to tackle doping, playing on the doping market has become an increasingly at-risk business. As a result, it is worthwhile to consider whether the criminal networks, which do not have to suffer from the consequences of the various doping scandals, and which are less concerned with criminal justice interventions – the risks of being investigated or sued are part of their risk assessment (Werb et al., 2011) – could benefit from anti-doping policy. The beneficiaries of the anti-doping crusade would then paradoxically be those against whom the anti-doping efforts should focus on. For criminologists, the displacement issue as an effect of the increased repression is commonplace (Johnson, Guerette, & Bowers, 2014). Yet, an important threat that comes out from the ongoing anti-doping policy is the risk of development of a competitive doping market, which is what the culture of tolerance towards doping has so far enabled to prevent. If one assumes, with economic theory, that the efficiency of markets is enhanced through competition, say Beckert & Wehinger (2013: 18), illegal markets are structurally inefficient. It would then be unfortunate if anti-doping efforts contributed to the emergence of competitive supply practices. In particular, one should try to avoid the side-effects allowing market-oriented dealers (for comparison with the cannabis market, see Decorte, 2010) to play a more active part to the cost of athletes, that is those anti-doping policy-makers claim to protect. Of course, the global supply of performance-enhancing drugs is all but restricted to athletes. In a WADA-funded study, Donati (2007) estimated the global production of EPO as six times higher than what is necessary to supply the therapeutic needs for patients worldwide. It is obvious that athletes alone cannot absorb this overproduction. Actually, the differentiation of the doping market in two clear-cut markets for athletes and other users is already a reality (Paoli & Donati, 2014: 104). According to law enforcement agencies,[14] the profit margin of the doping supply criminal activities would exceed the profit margin of other drug trafficking networks. In the context of proliferation of online pharmacies selling performance-enhancing drugs (Cordaro, Lombardo, & Cosentino, 2011; European Monitoring Centre for Drugs and Drug Addiction, 2016), and given the increasing development of the darknet markets (Aldridge & Askew, 2017; Van Buskirk, Roxburgh, Bruno, & Burns, 2013; Van Hout & Bingham, 2013), several international and national policy initiatives have started to tackle these issues.[15] Beyond the development of the doping market in (elite) cycling, these perspectives could (or should?) help to rethink how anti-doping policies are framed and shaped. May sports not be the good entrance door for anti-doping? From an academic point of view, there is also undoubtedly a need for further research on this very topical issue. As suggested by this book, interdisciplinary perspectives could then contribute to better evidence-based policy-making.

Notes

1 https://en.wikipedia.org/wiki/Festina_affair
2 Interviewees' names have all been changed.
3 http://velorooms.com/index.php?topic=8132.0
4 www.cyclisme-dopage.com/portraits/delmoral.htm
5 www.dopeology.org/people/Massimo_Besnati/
6 www.cyclisme-dopage.com/portraits/celaya.htm
7 www.dopeology.org/people/Jos%C3%A9_Ibarguren/
8 www.radsportkompakt.de/2012/11/20/hamilton-belastet-auch-deutschen-mediziner/
9 www.theguardian.com/sport/2015/jan/22/geert-leinders-life-ban-team-sky-doctor
10 www.dopeology.org/people/Andrei_Mikhailov/
11 www.dopeology.org/people/Manuel_Rodriguez-Alonso/
12 www.cyclismas.com/biscuits/is-there-a-doctor-in-the-house/
13 http://news.bbc.co.uk/sport2/hi/other_sports/cycling/9391538.stm#sa-link_location=TEMP&intlink_from_url=https%3A%2F%2Fwww.bbc.com%2Fsport%2Fcycling%2F17775015&intlink_ts=1533799500795-sa
14 www.police.be/fed/fr/downloads/file/Rapports+d+activites/Rapport-annuel-CMDH-2014.pdf
15 www.interpol.int/Crime-areas/Pharmaceutical-crime/Operations/Operation-Pangea

References

Aldridge, J. & Askew, R. (2017). Delivery dilemmas: How drug cryptomarket users identify and seek to reduce their risk of detection by law enforcement. *International Journal of Drug Policy*, *41*, 101–109.

Arlacchi, P. (1998). Some observations on illegal markets. In V. Ruggiero, N. South, & I. Taylor (Eds), *The New European Criminology. Crime and Social Order in Europe* (pp. 203–215). London: Routledge.

Athey, N. & Bouchard, M. (2013). The BALCO scandal: the social structure of a steroid distribution network. *Global Crime*, *14*(2–3), 216–237.

Beckert, J. & Dewey, M. (2017). The social organization of illegal markets. In J. Beckert & M. Dewey (Eds), *The Architecture of Illegal Markets. Towards an Economic Sociology of Illegality in the Economy*. Oxford: Oxford University Press.

Beckert, J. & Wehinger, F. (2013). In the shadow: illegal markets and economic sociology. *Socio-Economic Review*, *11*(1), 5–30.

Brissonneau, C. & Montez de Oca, J. (2018). *Doping in Elite Sport: Voices of French Sportspeople and Their Doctors, 1950–2010*. London: Routledge.

Christiansen, A.V. (2005). The legacy of festina: patterns of drug use in European cycling since 1998. *Sports in History*, *25*(3), 497–514.

Clinard, M. & Quinney, R. (1973). *Criminal Behavior Systems: A Typology*. New York: Holt, Rinehart & Winston.

Cloward, R.A. & Ohlin, L.E. (1960). *Delinquency and Opportunity: A Theory of Delinquent Gangs*. New York: Free Press.

Coakley, J. (2015). Drug use and deviant overconformity. In V. Møller, I. Waddington, & J. Hoberman (Eds), *Routledge Handbook of Drugs and Sport* (pp. 379–392). New York: Routledge.

Coomber, R. (2013). How social fear of drugs in the non-sporting world creates a framework for doping policy in the sporting world. *International Journal of Sport Policy and Politics*, 6(2), 171–193.

Coomber, R. & Moyle, L. (2014). Beyond drug dealing: developing and extending the concept of 'social supply' of illicit drugs to 'minimally commercial supply'. *Drugs Education, Policy and Prevention*, *21*(2), 157–164.

Coomber, R., Paylidis, A., Santos, G., Wilde, M., Schmidt, W., & Redshaw, C. (2015). The supply of steroids and other performance and image enhancing drugs (PIEDs) in one English city: Fakes, counterfeits, supplier trust, common beliefs and access. *Performance Enhancement & Health*, 3(3), 135–144.

Cordaro, F., Lombardo, S., & Cosentino, M. (2011). Selling androgenic anabolic steroids by the pound: identification and analysis of popular websites on the Internet. *Scandinavian Journal of Medicine & Science in Sports*, *21*(6), 247–259.

Decorte, T. (2010). The case for small-scale domestic cannabis cultivation. *International Journal of Drug Policy*, *21*(4), 271–275.

Desroches, F. (2007). Research on upper level drug trafficking: A review. *Journal of Drug Issues*, *37*, 827–844.

D'Hont, J. (2007). *Memoires van een wielerverzorger*. Leuven: Van Halewyck.

Dimeo, P. (2007). *A History of Drug Use in Sport, 1876–1976: Beyond Good and Evil.* London: Routledge.

Dimeo, P. (2014). Why Lance Armstrong? Historical context and key turning points in the 'Cleaning Up' of professional cycling. *The International Journal of the History of Sport*, *31*(8), 951–968.

Donati, A. (2007). *World Traffic in Doping Substances*. Lausanne: Agence Mondiale Antidopage. www.wada-ama.org/Documents/World_Anti-Doping_Program/Governments/WADA_Donati_Report_On_Trafficking_2007.pdf

Donati, A. (2012). *Lo sport del doping. Chi lo subisce, chi lo combatte*. Torino: Edizioni Gruppo Abele.

Dubin, C. (1990). *Commission of inquiry into the use of drugs and banned practices intended to increase athletic performance*. Ottawa: Canadian Government Publishing Centre.

European Monitoring Centre for Drugs and Drug Addiction (2016). *The internet and drug markets*. Luxembourg: EMCDDA, Insights 21, Publications Office of the European Union.

Fignon, L. (2010). *We Were Young and Carefree*. London: Yellow Jersey.

Fincoeur, B. (2016). *Le marché du dopage dans le cyclisme sur route belge et français: analyse de la demande, de l'offre et de l'impact de la lutte antidopage*. Doctoral thesis: KU Leuven.

Fincoeur, B., Frenger, M., & Pitsch, W. (2014). Does one play with the athletes' health in the name of ethics? *Performance Enhancement & Health*, 2, 182–193.

Fincoeur, B. & Paoli, L. (2014). Des pratiques communautaires au marché du dopage. Évolution de la distribution des produits dopants dans le cyclisme. *Déviance et Société*, 38(1), 3–27.

Fincoeur, B., van de Ven, K., & Mulrooney, K. (2014). The symbiotic evolution of anti-doping and supply chains of doping substances: How criminal networks may benefit from anti-doping policy. *Trends in Organized Crime*, *17*, 1–22.

Gaumont, P. (2005). *Prisonnier du dopage*. Paris: Grasset.

Hough, M., Warburton, H., Few, B., May, T., Man, L.H., Witton, J., & Turnbull, P. (2003). *A Growing Market: The Domestic Cultivation of Cannabis*. York: Joseph Rowntree Foundation.

Johnson, S.D., Guerette, R.T., & Bowers, K. (2014). Crime displacement: what we know, what we don't know, and what it means for crime reduction. *Journal of Experimental Criminology*, *10*(4), 549–571.

Kayser, B. & Kornbeck, J. (2018). Do public perception and the 'spirit of sport' justify the criminalisation of doping? A reply to Claire Sumner. *International Sports Law Journal*. Pre-publication online. https://doi.org/10.1007/s40318-018-0120-4

Kornbeck, J. (2013). *Inspiration from Brussels? The European Union and Sport*. Bremen: Europaeischer Hochschulverlag.

Kraska, P., Bussard, C., & Brent, J. (2010). Trafficking in bodily perfection: Examining the late-modern steroid marketplace and its criminalization. *Justice Quarterly*, *27*(2), 159–185.

López, B. (2013). Creating fear: the 'doping deaths', risk communication and the anti-doping campaign. *International Journal of Sport Policy and Politics*, 6(2), 213–225.

Marijon, E., Tafflet, M., Antero-Jacquemin, J., El Helou, N., Berthelot, G. Celermajer, D., Bougouin, G., Combes, N., Hermine, O., Empana, J.P., Rey, G., Toussaint, J.F., & Jouven, X. (2013). Mortality of French participants in the Tour de France (1947–2012). *European Heart Journal*, *34*(40), 3145–3150.

Mignon, P. (2003). The Tour de France and the doping issue. In H. Dauncey & G. Hare (Eds), *The Tour de France 1903–2003* (pp. 227–245). London: Cass.

Morselli, C. (2009). *Inside Criminal Networks*. New York: Springer.

Mouton, G. (2001). *Les Méthodes du Docteur Mouton*. Bruxelles: Editions Luc Pire.

Ohl, F., Fincoeur, B., Lentillon-Kaestner, V., Defrance, J., & Brissonneau, C. (2015). The socialization of young cyclists and the culture of doping. *International Review for the Sociology of Sport*, *50*(7), 865–882.

Paoli, L. (2016). The market for doping products: A quasi-illegal market and its suppliers. In N. Ahmadi, A. Ljungqvist, & G. Svedsater (Eds), *Doping and Public Health* (pp. 71–93). London: Routledge.

Paoli, L. & Donati, A. (2014). *The Sports Doping Market. Understanding Supply and Demand, and the Challenges of Their Control*. New York: Springer.

Paoli, L. & Reuter, P. (2008). Drug trafficking and ethnic minorities in Western Europe. *European Journal of Criminology*, *5*, 13–37.

Potter, G. (2009). Exploring retail-level drug distribution: Social supply, 'real' dealers and the user/dealer interface. In Z. Demetrovics, J. Fountain, & L. Kraus (Eds), *Old and New Policies, Theories, Research Methods and Drug Users Across Europe*. Lengerich: Pabst Science Publishers.

Roussel, B. (2001). *Tour de Vices*. Paris: Hachette.

Soulé, B. & Lestrelin, L. (2011). The Puerto Affair: Revealing the difficulties of the fight against doping. *Journal of Sport and Social Issues*, *35*(2), 186–208.

Van Buskirk, J., Roxburgh, A., Bruno, R., & Burns, L. (2013). *Drugs and the Internet*. Sydney: National Drug and Alcohol Research Centre.

van de Ven, K. (2016). 'Blurred lines': Anti-doping, national policies, and the performance and image enhancing drug (PIED) market in Belgium and the Netherlands. *Performance Enhancement & Health*, 4(3), 94–102.

van de Ven, K. (2017). The evolution of the production and supply of performance and image enhancing drugs (PIEDs) in Belgium and the Netherlands. In D. Siegel & H. Nelen (Eds), *Contemporary Organized Crime: Developments, Challenges and Responses*. New York: Springer.

van de Ven, K. & Mulrooney, K. (2017). Social suppliers: Exploring the cultural contours of the performance and image enhancing drug (PIED) market among bodybuilders in the Netherlands and Belgium. *International Journal of Drug Policy*, 40, 6–15.

Van Hout, M. & Bingham, T. (2013). Surfing the Silk Road: a study of users' experiences. *International Journal of Drug Policy*, 24(6), 524–529.

Voet, W. (2002). *Breaking the Chain. Drugs and Cycling: The True Story*. London: Random House.

Voy, R. (1991). *Drugs, Sport and Politics*. Champaign: Leisure Press.

Waddington, I. (1996). The development of sports medicine. *Sociology of Sport Journal*, *13*, 176–196.

Waddington, I. (2000). *Sport, Health and Drugs. A Critical Sociological Perspective*. London: Spon Press.

Waddington, I. & Smith, A. (2009). *An Introduction to Drugs in Sport: Addicted to Winning?* London: Routledge.

Werb, D., Rowell, G., Guyatt, G., Kerr, T., Montaner, J., & Wood, E. (2011). Effect of drug law enforcement on drug market violence: a systematic review. *International Journal of Drug Policy*, 22(2), 87–94.

Chapter 6

The peculiarities of the market for doping products and the role of academic physicians

Letizia Paoli

Doping consists of athletes' use of substances and methods[1] that are prohibited by sport bodies and state institutions to enhance their performance or evade detection. Since 2004, the World Anti-Doping Agency publishes an annual list of the prohibited substances and methods, which we in short call doping products. Since the Festina affair at the 1998 Tour de France,[2] it has become progressively clear that doping 'was part of the job' in elite cycling, as Lance Armstrong, former seven-times winner of the Tour de France, admitted himself (*Telegraph*, 2013). Subsequent scandals prompted by judicial and quasi-judicial investigations (e.g. Sanvito, 2018; McLaren, 2016a, 2016b; USADA, 2012) or media reports[3] as well as scholarly analyses (e.g. De Hon, Kuipers, & van Bottenburg, 2015; Ulrich et al., 2018) have shown that the use of doping products is not limited to elite cycling. These investigations indicate thousands of athletes worldwide in many, if not most, Olympic disciplines and across all levels of sport. Some of the doping substances are also used by non-competitive sportspeople for broader lifestyle or psychoactive purposes, such as growing muscle, reducing fat, or boosting aggressiveness, and are therefore also known as performance and image-enhancing drugs (for example, Koenraadt & van de Ven, 2017).

Given the size of the problem, my coauthor and I (e.g. Paoli & Donati, 2014; Paoli & Greenfield, 2017) conceptualised the use and supply of doping products (regardless of the users' type) as a market, applying the theories and tools developed by criminology to study illegal markets in a case study of the Italian market. Subsequent studies have confirmed the validity of the market perspective (e.g. Antonopoulos & Hall, 2016; Fincoeur, 2016). My original motivation for studying the Italian market for doping products (hereinafter, in short, doping market) was the assumption that there were similarities between the supply of doping products and that of other illegal drugs. However, in the course of the project on Italy and other projects on doping (see infra), my coauthors and I have identified two peculiarities of the doping market that distinguish it from other, more consolidated illegal markets:

1 The non-criminal background of the suppliers, and particularly the repeated involvement of (academic) physicians in doping practices;

2 The persistent protection offered by state agencies, sport bodies and their representatives to doping practices in elite sport.

To prove these peculiarities, I will use evidence from three recent research projects in Italy, Belgium, France, and Germany, briefly referring also to past and recent scandals and investigations concerning other countries. In particular, I will devote attention in this article to the persistent role of academic physicians in the supply of doping products to elite athletes and explore three sets of elements that might have promoted such a role.

The chapter is structured as follows. The first section presents my data sources. The second section considers the first of the two above-mentioned peculiarities and the third one zooms in on the role of academic physicians. The fourth section discusses the second peculiarity of the doping market. Some concluding remarks follow.

Data sources

To develop my argument, I have primarily relied on the data of three recent projects.

The first project is an empirical study of the supply and demand of doping products in Italy that I conducted with Alessandro Donati on behalf of the WADA (Paoli & Donati, 2014). Much of the data of that study was collected in close collaboration with the Carabinieri Command for Health Protection. This unit is still known – and will be referred to here – by the acronym NAS from its original name, Nuclei Anti-Sofisticazione. In that project, our first source was the 'NAS Investigations Database', which includes summary data for the 80 major anti-doping investigations conducted by NAS between 1999 and 2009. These investigations represent the vast majority of the anti-doping criminal investigations and the related criminal proceedings initiated in Italy in those years. The second source is a set of official documents related to 46 different criminal investigations, 36 of which were carried out by NAS and were thus included in the NAS Investigation Database and ten of which were conducted by other police forces and were thus new. The third source is a set of interviews with 26 NAS officers, seven prosecutors, one policy-maker, and one other expert on anti-doping testing. Donati and I also worked with various other published and unpublished materials. In particular, we conducted an extensive review of the three main Italian news agencies' – *Ansa*, *Agi*, and *Adnkronos* – doping-related media reports for the period January 1998 through February 2012.

The second project, entitled 'Doping and its Supply: Exploring the Market and Assessing the Impact of Anti-Doping Policies in Belgian and French Cycling' together with Bertrand Fincoeur (e.g. Fincoeur, 2016; Fincoeur & Paoli, 2014), tackles the supply of doping products in Belgium and France for cycling. Specifically, it was intended: (a) to empirically investigate the supply of doping products; (b) to reconstruct the implementation of anti-doping policies and specifically supply-side interventions and to assess their impact. The data collection included the analysis of policy documents, criminal proceedings, and teams' websites and other documents, 77 interviews with different policy-makers, law enforcement officers, and stakeholders and survey of 2776 competitive Flemish riders, who returned 767 valid questionnaires.

The third project is not a classical research project but consists of my chairmanship of, and my investigative work for, the Evaluierungskommission Freiburger Sportmedizin (hereinafter Freiburg Commission or simply Commission). The commission was established in 2007 by the University of Freiburg after the Belgian soigneur Jef D'Hont revealed that the Team Telekom/T-Mobile cycling team systematically used EPO and other doping products (Geyer, Gorris, & Ludwig, 2007) and that at least two Freiburg University sport physicians had since 1992 been involved in, and partially even coordinated, these doping practices. The Freiburg Commission was composed of eight German and foreign renowned scientists; I became its chair in 2010. Its main task was to evaluate the activities of the Freiburg University Sport Medicine, including its alleged involvement in doping practices since the 1950s. Over the years, it heard more than 100 witnesses, including (former) athletes, sport physicians, sport and university officials, law enforcement officers, and policy-makers. It also collected and analysed over 30,000 pages of documentation from more than 12 different local and national archives. Five commission's reports have since 2015 been published by the University of Freiburg, totaling more than 1500 pages (see Albert-Ludwigs-Universität Freiburg, 2017).

The non-criminal background and modus operandi of the suppliers

Our analyses in Italy, France, and Belgium indicate that the suppliers of doping products rarely have criminal records (Paoli & Donati, 2014; Fincoeur & Paoli, 2014; Fincoeur, 2016). In Italy, in particular, most suppliers known to NAS were male, Italian citizens and with few exceptions had a legitimate profession or occupation (see Table 6.1). On the basis of the most relevant professional and occupational delineations and rankings in the NAS Investigations Database and all the criminal proceedings, Paoli and Donati (2014) identified ten main types of illegal suppliers of doping products in Italy and grouped them in five over-arching categories: gym, health care, organised sport world (human) horse-racing, semi-professional sportspeople, other (see Table 6.1).

Even in Italy the evidence does not suggest a major role for organised crime, as most typically construed, in the supply of doping products. The analysis of the Italian criminal proceedings and the expert interviews indicate a very limited involvement of Southern Italian mafia groups in the production and distribution of doping products in Italy. Only one specific type of supplier is linked to Southern Italian mafia-type organised crime groups: the hijackers who steal

Table 6.1 Types of suppliers of doping products in Italy

Category	*Type*
Gym	Gym owners or managers and body-building instructors
	Owners or managers of dietary supplement shops
Health care	Pharmacists
	Physicians
	Hospital employees
	Employees, sale representatives of (para-) pharmaceutical companies
Organised sports world (human)	Staff members of sports teams
	Staff members of sports federations
Horseracing	Veterinary physicians, breeders, jockeys, and drivers
Semi-professional sportspeople	Elite athletes, and their family members
	Hard-core body-builders, including law enforcement, military and private security company staff, and their family members
Other	People with no distinctive profession or occupation

Source: Adapted from Paoli and Donati (2014), drawing data from reports in the NAS Investigations Database, criminal proceedings, and media sources.

doping substances from trucks and are often associated with Neapolitan camorra groups. Members of some camorra groups also play an important role in fixing horse races, which can be achieved by doping horses (see also Paoli & Greenfield, 2017).

Unlike illegal drug traffickers or dealers, the majority of the suppliers of doping products can hide their illegal transactions and their relationships with their 'doping partners' – their own suppliers, collaborators, and customers or patients – behind the legitimate roles they play in their businesses, organisations, or professions. The embeddedness of doping-related supply-side activities in legitimate professions, roles, and institutions mostly makes the development of separate illegal enterprises to run these activities unnecessary. This embeddedness is suggestive of white-collar crime (Sutherland, 1983), and the related and partially overlapping concepts of occupational, corporate (Clinard & Quinney, 1973), and organisational crime (Schrager & Short, 1978) – rather than organised crime.

Reflecting this white-collar background, the suppliers of doping products are also rarely reported to use physical violence. The evidence on corruption is mixed, depending partly on how one defines corruption. In none of the countries studied have we found evidence of bribery. We have found, instead, ample evidence of 'abuse of public or private office' albeit not necessarily 'for personal gain' (OECD, 2008: 22). Particularly in elite sports, different types of suppliers – e.g. physicians, pharmacists, coaches, and sports federation officials – appear to abuse their positions and the athletes' and the latter's parents' trust by prescribing, selling, or administering the athletes doping products and convincing them of the necessity and harmlessness of doping products (see the next section also). However, these abuses typically do not occur 'for personal gain' – or at least not fully so – but in the name of a misconceived public or team good.

The role of academic physicians

As the typology suggests and the analysis of the doping supply in Belgian and French cycling (Fincoeur & Paoli, 2014) and the Freiburg Commission's investigations confirm, physicians – in many cases, university physicians – have also been repeatedly active as suppliers of doping products in the elite segment of the market. This trend is part of the broader involvement of physicians in the treatment of elite athletes since World War II: as Waddington (2000: 141) notes

> the growing involvement of practitioners of sports medicine in high-performance sport, especially from the 1950s, has increasingly involved them in the search for championship-winning or record-breaking performances, and this had led them in the direction not only of developing improved diet or mechanical and psychological techniques but, on occasions, it has also led them ... to play an active part in the development and use of performance-enhancing drugs.
>
> (Waddington, 2000: 141)

The father of Italian 'doping physicians' is undoubtedly Prof. Francesco Conconi, a professor of biochemistry at the University of Ferrara since 1967, long-time head of its Centro di Studi Biomedici applicati allo Sport and rector of the same university from 1998 to 2004.[4] In the late 1970s, Conconi started providing a variety of doping products to Italian elite athletes, primarily in track and field, cycling, swimming, pentathlon, rowing, and ski sports, with the tacit support of CONI, the Italian Olympic Committee (see section 4). By the early 1990s, Conconi had extended his services to elite riders working in private teams, treating a large number of 'stars', such as Marco Pantani, Claudio Chiappucci, and Gianni Bugno. In those same years he was a member of the Medical Committee of the International Olympic Committee (IOC), the President of the Medical Commission of the Union Cycliste Internationale (UCI) and received large amounts of funding from the IOC – supposedly to develop an EPO test, which he never delivered. At the end of 1990s, the Ferrara Prosecutor's Office indicted Conconi and two of his assistants of the crime of sporting fraud. Despite 'the seriousness and convergence of all the evidence' (Tribunale di Ferrara, 2003: 46), however, the inefficiency of the Italy judicial system and the defendants' procedural tactics (e.g. Toti, 2003) left the Ferrara judge no other choice but to dismiss the case in 2003 due to the statute of limitations.

In Germany, Conconi's pendant was represented by Profs. Armin Klümper and Joseph Keul, two former top sports physicians of the University of Freiburg, which in the 1970s and 1980s treated up to 80–90% of the West German elite athletes (e.g. Strepenick, 2016). Thanks to the Freiburg Commission's work, it has become clear that the Freiburg University sport physicians were long in charge of making – with all means, including the use of harmful doping products – West German athletes 'competitive' vis-à-vis those from East Germany and other nations of the former Soviet bloc that had organised a centralised system of 'state doping' (Berendonk, 1992; Spitzer, 2013).

Documents revealed by the Commission show that Armin Klümper in the 1970s and 1980s systematically provided the German Cycling Federation, i.e. an entire sports federation, with anabolic steroids – possibly including youth and junior teams. These documents also show that the Freiburg doctors have doped not only cyclists, but also track and field athletes, soccer players, wrestlers, canoeists, as well as other athletes in Olympic sports disciplines (e.g. Singler, 2016a; Singler & Treutlein, 2017a).

Despite being for more than a decade the senior Olympic doctor of the Federal Republic of Germany, Keul tolerated – and probably even encouraged – the administration of anabolic steroids to athletes, including women athletes, despite the proven serious harms of such substances (Singler & Treutlein, 2017b). As chair of the Freiburg University Sport Medicine Department, he also directed his team to study the effects of new and old performance-enhancement substances, often trying to minimise or even deny both their performance enhancement and side-effects in his public statements and even some publications, so that these substances could remain available for the West German athletes.

Freiburg physicians' doping practices did not end with Germany's Reunification in 1990. The 2007 Team Telekom/T-Mobile scandal and the Commission's investigations indicate that doping continued almost uninterrupted in Freiburg until 2007 (Singler, 2016a). As they themselves admitted (see Spiegel, 2007), two members of the Freiburg University Sport Medicine Department, Lothar Heinrich, and Andreas Schmid, supervised and partially even organised the doping practices of the Team Telekom/T-Mobile cycling team, no doubt contributing to the Tour de France victories of Bjarne Riis and Jan Ullrich in 1996 and 1997, respectively.

Media investigations in 2017 further showed that many track and field athletes straddling the past and current century consulted Heinrich. After these revelations, the University of Freiburg confirmed that it held blood samples of Haile Gebrselassie, an Ethiopian long-distance track and road running athlete, who had won two Olympic gold medals and four World Championship titles (e.g. SWR, 2017).

Before looking for possible explanatory elements, it is worthwhile recalling how extraordinary the involvement of university physicians in doping practices is considering, on the one hand, the high, 'above suspicion' (van de Bunt, 2010:

441) of the academic physician and, on the other, the more and more illegal status of the doping practices. As for the latter, the use of an increasing number of doping products has since the 1960s progressively been prohibited under sports rules and criminalised by many western states, including France, Belgium, and Italy. Moreover, even before the adoption of explicit anti-doping provisions in criminal law (in Germany, for example, a specific anti-doping bill was adopted only in 2015), doping practices can be subsumed under broader crimes, such as acts of bodily harm, to the extent that they are harmful to the athletes' health. They also breach the Hippocratic Oath, which has been historically taken by physicians and is often summarised in the Latin phrase 'primum non nocere' (first do no harm). The Hippocratic Oath has been reformulated in contemporary times in the Physician's Pledge of the Declaration of Geneva, which was adopted by the General Assembly of the World Medical Association in Geneva in 1948 (WMA, 2017).

In addition to the growing sophistication of doping practices – Fincoeur (2016: 206) speaks of 'medicalisation of doping' – three sets of elements can be singled out to explain the repeated participation of academic physicians in doping practices. I discuss the first two elements in this section and the third element in the following one, because it coincides with the second peculiarity of the doping market.

The first element consists of the physicians' ambition, which constitutes their personal motivation and can encompass several specific objectives: prestige and fame, personal wealth, and/or funding for one's research institute. The investigations of the Freiburg Commission provide much details on this first element. In the last three decades of the twentieth century, Keul and Klümper enjoyed considerable notoriety within the sports world and general public. Both were among the most famous physicians of the Freiburg Faculty of Medicine, although they 'only' were, respectively, the head of the Sport Medicine Department, a comparatively small university department, and the Sport Traumatology Ambulance, an even smaller ad hoc institute.

The provision of doping products and their tasks in elite sports brought Keul and Klümper in contact with many well-known athletes and let them profit from the latter's fame. From 1980 to 2000 Keul was the senior physician of the (West) German Olympic team and the medical doctor of West German Davis Cup team, in years in which Steffi Graf and Boris Becker were world stars. Klümper was the preferred sport physician of many top athletes as well as preferred orthopedist of the sport, economic, and political elite in Freiburg and the whole state of Baden-Württemberg. In both these circles, Klümper was known as 'the Doc' to court. As a witness told the Freiburg Commission: 'Klümper was only called Doc. "I go to the Doc," "Have you seen the Doc?" (…) He was a guru, a real guru' (Singler & Treutlein, 2017a: 22). When Klümper was sentenced to pay high monetary sanctions in tax and criminal proceedings, some of the most famous West German athletes, including Karl-Heinz Rummenigge and Uli Hoeneß, collected over 250,000 DM to help him pay the sanctions (Singler & Treutlein, 2017a: 172).

As for the personal wealth, both Keul and Klümper issued private invoices to their patients – even if Klümper did not even had the right to do so – and thus considerably enhanced their regular university salaries. Faced with an investigation for prescription fraud, Klümper reported to the German tax authorities that he had 'forgotten' to declare income for 1329 million DM between 1971 and 1981 – a considerable sum at the time (Singler & Treutlein, 2017a: 168). Both obtained generous financial support for their institutes from politicians and government agencies – in Klümper's case despite the opposition of some of his colleagues at the Freiburg Faculty of Medicine (Singler & Treutlein, 2017a, 2017b).

Personal ambition is not unique to sport physicians and in itself cannot explain the persistent involvement of sport physicians in doping practices. The second plausible explanatory element has to do with the ambiguities in the sport medicine's mission. Having its roots in occupational medicine in Fordist factories and in wartimes, one of sport medicine's main focuses has historically been to enhance top athletes' performance even to the detriment of the latter's long-term (and sometimes even short-term) health. Keul, for example, understood himself above all as a 'performance physician' (Singler & Treutlein, 2017b: 161): 'Where is it written that we should prevent harm?', he asked in a TV-programme 'Kontrovers' in 1976. 'This is a general medical task, which has nothing to do with sport medicine' (Singler & Treutlein, 2017b: 161). In the second half of the 1970s, when anabolic steroids had already been banned by the International Amateur Athletic Federation (in 1970), the Germany Athletic Federation (in 1971) and the IOC (in 1974), Keul and his acolytes still invested considerable time and energy in convincing sports functionaries, government officials, and politicians that anabolic steroids were not harmful. This strategy is evident in the letter that Keul and Herbert Reindell[5] wrote in 1976 to Willi Daume, the president of the National Olympic Committee. In that letter Keul and Reindell argued that the prohibition of anabolic steroids 'from a medical perspective, at least for men' was questionable, 'as no disease or harm is up to now known' (Singler & Treutlein, 2017b: 161). In the same year, the Consortium of German Sport Federation Physicians called for a 'de facto tolerance for anabolic steroid and substances that do not really cause harm', in a symposium in Freiburg that took place together with the conference of the German Sport Physicians' Society (Singler & Treutlein, 2017b: 163).

Only recently the German Society for Sport Medicine (the follow-up organisation of the German Sport Physicians' Society) has started facing the longstanding ambiguities on its mission and published an editorial in its own journal in which it explicitly rejected the prescription of steroids to athletes for either performance enhancement, 'substitution or 'therapy', the conduction of studies on the effects and side-effects of steroids among active athletes and the trivialisation of such side-effects (DGSP, 2015). The list of the signatures, however, did not include some famous German sports physicians, such as Wilfried

Kindermann, one of the Keul's most influential pupils and his successor as senior physician of the German Olympic team.

Doping protection by sport bodies and state authorities

The three selected research projects as well as several past and ongoing scandals (see below) document the 'protection' long provided by officials and staff members of sport authorities and key sport federations, some of whom were civil servants and even government officials, to doping elite athletes and the latter's suppliers. This protection constitutes the second peculiarity of the doping market as well as the third and most important element to explain academic physicians' repeated role as doping suppliers.

Among the countries in which I have carried out empirical investigations, the proof of government protection is most solid in Italy. There, as Italian criminal investigations and the resulting scandal indicate, the representatives of national sports bodies, including some very high-ranking officials, exercised their roles as 'protectors' quite openly until the late 1990s. A fine line might separate individuals from their institutions, but a request filed in October 2000 by the Prosecutor's Office of Ferrara in the proceedings against Conconi provides evidence of high-ranking individual involvement so much so that it might be difficult to argue against institutional complicity. After reconstructing the relationships between CONI and Conconi since the late 1970s, in fact, Prosecutor Soprani came to the conclusion that Conconi had set up a 'criminal organisation' (article 416 of the Italian criminal Code, CP; Procura della Repubblica di Ferrara, 2000: 42) together with three CONI Presidents – Franco Carraro (CONI President from 1981 to 1986), Arrigo Gattai (CONI President from 1987 to 1994), Mario Pescante (CONI Secretary General from 1981 to 1994 and CONI President from 1995 to 1998) – and the head of the Research and Documentation Section of the CONI School of Sport, Gianfranco Carabelli. This criminal association had allegedly the purpose of distributing drugs in a dangerous way to public health (article 445 CP) and was active throughout the 1980s (ibid.; see also Capodacqua, 2000). Pescante and Conconi were regarded as the promoters of the criminal organisation. As too much time had elapsed between the alleged activities and the prosecution, Soprani had to dismiss the case but insisted that his request 'does not diminish the social and criminal non-value of the activities proved' (Procura della Repubblica di Ferrara, 2000: 56). Despite these charges, Pescante became Italy's undersecretary for sports less than a year after the prosecutor's request was filed.

In Germany, the judicial evidence of government and sports federations' direct involvement in doping practices is less clear-cut. Perhaps because they are subjected to ministerial control, German prosecutors have rather focused on doping in the former German Democratic Republic, neglecting the investigation of West German doping and its protection networks. Nonetheless, in

Germany too, the police and judicial documents analysed by the Freiburg Commission and other sources clearly show federal, regional, and local politicians and government entities long gave their unofficial, but decisive, support to the doping practices of Klümper, Keul, and Co. These sources also indicate that a variety of other public entities, including the Freiburg University leadership and the local prosecutor's office and courts, long showed benign neglect for such practices and did not properly exercise their supervisory responsibilities.[6] The speech held in 1976 by Gerhard Groß at the inauguration of the Keul's new Sport Medicine Department's building is illustrative of the stance of many West German politicians and government representatives of that epoch. Speaking on behalf of the Federal Ministry of the Interior, of which he was a civil servant, Groß stated:

> The keyword medical performance enhancement leads me to spend a moment on this topic.... I know that Freiburg, too, has repeatedly spoken about it – if, dear professor Keul, I can identify Freiburg with your person. If no danger or harm to health is caused, you consider such performance enhancement means acceptable. The Federal Ministry of the Interior shares this view. Our athletes cannot be deprived of means that have been tested in other states as a successful training and competition support and have proven themselves to be harmless in year-long praxis. This stance is necessary if we want to keep the pace with the top of the sport movement – and that's what we want.
>
> (Singler & Treutlein, 2017b: 160)

In supporting doping, many West German sports officials and politicians were probably even convinced of operating for a higher national interest. In those years East German athletes were extraordinarily successful in international sports competitions due to a systematic top-down doping programme (Spitzer, 2013). Such a programme was not yet known to the broad public, but West German sport insiders were already aware of its existence. In those years, securing the 'equality of chances' of West German athletes versus their East German counterparts seemed to be a valuable policy goal. Even Wolfgang Schäuble, who later became Minister of the Interior and as such responsible for German elite sports, was influenced by Keul's trivialisation of steroid harm. In a parliamentary hearing of the Bundestag's Sport Commission, Schäuble stated:

> We advocate only the most limited use of these drugs and only under the complete control of the sports physicians – because it is clear that there are disciplines in which the use of these drugs is necessary to remain competitive at the international level.
>
> (Deutscher Bundestag 1977: 102)

In assessing these stances, we must consider that in the Cold War era, sport was mostly considered as 'war minus the shooting', referring to George Orwell's famous quote. However, repeated, more recent scandals show that politicians' support of doping practices has not ended with the Cold War – nor affects only 'corrupt' Mediterranean countries, such as Italy, or post-Soviet authoritarian countries, such as Russia (e.g. McLaren, 2016a, 2016b). The sports federations of several western countries, as represented by high-level officials, have until recently regarded doping as a de facto legitimate practice or, even if they increasingly have had 'doubts' about its formal legitimacy, they have still supported or tolerated it in the pursuit of the higher goal of sports success. A good case in point here is the 2001 Lahti scandal. A few days before the start of the 2001 Nordic World Championships in Lahti, Finland, the team physician of the Finnish national ski team mistakenly left his bag containing plasma expander, bloody needles, and intravenous tubes at a petrol station. A scandal burst when six Finnish skiers tested positive for plasma expander a few days afterwards and the bag was linked to the team physicians and positive tests. Most probably, the athletes had taken EPO, then used plasma expander to lower their hematocrit levels before the races. A Doping Enquiry Taskforce (2001: 3) set up by the Finnish Ministry of Education to investigate the scandal concluded: 'What made the Lahti doping cases serious was not only the large number of perpetrators, six, but also that doping had taken place under the auspices of Finnish Ski Federation coaching'. In 2008, Kari-Pekka Kyrö, the former coach of the Finnish national team and the only person sentenced for the 2001 scandal, finally admitted that 'in the 1990s there was a pharmacological programme in the Finnish Ski Federation' and that Finnish skiers systematically took EPO, GH, and plasma expander (Hahn & Häyrinen, 2008).

The scandal affecting the Austrian Ski Federation that burst at the 2006 Turin Olympic Games also suggests that doping has continued to be tolerated at the highest sports levels in western countries even in the current century. This federation hired and protected the trainer Walter Mayer, even after he had been suspended by the IOC, allowed the doping of many of its biathlon and cross-country athletes under Mayer's supervision and even set up two haematological 'laboratories' to check the athletes' blood values at their training location in Austria and at their premises at the Olympic Village in Turin. After these events became public thanks to the intervention of Italy's law enforcement agencies, the IOC Disciplinary Commission concluded that the whole Austrian Olympic Committee had

> breached its obligations under the Olympic Charter, the IOC Code of Ethics and applicable anti-doping regulations … 1. through its responsibility for the conduct of the Austrian Ski Federation, as well as for the anti-doping rule violations committed by its athletes and support staff at the Torino Olympic Games …; 2. by failing to prevent Mr. Mayer from participating in the Torino Olympic Games in breach of the IOC's decision against Mr. Mayer after the 'Blood Bag Affair'…; and 3. by failing to

> implement appropriate organisational changes in an attempt to prevent a repeat of the problems experienced in 2002.
>
> (IOC, 2007)

Even in unified Germany, the repeated emphasis placed on the medals to be won by German athletes in international competitions suggests that politicians and government bodies are more interested in the final results than in the methods with which such results are achieved. As recently as 2016, the Federal Minister of the Interior Thomas De Mazière prompted German elite sport 'in the tradition of the two German states' to win 'at least 30% more medals' (FAZ, 2015). Moreover, German sport authorities have shown a surprising eagerness in involving East German trainers and functionaries in the federal sport federations right after Germany's unification in 1990 – a practice that virtually has no parallel in other policy fields (Treutlein, 2017). As other governments, the German federal government also generously funds elite sports with almost 170 million euro in 2017, more than a third of which goes directly to national sports federations (BMI, n.d.). Although no precise figures are available, the funds invested in non-competitive sports are comparatively much smaller, even if such funds could have tangible beneficial effects on a comparatively much larger share of the population.

Doping practices have been tolerated not only by single national governments and their representatives but also by the very bodies that are supposed to govern the world of sports, starting from the IOC. At least until the current century, the IOC did not make a credible effort to implement their own sports rules and anti-doping tests. Its mild treatment of Russian athletes at the 2016 Rio and 2018 Pyeongchang Olympics suggests a persistent lack of enthusiasm among senior members of the IOC for an intensive anti-doping programme and for sanctioning its state protectors. Even Dick Pound (2011), former IOC vice-president and founding president of WADA, is very critical:

> The response to doping in sport, on the part of sports authorities and governments, did not come until long after the phenomenon was recognized as a serious problem in virtually every sport. Years and years and years of endemic doping in cycling passed almost without notice and, when it was noticed, it was denied or passed off as an isolated aberration. The growing use of anabolic steroids, stimulants and other doping methods in other sports were met with institutional denial, individual lies and inconsequential sanctions. Testing was introduced with enormous reluctance and testing programs were normally limited to in-competition tests, in which a positive test was, in effect, failure of an intelligence test as much as a doping test.
>
> (Pound, 2011)

It is plausible that the IOC's longstanding neglect of doping has been driven by its growing concern with commercial issues, since effective controls would expose numerous famous athletes and alienate Olympic corporate sponsors (e.g. Hoberman, 2001: 245). This critical view of the IOC is reinforced by persistent allegations of suppressed positive test results at several Olympic Games during the 1980s and, more recently, at the 2008 Olympic Games in Beijing and the 2014 Winter Olympic games in Sochi (McLaren, 2016a, 2016b; Independent Commission, 2015; Rumsby, 2017).

Important sport federations do not have a better track record than the IOC in enforcing anti-doping rule. Some – for example the UCI – were too long afraid to question their 'heroes', such as Lance Armstrong, and thus lose public support and ruin their business model (Cycling Independent Reform Commission, 2015). Others federations, such as the International Association of Athletics Federations (IAAF; e.g. Independent Commission, 2015) were also too misgoverned and corrupt to enforce a strict policy on doping.

Concluding remarks

Drawing on the findings of three research projects, I have argued in this chapter that the doping market is characterised by two startling peculiarities: the suppliers' non-criminal background, and particularly the repeated involvement of academic physicians in doping practices, and the persistent protection offered by state agencies, sports bodies, and their representatives to doping practices in elite sport. These peculiarities imply a veritable policy conundrum. Despite their official prohibition by sports rules and legal codes, doping practices have long been perceived as legitimate and actively encouraged or at least tolerated by the very bodies that were supposed to suppress them.

On a more positive note, the analyses also suggest that criminal law enforcement can help to effectively tear down the 'walls of secrecy and silence' (van de Bunt, 2010) surrounding illegal or otherwise prohibited practices. In particular, the Italian experience in dealing with both the Conconi's affair and Austrian Ski Federation's doping scandal at the 2006 Turin Olympic Games show the value added of independent prosecutors who are not conditioned by the executive power (if only the Italian judicial system were a bit more efficient! See Paoli & Donati, 2014). French law enforcement authorities also played an essential role in revealing and investigating the Festina affair (e.g. Fotheringham, 2016).

More generally, the analyses also show that the athletes, as well as their suppliers and protectors, within the elite sports world are sensible to deterrent measures, because they, as most white-collar criminals, have a lot to lose. And even if the perpetrators' behaviour does not change in the short term, criminal investigations can at least disclose illegal or otherwise prohibited practices, thus contributing to their delegitimation among the general public. Criminologists, like me, are mostly sceptical of the application of criminal law, as we are all too well aware of the many serious harmful, intended and unintended, consequences that often accompany it. Whereas these criticisms are well founded, the present analyses indicate that the enforcement of criminal law has a positive, if small, role to play.

Given the dependence of the elite sport doping on state and sport bodies' protection and funding, the analyses also indicate that governments have more leverage in securing anti-doping compliance in elite sports than they do in other 'semi-illegal' markets (e.g. Paoli & Greenfield, 2017), simply because most national sports federations, with the exception of the football federations and a few others, depend on government funding. As Bette (2011: 169–170) argues, 'a lot could be achieved with money that you either make available to sports organisations or withdraw in case of observed deviance or lack of cooperation' (see also Grix & Carmichael, 2012). Through their funding, government bodies could easily create incentives for serious anti-doping interventions, for example, by making the allocation of funding dependent on the implementation of specific anti-doping interventions and demanding the reimbursement of funding if these interventions are not implemented. Investigating the 2001 Lahti scandal, the Doping Enquiry Taskforce (2001: 3) set up by the Finnish Ministry of Education argued that 'a federation is always responsible for its own activities', and proposed that the ministry 'refrain from paying one million FIM of the 4.52 million granted to the Ski Federation for 2001 because of the failure to comply with the conditions for government aid. In addition, future aid should be dependent on the anti-doping action of the Federation in the coming years'. The Ministry of Education enforced the Taskforce's suggestions.

In other words, effective supply-side interventions, including but not limited to criminal prosecution, are possible. These interventions can reduce both the supply and use of doping products, especially in the organised sports world, but they presuppose a political will that many governments and sports ruling bodies have yet to show consistently.

Notes

1 Doping substances include, among others, anabolic steroids, stimulants, erythropoietin (EPO), growth hormones. Doping methods primarily consist of blood transfusions (see WADA, 2015).
2 The affair began when the French customs seized a large haul of doping products in a car belonging to the Festina cycling team just before the start of the race. The subsequent criminal investigations revealed that many riders from the Festina and other teams made use of EPO – so that several teams withdrew from the race (see, e.g. Fotheringham, 2016).
3 E.g. *Geheimsache Doping: Wie Russland seine Sieger macht*, the 2014 German ARD documentary that provided proofs of systematic state-organised doping in Russia.
4 See his personal webpage at http://docente.unife.it/francesco.conconi/curr
5 Reindell was Keul's and Klümper's PhD supervisor, as well as Keul's predecessor as head of the Freiburg University Sport Medicine Department and as senior physician of the West German Olympic team. At the time of the letter, in 1976, he was also the President of the German Sport Physicians' Society (see Singler and Treutlein, 2016).
6 The Commission's analyses further show that the internal and external weaknesses in the Freiburg University Sport Medicine's governance also allowed numerous instances

of scientific misconduct and breaches of scientific integrity, such as plagiarism, data manipulation, and falsification in scientific activities and publications (e.g. Köppelle, 2014).

References

Albert-Ludwigs-Universität Freiburg. (2017). Sportmedizin und Doping: Aufklärungsarbeit der Universität Freiburg. Available: www.uni-freiburg.de/universitaet/einzelgutachten

Antonopoulos, G.A. & Hall, A. (2016). 'Gain with no pain': Anabolic-androgenic steroids trafficking in the UK. *European Journal of Criminology*, *13*(6), 696–713.

Berendonk, B. (1992). *Doping: von der Forschung zum Betrug*. Hamburg: Rowohlt.

Bette, K. (2011). *Sportsoziologische Aufklärung: Studien zum Sport der modernen Gesellschaft*. Bielefeld: transcript.

BMI, Bundesinnenministerium (n.d.). Die Finanzierung des Sports. Available: www.bmi.bund.de/DE/themen/sport/sportfoerderung/finanzierung-des-sports/finanzierung-des-sports-node.html

Capodacqua, E. (2000). Accuse choc da Ferrara: il Coni dietro al doping. *La Repubblica*. Available: www.repubblica.it/online/sport/pantapro/con/con.html?ref=search

Clinard, M. & Quinney, R. (1973). *Criminal Behavior Systems: A Typology*. New York: Holt, Rinehart and Winston.

Cycling Independent Reform Commission (2015). *Report to the President of the Union Cycliste Internationale*, written by D. Marty, P. Nicholson, & U. Haas. Available: www.uci.ch/mm/Document/News/CleanSport/16/87/99/CIRCReport2015_Neutral.pdf

De Hon O., Kuipers H., & van Bottenburg M. (2015). Prevalence of doping use in elite sports: a review of numbers and methods. *Sports Medicine*, 45(1), 57–69.

Deutscher Bundestag, Ed. (1977). *Stenographisches Protokoll über die Anhörung von Sachverständigen in der 6. Sitzung des Sportausschusses am Mittwoch, dem 28. September 1977*. Bonn.

Doping Enquiry Taskforce (2001). Report. 23 May. Available: www.minedu.fi/export/sites/default/OPM/Julkaisut/2001/liitteet/opm_57_doping_en.pdf?lang=fi

DGSP, Deutschen Gesellschaft für Sportmedizin und Prävention (2011). Doping im Leistungssport in Westdeutschland: Stellungnahme der Hochschullehrer der deutschen Sportmedizin und des Wissenschaftsrates der Deutschen Gesellschaft für Sportmedizin und Prävention (DGSP). *Deutsche Zeitschrift für Sportmedizin*, 62(11), 343–344.

FAZ, Frankfurter Allgemeine Zeitung (2015). *Sportminister de Maizière: Wir müssten mindestens ein Drittel mehr Medaillen bekommen*. 16 April. www.faz.net/aktuell/sport/sportpolitik/sportminister-de-maiziere-fordert-ein-drittel-mehr-medaillen-13706187.html

Fincoeur, B. (2016). *Le marché du dopage dans le cyclisme sur route belge et français: analyse de la demande, de l'offre et de l'impact de la lutte antidopage*. KU Leuven: Unpublished PhD thesis.

Fincoeur, B. & Paoli, L. (2014). Des pratiques communautaires au marché du dopage. Evolution de la distribution des produits dopants dans le cyclisme. *Déviance et Société*, 38(1), 3–27.

Fotheringham, A. (2016). *The End of the Road: The Festina Affair and the Tour that Almost Wrecked Cycling*. London: Fotheringham.

Geyer, M., Gorris, L., & Ludwig, U. (2007). Der einzige Zeuge. *Der Spiegel*, 30 April. Available: www.spiegel.de/spiegel/a-480024.html

Grix, J. & Carmichael, F. (2012). Why do governments invest in elite sport? A polemic. *International Journal of Sport Policy and Politics*, 4(1), 73–90.

Hahn, T. & Häyrinen, R. (2008). Doping im finnischen Skisport. Die schmutzigen Neunziger. *Süddeutsche Zeitung*. 25 June. Available: www.sueddeutsche.de/sport/doping-im-finnischen-skisport-die-schmutzigen-neunziger-1.203060

Hoberman, J. (2001). How drug testing fails. The politics of doping control. In W. Wilson & E. Derse (Eds), *Doping in Elite Sport* (pp. 241–274). Champaign: Human Kinetics.

Independent Commission (2015). The Independent Commission Report #1: Final Report. 9 November. Available: https://Wada-Main-Prod.S3.Amazonaws.Com/Resources/Files/Wada_Independent_Commission_Report_1_En.Pdf

IOC, International Olympic Committee (2007). Summary of the IOC Disciplinary Commission Recommendations Regarding the National Olympic Committee of Austria (Österreichisches Olympisches Comité – ÖOC). Available: www.olympic.org/Documents/Reports/EN/en_report_1183.pdf

Koenraadt, R. & van de Ven, K. (2017). The Internet and lifestyle drugs: an analysis of demographic characteristics, methods, and motives of online purchasers of illicit lifestyle drugs in the Netherlands. *Drugs: Education, Prevention and Policy*, 1–11.

Köppelle, W. (2014). Freiburger Plagiatsaffäre: Den Bock zum Gärtner gemacht? Säubermänner mit dreckigen Westen am Uniklinikum. *Laborjournal*, *12*, 12–19. Available: www.laborjournal-archiv.de/epaper/LJ_14_12/files/assets/common/downloads/Laborjournal_2014_12.pdf

McLaren, R.H. (2016a). The independent person report. Part I. 18 July. Available: www.wada-ama.org/en/resources/doping-control-process/mclaren-independent-investigation-report-part-i

McLaren, R.H. (2016b). The independent person report. Part Ii. 9 December. Available: www.wada-ama.org/en/resources/doping-control-process/mclaren-independent-investigation-report-part-ii

OECD, Organisation for Economic Co-Operation and Development (2008). *OECD Glossaries – Corruption: A Glossary of International Standards in Criminal Law*. Paris: OECD.

Paoli, L. & Donati, A. (2014). *The Sports Doping Market: Understanding Supply and Demand, and the Challenges of Their Control*. New York: Springer.

Paoli, L. & Greenfield, V.A. (2017). The supply of doping products and the relevance of market-based perspectives: Implications of recent research in Italy. In J. Beckert & M. Dewey (Eds), *The Architecture of Illegal Markets* (pp. 245–267). New York: Oxford University Press.

Pound, R.W. (2011). WADA – A success story? Presentation made at the Freiburg Symposium 'Sports Medicine and Doping', Freiburg, 12–14 September. Available: www.uni-freiburg.de/universitaet/einzelgutachten.

Procura della Repubblica presso il Tribunale di Ferrara (2000). Richiesta di archiviazione parziale. Procedimento penale control Pescante Mario + 13 altri. N. 893/99/21 R.G. notizie di reato/Mod. 21.

Rumsby, B. (2017). IOC accused of failing to investigate positive drugs tests – including by Jamaican sprinters – from 2008 Olympics. *Telegraph*. 3 April. Available: www.telegraph.co.uk/athletics/2017/04/03/ioc-accused-failing-investigate-positive-drugs-tests-including/

Sanvito, N. (2018). Sentenza Schwazer/Donati: 'Un'ora dopo la deposizione, deciso il controllo antidoping'. Dimissioni IAAF?. *Il Sussidiario*. 25 January. Available: www.ilsussidiario.net/News/Calcio-e-altri-Sport/2018/1/25/SENTENZA-SCHWAZER-Donati-Un-ora-dopo-la-deposizione-deciso-il-controllo-antidoping-Dimissioni-IAAF-/803511/

Schrager, L.S. & Short, J.F. (1978). Toward a sociology of organizational crime. *Social Problems*, *25*(4), 407–419.

Singler, A. (with assistance of L. Heitner) (2016a). Doping beim Team Telekom/T-Mobile: Wissenschaftliches Gutachten zu systematischen Manipulationen im Profiradsport mit Unterstützung Freiburger Sportmediziner. Available: www.uni-freiburg.de/universitaet/einzelgutachten

Singler, A. (2016b). Systematische Manipulationen im Radsport und Fußball: Wissenschaftliches Gutachten zu neuen Erkenntnissen zum Doping in der Bundesrepublik Deutschland im Zusammenhang mit dem Wirken von Armin Klümper. Available: www.andreas-singler.de/doping-forschung/

Singler, A. & Treutlein, G. (2010). *Doping im Spitzensport. Sportwissenschaftliche Analysen zur nationalen und internationalen Leistungsentwickung* (5th ed.). Aachen: Meyer & Meyer.

Singler, A. & Treutlein, G. (2016). Herbert Reindell als Röntgenologe, Kardiologe und Sportmediziner: Wissenschaftliche Schwerpunkte, Engagement im Sport und Haltungen zum Dopingproblem. Available: www.uni-freiburg.de/universitaet/einzelgutachten

Singler, A. & Treutlein, G. (with assistance of L. Heitner) (2017a). Armin Klümper und das bundesdeutsche Dopingproblem: Strukturelle Voraussetzungen für illegitime Manipulationen, politische Unterstützung und institutionelles Versagen. Available: www.uni-freiburg.de/universitaet/einzelgutachten

Singler, A. & Treutlein, G. (with assistance of L. Heitner) (2017b). Joseph Keul: Wissenschaftskultur, Doping und Forschung zur pharmakologischen Leistungssteigerung – Wissenschaftliches Gutachten im Auftrag der Albert-Ludwigs-Universität Freiburg. Available: www.uni-freiburg.de/universitaet/einzelgutachten

Spiegel, Der. (2007). *T-Mobile Ärzte outen sich als Doping-Helfer*. 23 May. Available: www.spiegel.de/sport/sonst/t-mobile-aerzte-outen-sich-als-doping-helfer-a-484633.html

Spitzer, G. (2013). *Doping in der DDR: Ein historischer Überblick zu einer konspirativen Praxis. Genese – Verantwortung – Gefahren*. Köln: Strauss.

Strepenick, A. (2015). Das Dopingparadies: Freiburger Sportmediziner haben vier Jahrzehnte lang gedopt. Der eigentliche Skandal: Der Staat, Sportpolitiker und Funktionäre ließen sie gewähren – eine Spurensuche. *Die Zeit*. 23 March. Available: www.zeit.de/sport/2015-03/freiburg-doping-kluemper-uni

Sutherland, E.H. ([1949] 1983). *White-Collar Crime: The Uncut Version*. New Haven: Yale University Press.

SWR (2017). Doping-Verdacht in Freiburg Uni bestätigt Kontakt zu Gebrselassie. www.swr.de/sport/doping-verdacht-in-freiburg-uni-bestaetigt-kontakt-zu-gebrselassie/-/id=1208948/did=20035816/nid=1208948/1errajd/index.html

Telegraph (2013). Lance Armstrong Oprah interview: 'I doped during all seven Tour wins'. Available: www.telegraph.co.uk/sport/sportvideo/9810214/Lance-Armstrong-Oprah-interview-I-doped-during-all-seven-Tour-wins.html

Toti, G. (2003). Caso Conconi, indietro tutta. *Corriere della Sera*. 26 March: 46. Online available: http://archiviostorico.corriere.it/2003/marzo/26/Caso_Conconi_indietro_tutta_co_0_030326239.shtml

Treutlein, G. (2017). Hinsehen statt Wegsehen. *Doping*, *4*(2), 108–112.

Tribunale di Ferrara. 2003. Sentenza nei confronti di Conconi Francesco + altri. No. 893/99 RGNG. 19 November.

Ulrich, R., Pope, HG Jr., Cléret, L., Petróczi, A., Nepusz, T., Schaffer, J., Kanayama, G., Comstock, R.D., & Simon, P. (2018). Doping in two elite athletics competitions assessed by randomized-response surveys. *Sports Medicine*, *48*(1), 211–219.

USADA, U.S. Anti-Doping Agency. (2012). Members of the United States Postal Service Pro-Cycling Team doping conspiracy, Dr. Garcia Del Moral, Dr. Ferrari and trainer Marti receive lifetime bans for doping violations. 10 July.

van de Bunt, H. (2010). Walls of secrecy and silence: The Madoff case and cartels in the construction industry. *Criminology and Public Policy*, 9(3), 435–453.

van de Ven K., & Mulrooney K.J. (2017). Social suppliers: Exploring the cultural contours of the performance and image enhancing drug (PIED) market among bodybuilders in the Netherlands and Belgium. *International Journal of Drug Policy*, *40*, 6–15.

WADA, World Anti-Doping Agency (2015). *World Anti-Doping Code*. Available: www.wada-ama.org/en/resources/the-code/world-anti-doping-code

Waddington, I. (2000). *Sport, Health and Drugs. A Critical Sociological Perspective*. London: Spon Press.

WMA, World Medical Association (2017). Declaration of Geneva. The Physician's Pledge. Available: www.wma.net/policies-post/wma-declaration-of-geneva

Part II

Threats on cycling and opportunities for anti-doping

Chapter 7

Doped humans and rigged bikes – and why we (wrongly) get more upset about the bikes

Ask Vest Christiansen

Cyclists are cheaters

In October 2017, I visited Mallorca in the Mediterranean. During the last decade, the beautiful island has become a cycling Mecca not only for professional cyclists but even more so for recreational ones who want to try themselves out on the well-kept scenic roads in the mild climate. While I was sipping coffee at a café one afternoon, I could not avoid overhearing the conversation among a group of British lycra-dressed cyclists at the neighbouring table. The discussion was about Chris Froome. A woman speculated what would happen if the four-time Tour de France winner was caught doping, when her friend interrupted in a lecturing tone: 'Debbie, I have to correct you on this: It is not a question of "*if* he is caught", it is "*when* he is caught"'. The group laughed in apparent agreement. (Little did they know, at this point, Froome already had an 'adverse analytical finding' for salbutamol, taken after stage 18 of Vuelta a España 2017).

The anecdote exemplifies a mistrust in elite cycling that became widespread among large segments of the public after the doping scandals in the late 1990s and mid-2000s. Even if those large-scale scandals happened some years ago, the doping stigma has not left the sport. People who dare to look through the commentaries following online articles on even the most insignificant doping case in cycling are guaranteed to find a number of cranky comments on the sport's ingrained immorality. In other words, it seems as if elite cycling culture is more prone to cheating, and hence morally corrupt, than others. However, the truth is more complicated. Although doping has been prevalent in the sport since its creation (and banned since the 1960s), I will argue that cyclists' moral compass show no greater error than it does for other elite athletes or people in general. In fact, cyclists react very strongly against rule breaking that they regard as a transgression to the constraints specific to the sport.

The questions I will address in this chapter are whether professional cyclists' morality concerning cheating differs from that of other people, and how potential limits of accepted cheating within the cycling culture are constructed. With the point of departure in a common understanding of cheating and dishonest behaviour, I will first present research on how people generally respond to opportunities to cheat, with the purpose of establishing how cheating operates normally, and what may cause people to cheat more or less. Afterward, I will assess how this knowledge fits with what has been observed concerning doping in cycling, and compare the apparent widespread acceptance of doping in the 1990s and early 2000s with cyclists' strong reactions against the use of so-called motor-doping, or technological fraud (as the UCI has termed it). With this, I will finally seek to demonstrate that these different moral positions result from an embedded culture that distinguishes what it considers the necessary conditions for a sporting performance to be valid and at the same time blinds its members from seeing its own idiosyncrasies on what counts as fair and what crosses the line.

The Simple Model of Rational Crime

When experts comment on why athletes choose (not) to dope, a common answer is that athletes most likely make up their mind by weighing the pros against the cons. This answer implicitly builds on a model of human decision-making process known as *Rational Man*, or when specifically concerned with dishonest or illegal behaviour, the *Simple Model of Rational Crime* (SMORC). University of Chicago economist Gary Becker, a Nobel laureate, developed the SMORC, which suggests that people commit crimes based on a rational analysis of each situation. The essence of Becker's theory is that decisions about honesty, like most other decisions, are based on a cost–benefit analysis. In other words, for a given behaviour or action we consciously calculate the expected positive gains against the expected negative consequences, i.e. the risk of getting caught and the associated punishment and, if the former outweighs the latter, then we go for it. Otherwise, we do not. It therefore also assumes that if the risk of being caught and punished is negligible and there are only positive gains of a specific type of behaviour, we will always go for it. Similarly, it assumes that if the potential negative consequences are enormous and the gains are less, then we will never choose that behaviour. As professor of Behavioural Economics, at Duke University, Dan Ariely, points out, if the SMORC model accurately describes people's behaviour, society basically has two means to deal with dishonesty:

> The first is to increase the probability of being caught (through hiring more police officers and installing more surveillance cameras, for example). The second is to increase the magnitude of punishment for people who get caught (for example, by imposing steeper prison sentences and fines).
>
> (Ariely, 2012: 4–5)

Two examples may illustrate why the SMORC is likely an incomplete theory: (1) In the summertime, I like to stop at the small stands by the roadside to buy strawberries and potatoes. Such stands are found frequently in the countryside in Denmark and are usually unmanned and not under surveillance. Payment is done by putting cash in the box provided (or, these days, by making the transaction with your mobile phone). Since the behaviour would have only pros and no cons, the SMORC predicts that I should simply stop the car, grab a bag of potatoes, and happily move on without paying. However, I do not. Some people likely do, but most do not, otherwise the stands would not be there. (2) In the state of Louisiana, USA, there is the death penalty for homicide. It is hard to imagine a consequence more dire than losing your life. Does this mean that there are no homicides in Louisiana? No! In fact, apart from the District of Columbia, Louisiana has the highest rate of homicide per 100,000 inhabitants in the USA, namely 10.3. Compare this to a rate of 0.7 in Denmark where there is no death penalty (Justitsministeriets Forskningskontor, 2014; Wikipedia, 2018). The SMORC thus seems to underestimate the prevalence of both moral and immoral behaviour. There thus seems to be something inherently wrong with the SMORC as the framework for understanding socially unacceptable behaviour, whether it is killing, stealing, or doping. So, if the SMORC is incomplete what forces is it then that spur us to act dishonestly and what is it that keep us honest? This is what Ariely has studied in a simple but very effective design.

A little dishonesty is okay

Together with his colleague, Nina Mazar, Ariely developed what they call the matrix task.[1] Participants sit at separate desks and receive a sheet of paper with 20 matrices each containing 12 fields with a three-digit number in each field (numbers like 1.69; 4.81; 8.32; 5.19). Their task is then for each of these matrices to find the two numbers that add up to 10 (e.g. 4.81; 5.19). When the experimenter says 'begin', participants turn over their sheet of paper and do as many of the math puzzles they can in five minutes. When the time is up, they count their correct answers, go to the experimenter, get their answers checked, and are paid one dollar for each correct answer. In the control condition, where there is no possibility of cheating, they found that people on average solve four of the 20 matrices in five minutes. However, the clever part of the experiment is the test situation. Here, when the five minutes are up, participants are asked to count how many correct answers they have, then go to the shredder in the back of the room, shred their test, go back to the experimenter, tell her how many correct answers they had, and collect their payment. This obviously opens the possibility for cheating, since participants can now tell the experimenter how many correct answers they have and collect their reward without documentation. Since there is a nice reward, no risk of being caught and punished, all rational participants should, according to the SMORC, go and tell the experimenter that they solved all 20 puzzles and collect their money. However, this was not what Ariely and his colleagues found. As in the control condition, people on average solved four problems but now reported solving six. Interestingly, while nearly 70% of the more than 40,000 people that have taken the test have cheated, only 20 people were 'big cheaters' who claimed to have solved all 20 problems. They cost the experiment 400 dollars. They also found more than 28,000 'little cheaters' who cost the experiment 50,000 dollars. Furthermore, the amount of cheating was the same regardless of whether the payment for each correct puzzle was 25 cent, 50 cent, 1 dollar, 2 dollars, or 5 dollars. In fact – and once again contrary to the prediction of the SMORC – cheating was slightly lower when participants were paid the highest, 10 dollars, for each correct answer.

With this knowledge, Ariely and his group adjusted the matrix task in a number of ways with the purpose of examining what would cause cheating to increase and what would cause it to decrease. For instance, when an actor was placed in the room with the test-participants, and he, only one minute into the test, stood up and declared that he had solved all 20 matrices, walked up to the experimenter, and collected his 20 dollars, cheating among all participants went up. Cheating also went up when participants prior to the matrix task had either starved or undergone a number of intellectually demanding test and were thus depleted when they took the test (Ariely, 2012: 103–112). On the other hand, cheating went down when participants prior to the test were requested to sign a document stating that they understood that the experiment fell under the university's honour code. The same pattern was observed when participants were asked to write down the Ten Commandments or swear on the Bible prior to test. In other words, whereas depletion and witnessing others' dishonest acts increased cheating, being reminded of values decreased cheating.

Moreover, the results display a universal pattern. When the experiment was replicated in countries with different cultures (and different rates of corruption) such as Turkey, Italy, Canada, Columbia, United Kingdom, Israel, and China, the amount of cheating was the same as in the USA. This does not mean that culture does not influence cheating. Rather, since the matrix task is abstract from culture, it reveals 'a basic human capacity to be morally flexible and reframe situations and actions in ways that reflect positively on ourselves' (Ariely, 2012: 242).

Based on a vast variety of experiments Ariely and his collaborators have done on what causes, decreases, and increases dishonest behaviour, Ariely concludes: 'Our sense of our own morality is connected to the amount of cheating we feel comfortable with. Essentially, we cheat up to the level that allows us to retain our self-image as reasonable honest individuals' (Ariely, 2012: 22–23). In other words, the forces that govern dishonesty are much more complex than predicted by the SMORC, since it does not say anything about moral consciousness, self-image, or emotional irrationality.

As an alternative thesis that can better accommodate their findings, Ariely suggests that human behaviour is driven by two opposing motivations: on the one hand side, we want to view ourselves as good, honest, decent people, who can look in the mirror and feel good about ourselves. On the other hand, we want to benefit from cheating when we can. There is thus a delicate balance between the contradictory desires to maintain a positive self-image and to benefit from cheating. To balance such opposing motivations, we allow a certain amount of flexibility in our behaviour before our self-image is affected. Thus, when we cheat, we rationalise our behaviour, by telling ourselves that in this context, with these circumstances it is okay to cheat by this degree, without being immoral. Therefore, culture still matters and the specific cultural context where our daily activities take place can influence dishonesty in two main ways: 'it can either take particular activities and transition them into and out of the moral domain, and it can change the magnitude of [how much flexibility] is considered acceptable for any particular domain' (Ariely, 2012: 242).

It was like air in the tyres

Ariely's findings fit surprisingly well with not only the doping stories coming out from cycling these last 10–15 years, but also what is seen in every race of the season. As with the matrix task, we also here find a lot of little cheaters, and fewer big cheaters. There are many sticky bottles,[2] some cheat with Therapeutic Use Exemptions (TUE) and cortisone injections, but (these days most likely) few full-scale-team-organised-blood-bank-EPO-programmes. Also in agreement with Ariely, when revelations about doping have come out, they have often fitted a uniform rationalisation template: 'I just did what everybody else was doing' or 'I did not want to get dropped by less talented riders'. Such rationalisations have often been delivered along with explanations of complete physical and mental depletion. In his autobiography *The Secret Race* American Tyler Hamilton, has an illuminating description of his first three years as a professional rider.

> Here's an interesting number: one thousand days. It's roughly the number of days between the day I became professional and the day I doped for the first time [...] First year, neo-pro, excited to be there, young pup, hopeful. Second year, realization. Third year, clarity – the fork in the road. Yes or no. In or out. Everybody has their thousand days [...] One thousand mornings of waking up with hope; a thousand afternoons of being crushed. [...] Willpower might be strong, but it's not infinite.
>
> (Hamilton & Coyle, 2012: 46)

Ariely's studies confirm how depletion affects decisions:

> As it turned out, the more taxing and depleting the task, the more participants cheated [...] if you wear down your willpower, you will have considerably more trouble regulating your desires, and that difficulty can wear down your honesty as well.
>
> (Ariely, 2012: 106)

Moreover, a number of riders have spoken about experiences of a natural hierarchy they felt was being distorted. Hamilton thus describes how the change in his friend Marty Jemison's performance in 1997 was a driver for his decision to use erythropoietin (EPO):

> The main thing I knew about Marty, though, is that I could usually beat him. [...] The gap between our abilities was as stable and reliable as our height. But in the spring of 1997, the pattern reversed. [...] Marty started doing better than me, and it made me nervous. Was he doing something? Did I need to do something too? [...] Marty used to be a few groups behind me; now he was a few groups ahead. [...] This was bullshit. This was not fair. In that moment, the future became clear. Unless something changed, I was done.
>
> (Hamilton & Coyle, 2012: 54–55)

The Danish professional cyclist Michael Rasmussen tells a comparable story in his autobiography, *Yellow Fever*. After having dominated the mountain bike sport the year before, he had a lousy 1998 season. With his almost obsessed dedication, persistent ambition and self-image as one of the sport's most talented riders he could not accept that he now could not follow riders he used to crush. If that meant he had to take EPO to regain his position, then that was what he would do:

> At the time, I had no well-developed feeling that I was doing something banned. The only thing on my mind was how miserable a season I had had. I was 24 years old and I came from being one of the world's best to now fooling around with the chubby girls in class. I had to get back to my level. At all costs. This was the way out.
>
> (Rasmussen & Wivel, 2013: 55)[3]

Maybe Rasmussen did not have a clear concept of what was banned, but when he contemplates over the ease by which his Italian teammates used drugs it is clear that he knew doping was immoral: 'I was stunned at how good they felt doing what they did. For them, it was as natural as shaving in the morning' (Rasmussen & Wivel, 2013: 52). In line with this, Ariely also found that witnessing others' dishonest acts increases dishonesty. Thus, riders adopt to the surrounding culture, hence doping can become a normal and necessary part of the trade. This was highlighted in Lance Armstrong's famous interview with Oprah Winfrey in 2013. Winfrey asked him if it was correct that to win and keep winning, he had to use banned substances:

> Yes, but – and I'm not sure that this is an acceptable answer – but that's like saying we have to have air in our tyres or we have to have water in our bottles. That was, in my view, part of the job.
>
> (Mahon, 2013)

Such stories on how the initial resistance was suppressed and doping became normalised, likely express an experience common to riders of Armstrong's generation. In line with this, Ariely's group also found that a little bit of cheating became a substantial amount of cheating as the experiment went on and participants got used to the situation or, as noted above, when participants were physically and mentally depleted before the test. After a while participants reach their 'honesty threshold', as it seems: 'for many people there was a very sharp transition where at some point in the experiment, they suddenly graduated from engaging in a little bit of cheating to cheating at every single opportunity they had' (Ariely, 2012: 130). Scottish rider David Millar puts it this way: 'I went from thinking one hundred percent that I would never dope to making a decision in ten minutes that I was going to do it' (Hamilton & Coyle, 2012: 40). For Rasmussen the real transgression was learning to take injections even if they at first only contained vitamins and iron. It was the penetration of the skin that was the moral barrier. As soon as he accepted and learned the practice any liquid could flow from the ampoule: 'vitamin C, EPO, diesel oil, anything basically. I had crossed to the other side' (Rasmussen & Wivel, 2013: 54).

Riders rationalise their behaviour by saying: 'everybody does it', 'there is a greater good to take care of', or 'others will benefit from what I am doing'. Over time, such rationalisations can push the initial moral barrier aside. Rather than pointing to a flaw in the individual rider's character, Hamilton's, Rasmussen's, and Armstrong's stories are expressions of an elite cycling culture that had developed an alternative norm. This element was perhaps disregarded by the group at the café in Mallorca. Nevertheless, with the then accepting attitude towards traditional pharmacological doping it is noteworthy how strong the world of cycling reacted against the use of so-called motor-doping that surfaced as a potential problem for the sport around 2010.

'They should suspend them for life'

Though rumoured for several previous years, 2017 saw the second and third case of verified motor-doping, or technical fraud as the Union Cycliste Internationale (UCI) has termed it. The topic began to attract public attention in 2010 when Swiss rider Fabian Cancellara came under suspicion after, with surprising strength, he rode away from his competitors in the spring classics Tour of Flanders and Paris-Roubaix (Bufalino, 2010). Some years later Canadian Ryder Hesjedal also came under scrutiny when after a crash in the Vuelta a España 2014 his back wheel kept spinning in what was considered a very suspicious manner (Squillari, 2014). However, it was a young woman, Femke Van den Driessche, who became the first competitive cyclist to be found using a motorised bike. The bike with the hidden motor was found in her pit at the junior world cyclocross championships, an offence that saw the Belgian national junior champion cop a six-year ban from the UCI (Cyclingnews, 2016). At the time of writing, she was still the only high-ranked racer to be caught since the two discovered cases of hidden motors in bikes in 2017 were both amateurs past their prime. In July, 53-year-old Italian Alessandro Andreoli was caught out in a race in Italy following a tip-off to organisers. In October of the same year, 43-year-old French amateur Cyril Fontayne was busted with a motorised bike after being deliberately targeted because of dramatic recent improvement in his results.

Looking at the reactions to these cases, one thing is immediately clear: they are not only strong and condemning, but also much stronger than we have seen with pharmacological doping. For instance, the *GCN Show* by Global Cycling Network, which has more than 1.2 million subscribers, opened their episode no. 238, after Andreoli was caught, in this way:

> This week we are pouring scorn on the second idiot to be caught using a hidden motor in a bike race [...]. We are going to start this week's show with some frustrating and frankly ridiculous news. The spectre of motorised doping has unfortunately reared its ugly head again for only the second time. But thankfully it has not come from within the pro-peloton. On this particular occasion, the alleged offender is a 53-year-old amateur cyclist who was participating in a race near Brescia in Italy. [...] It is absolutely ridiculous, though. I really did think that the Femke Van den Driessche-case would be the first and the last. I would personally think that he [Andreoli] should be banned for life.
>
> (Global Cycling Network, 2017)

The outrage extended beyond just the commentators. Winner of all three grand tours (Tour de France, Giro d'Italia, and Vuelta a España), Italian Vincenzo Nibali, joined the conversation: 'For me it is tantamount to stealing', he said, and added that he considered it worse than traditional doping:

> Stealing is always stealing. But the so-called technological doping I find more subtle. An athlete, even doped – and in the past there have been cases – can always have a bad day. It's different here. Push a button and go stronger, crush him again and go slowly. The rider has nothing to do with it anymore... unfortunately, as in other sports, I think there will always be someone who will try to circumvent the rules. Exemplary punishment is needed.
>
> (Stokes, 2016)

All-time cycling legendary, Eddy Merckx, also spoke freely about the matter:

> For me, they should suspend them for life. This is the worst that they can do, they should just race motorbikes then. For me, it's worse than doping. It gives you 50 watts more, or 100, it depends on the motor. It's no longer cycling at that point, it's motor racing.
>
> (Brown, 2016)

Interestingly, also some of the most stigmatised and demonised athletes of the sport came out to express their contempt. Riccardo Riccò, who in 2012 received a 12-year ban after his second doping offence, said he would rather see cyclists dope than use hidden motors in races: 'I prefer chemical doping to motors', he said. 'At least you have to have the courage to bet on yourself. With motors, it's another sport. I would never be able to use them. I'd feel like crap' (Brown, 2017). Finally, also Lance Armstrong expressed explicit disdain and indignation to even be asked the question, when Ger Gilroy of the Irish *Off the Ball* radio show wanted to hear whether he had been using a hidden motor in his bike during his professional career: 'Are you out of your mind? I know it's topical but are you crazy?' (Cyclingnews, 2017b). People like Riccò and Armstrong are very much aware that they have cheated, and being dishonest about what they have achieved in cycling. In addition, they both know that they did not only cheat a little but a lot. Still, they express a clear moral distinction between what they did and cheating with engines in bicycles. Let us explore why cheating in the category of Riccò and Armstrong, which most people consider unacceptable, is perhaps still easier to accept than cheating with engines.

Validity in sport

The more or less explicit assumption of the comments above is that motor doping turns cycling into a different sport. They are thus implicitly referring to limits of the sport that are transgressed with this particular type of enhancement. In other words, they address the question of validity, and thus suggest that some basic principles need to be upheld in order to talk about participating in a sport, not to mention winning it. In sport, the question of validity can be determined by the answer to both:

1 What is it we intend this competition to measure?
2 What does the competition actually measure?

Therefore, if we want to find out who can ride a bicycle the fastest, we need to set up a competition that can measure this. For (1) we have to establish the relevant terms and conditions for that measurement, i.e. the competition, and then for (2) find out whether the competition did in fact measure who was the fastest to ride a bicycle (Christiansen & Møller, 2016). (1) Is the business of rulemaking, (2) is overseeing that athletes play by the rules and evaluating the competition.

As the first necessary precondition in (1) we may stress that by the question 'who can ride a bicycle the fastest', we mean: which *human being* can ride a bicycle the fastest. (1) Thus contains two entities: human beings and bicycles. We therefore need to establish what can be accepted and not accepted as human beings and bicycles in order to make a proper assessment of the validity of the competition. However, for us to understand the riders' unambiguous judgement of technical fraud, we do not need to apply advanced knowledge on biomedicine or cognition to define the human being, or technical discussions and UCI regulations on frame geometry to define the bicycle. Instead, we can utilise a simple version of philosopher Edmund Husserl's eidetic variation. Eidetic variation is the imagining of variations in the properties of instances of a particular species or phenomenon in order to obtain knowledge of its essence (Smith & Smith, 1995: 331–332). If we apply this to the riders' different assessment of enhancement from motors and drugs, we can reach a probable understanding of their judgement. It thus seems to be a sensible preposition to claim that a human being that takes EPO is still a human being, even if he or she violates the rules of the sport. On the other hand, a bicycle to which we add an engine is no longer a bicycle, but more like a scooter or, as Merckx put it, indeed a motor bike. Consequently, using EPO does not violate the first necessary precondition for the sport competition to be valid, since a human being using EPO is still a human being, whereas using an engine on your bike does violate the first necessary precondition for the sport, since a bicycle with an engine is no longer a bicycle.

In light of this, the riders' much stronger reactions against technical fraud, compared to traditional doping are understandable. The question is whether their position is tenable.

Cheating in cycling – revisited

The above analysis suggests that it is not just because of arbitrary cultural perceptions, that Riccò would 'feel like crap' to use an engine, and that Armstrong considered the interviewer to be 'crazy' to even think of posing the question, but that there is a fundamental cause to it. A qualitative difference between that and other kinds of cheating, which makes the suggested lifetime bans reasonable.

However, seeing the competition from a bird's eye view, it is not self-evident that a 'rigged bike' invalidates the competition more than a 'rigged body'. In this regard, there is an element of sophism in the above argument. To quantify exactly how much of an advantage say EPO vs. a 50- or 100-watt engine gives and under what race circumstances is beyond the scope of this article. However, it is evidently easier to test bikes for motors than humans for drugs, and if a motor is found in a bike, it is much easier to prove intent than if a drug is found in a person's urine. In that sense, adding a motor to a bike is a less subtle way of cheating. But it is not evident that we should get more upset over cheating that lacks subtlety than cheating that exploits it.

Further, in terms of what it does to the validity of the competition, cheating with a motor is perhaps not that different from the infamous 'sticky bottle' or 'magic spanner'. It is not a difference of kind but of degree. It is true that the 'bottles' and 'spanners' are usually utilised behind the pack or breakaway, but both those and the motor assists the rider by producing extra watts for a short period, thus allowing him to move more quickly up the road. A thought experiment may illustrate how similar the two can be. Think of a sprinter in a stage race that hides a motor in his bike. He only uses the motor to get over the climbs so he can make the time cut. Compare this to a sprinter that grabs the sticky bottle up half of Alpe d'Huez to make the same time cut. The reaction to the former would be as fierce as we have seen above, while the latter would go ignored.

However, riders do not see it this way. Vincenzo Nibali, for instance, who views the use of motor assistance to be 'tantamount to stealing', was the protagonist of an episode in the Vuelta a España 2015, where, after a crash, he held on to his team car and was pulled up the road with speeds so high, that the group he left appeared to stand still (Elite Physiques, 2015). Nibali was disqualified from the race, but although the pull was significant enough to bring him back into contention had he not been found out and disqualified, he thought the reactions against his behaviour were too unforgiving. On Facebook, he said:

> It does not mean that it is not wrong, and I should not go unpunished. Just that the punishment is too severe. I thought I would get a hefty fine and kicked down in the classification. I would have accepted a penalty of ten minutes. After all; I am not the first or the last in this type of story.
>
> (Global Cycling Network, 2015)

He clearly knew it was wrong and was willing to risk the penalty, but just kept his fingers crossed. A similar incident with a rider that moved up the road assisted by an engine in a car took place at Paris-Nice in 2017. This time it was Frenchman Romain Bardet who, after a crash, several times had his bike serviced from the car with a 'magic spanner' allowing him to get back up with the chasing group, so he could still play a role in the race. However, Bardet too was disqualified and fined 200 Swiss Francs (Cyclingnews, 2017a).

Neither Nibali nor Bardet expressed content over their punishment although the sanctions were much more lenient than what they and their colleagues have proposed for riders who are assisted by engines located not in cars but in bikes. Such perceptions resonate with the findings from Ariely's research: cheating that can be rationalised within the groups' cultural confinement is somewhat accepted, cheating that cannot is frowned upon. Thus, while utilising the performance benefits of 'sticky bottles' and drugs has a long history in the sport, which has allowed them to be accepted to a certain degree, cheating with motors is new and perceived as extremely provocative.

With traditional doping and 'sticky bottles', it is thus still possible for the riders to see themselves as participating in the same sport as everyone else, and by that benefit from the performance-enhancing effects while still being able to look in the mirror and feel good. Cheating can be rationalised and a potential victory is still viewed as representative. For riders cheating with motors, the cycling community regard the rider to no longer be participating in the same sport and their potential victories are thus not seen as representative. The point is not whether this is logically correct reasoning, but that the riders accept it as such.

Conclusion

Doping has a long history in cycling. However, as we have seen, patterns of cheating among professional cyclists are similar to that of people in general, which suggests that they are no more morally corrupt than others are. Moreover, riders' reactions against technological fraud illustrate that there is a strong moral fibre in cycling that people disregard when they assert that immorality is ingrained in professional cycling. On the other hand, the riders' reactions also demonstrate how a specific culture, based on socio-cultural rationalisations rather than logical analysis of the phenomena in question, legitimises certain kinds of dishonest behaviours while rejecting others. To navigate such a culture, one must understand what – to use an oxymoron – constitutes legitimate rule-breaking, and thus know the necessary cultural conditions for a sporting performance to be perceived as valid.

Notes

1 This section draws on Ariely (2008, 2012).
2 A rider approaches his team's car to receive a bottle from the director. When the rider grabs the bottle, he holds his grip for a short while – the bottle 'sticks' to the rider's hand – and thus receives a quick boost of speed. As well as the sticky bottle, cycling also occasionally makes use of the 'magic spanner', which involves the mechanic in a team car 'making repairs' to a rider's bike while he holds on, in effect pulling him along with the vehicle.
3 AVC translated all quotes from Rasmussen's book.

References

Ariely, D. (2008). *Predictably Irrational: The Hidden Forces that Shape our Decisions* (1st ed.). New York: Harper.

Ariely, D. (2012). *The (Honest) Truth about Dishonesty. How we Lie to Everyone – Especially Ourselves*. New York: Harper Collins Publishers.

Brown, G. (2016). Merckx calls for lifetime ban on motorized doping. *Velonews*. Retrieved from www.velonews.com/2016/02/news/merckx-calls-for-lifetime-ban-on-motorized-doping_394367

Brown, G. (2017). Riccardo Riccò: Better to have doping than motors in cycling. *Velonews*. Retrieved from www.velonews.com/2017/12/news/riccardo-ricco-better-doping-motors-cycling_453986

Bufalino, M. (2010, 29 May). Bike with engine (doped bike) and Cancellara (Roubaix – Vlaanderen). Retrieved from www.youtube.com/watch?v=8Nd13ARuvVE

Christiansen, A.V., & Møller, R.B. (2016). Who is more skilful? Doping and its implication on the validity, morality and significance of the sporting test. *Performance Enhancement & Health*, 4(3–4), 123–129. doi:10.1016/j.peh.2016.04.002

Cyclingnews. (2016). Van den Driessche handed six-year ban for mechanical doping. *CyclingNews*. Retrieved from www.cyclingnews.com/news/van-den-driessche-handed-six-year-ban-for-mechanical-doping/

Cyclingnews. (2017a). Bardet disqualified from Paris-Nice. *CyclingNews*. Retrieved from www.cyclingnews.com/news/bardet-disqualified-from-paris-nice/

Cyclingnews. (2017b). Mechanical doping: A brief history. *CyclingNews*. Retrieved from www.cyclingnews.com/features/mechanical-doping-a-brief-history/

Elite Physiques. (2015, 24 August). Vincenzo Nibali Caught Cheating in Vuelta a Espana – Gets DQ'd. Retrieved from www.youtube.com/watch?v=7E4vRtC7IcY

Global Cycling Network. (2015, 25 August). Is This Really Cheating?! + The War On The Roads Continues | The GCN Show Ep. 137. *GCN Show*. 137. Retrieved from cwww.youtube.com/watch?v=KOhNu04aybY

Global Cycling Network. (2017, 01 August). Hidden Motors: Who's Mechanical Doping Now? | The GCN Show Ep. 238. *GCN Show*. 238. Retrieved from www.youtube.com/watch?v=5RsFWlvJjOg&list=PLUdAMlZtaV11hWi7uwv3oJzpBNUZitfMi&index=24

Hamilton, T. & Coyle, D. (2012). *The Secret Race: Inside the Hidden World of the Tour de France: Doping, Cover-ups, and Winning at all Costs*. London: Bantam.

Justitsministeriets Forskningskontor. (2014). *Drab i Danmark 2008–2011 (Research Unit of the Department of Justice – Homicide in Denmark)*. Retrieved from København: www.justitsministeriet.dk/sites/default/files/media/Arbejdsomraader/Forskning/Forskningsrapporter/2014/Drab%20i%20Danmark%202008-2011.pdf

Mahon, D. (2013). Full Transcript: Lance Armstrong on Oprah. Retrieved from https://armchairspectator.wordpress.com/2013/01/23/full-transcript-lance-armstrong-on-oprah/

Rasmussen, M., & Wivel, K. (2013). *Gul feber (Yellow Fever)*. København: People's Press.

Smith, B. & Smith, D.W. (1995). *The Cambridge Companion to Husserl* (Reprint. ed.). Cambridge: Cambridge University Press.

Squillari, N. (2014). Ryder Hesjedal's motor in bike? Stage 7 Vuelta a Espana 2014. Retrieved from www.youtube.com/watch?v=ynLMfzLTc8M

Stokes, S. (2016). Hidden motors: Nibali, Bugno call for draconian bans, CPA threatens legal action against those caught. *Cycling Tips*. Retrieved from https://cyclingtips.com/2016/04/hidden-motors-nibali-bugno-call-for-draconian-bans-cpa-threatens-legal-action-against-those-caught/

Wikipedia. (2018). Murder in the United States by state. In N/A (Ed.), *Wikipedia*.

Chapter 8

Everyone was doing it

Applying lessons from cycling's EPO era

John Gleaves

Professional cycling's 1994 Flèche Wallonne has come to mark the sport's entry into the full-blown EPO era. The Gewiss-Ballan professional cycling team had already dominated that season's spring classics, but at Flèche Wallonne, the team performed the impossible. With 72 kilometres left to race, the peloton approached their second ascent of the famous Mur de Huy, a steep climb averaging 9.3% for over one kilometre. At the base of the climb, three Gewiss-Ballan riders – Moreno Argentin, Evgeni Berzin, and Giorgio Furlan – assumed control of the peloton. The trio, using no violent acceleration, simply rode away from the rest of the field. For the next 70 kilometres, the three teammates held off the chasing peloton to sweep the podium.

In professional cycling, rarely does one team place two riders on a podium. Even rarer to place three. But to have three riders from the same team win in a breakaway? It was simply unprecedented. Afterwards, some riders lamented a tactical miscalculation that permitted the Gewiss-Ballan riders to go clear. Indeed, no one thought three riders could hold off the rest of the field working together for such a distance. Yet the tactical post-mortem masked what everyone else in professional cycling had come to realise – these were different times. Rumours of certain cyclists experimenting with the prohibited pharmaceutical drug Epogen, a synthetic form of erythropoietin (EPO) that boosts red blood cells, had been circling in the media since the drug's approval in 1989. Miraculous improvements by individual riders fuelled speculation that EPO use existed to some degree. Now people wondered if the Gewiss-Ballan team had managed to systematically employ EPO for their entire stable of riders.

Two days later, the world received a hint. On 22 April 1994, *L'Equipe* journalist Jean-Michel Rouet provided the curious peloton their answer. In an interview with the Gewiss-Ballan team doctor, Michele Ferrari, Rouet inquired about the magical performances emerging from the Italian team. Sensing the trap, Ferrari responded that 'the recipe is not pharmacological', though he added, 'But if I was a rider and knew that there was a non-detectable product capable of increasing performance, I would use it' (Rouet, 1994). Ferrari concluded with the now-infamous comment that, 'EPO is not dangerous, it is its abuse that is. It is also dangerous to drink ten litres of orange juice' (Rouet,

1994). After reading these comments, few in the professional peloton doubted the source of Gewiss-Ballan's dominance.

Ferrari's comments also pointed to the increasing realisation among professional cyclists. Without a means to test for EPO, which would not be employed until the 2000 Sydney Olympics, cyclists could use the drug intended to treat anemia with little risk of punishment despite its formal prohibition under cycling's anti-doping rules. Eventually, EPO use spread throughout professional cycling to become nearly universal. Jonathan Vaughters, a professional cyclist who raced from 1994–2003, noted that, 'By 1996, in big races like the Tour de France, I think doping was very close to 100 percent prevalent' (Lindsey, 2012).

Today, as cycling still deals with the effects of the EPO era, the misuse of therapeutic use exemptions (TUEs) threatens to draw not just cycling but many elite sports into new anti-doping controversies. Evidence of TUE misuse has emerged from professional riders and with leaked documents from the World Anti-Doping Agency's TUE application programme. These documents entangled British Tour de France winner Bradley Wiggins in a controversy around abusing the TUE system (House of Commons & Digital, 2018). Yet Renee Anne Shirley, a former head of the Jamaican Anti-Doping Commission who became a whistleblower, believes, 'The TUE situation with Wiggins is just the tip of the iceberg'. Indeed, Shirley claims that as of 2017, 'The TUE system is one of the main areas of abuse right now' (Benson, 2017). Whether Shirley's speculation is indeed correct, the lessons from cycling's admittedly uncomfortable EPO era coupled with the ethical justification for continuing the TUE programme can provide useful insights into potential administrative responses and reforms.

The right ingredients

Any formal dates marking cycling's 'EPO era' will be subject to interpretation and challenges. However, some turning points can provide a useful guide. The 1994 season and the reactions following the Flèche Wallonne race described above provide a good starting point where many riders indicated EPO went from experimental to standard for top-tier professional cyclists. When it ends is less clear. From 1994 to the 2001 season, professional cycling had no EPO test. The EPO test did not appear to dramatically reduce EPO use, though some riders began opting for blood transfusions during stage races. A more significant reduction appears to correspond with the introduction of the Athletes' Biological Passport introduced in 2008, but anti-doping punishments for including Floyd Landis in 2006 and investigations such as Operacion Puerto in 2006 and the Freiburg Investigation in 2007 had put cycling on edge (CIRC, Marty, Nicholson, & Haas, 2015). For this reason, 2005 appears to mark the end point for widespread and unchecked EPO use in professional cycling.

Cycling is not the only sport where athletes doped. Nor is cycling the only sport with doping scandals. History offers plenty of examples from, Major

League Baseball and BALCO to state-sponsored doping programmes in East Germany and Russia. What makes cycling's EPO era unique, however, is the degree to which nearly every athlete from nearly every professional team used the same banned drug, EPO, at some point in their career. Its use was so normal that cyclists on opposing teams would share their supply of EPO with each other. Teams would not only expect the riders to use EPO but many would purchase and supply their riders with the product. Riders have estimated that at major races like the Tour de France, every single rider boosted their haematocrit. What let cycling get to this point?

Historical analysis of rider interviews, court documents, and public comments reveal five key ingredients for professional cycling's EPO era.[1] Without any one of these, EPO use would not have become ubiquitous in professional cycling.

Professional cyclists:

1 Perceived little risk of punishment or health for the behaviour;
2 Received support from licenced medical professionals to engage in the behaviour;
3 Believed refraining from the behaviour would not stop others from doing it;
4 Believed refraining from the behaviour placed one at a disadvantage;
5 Did not believe engaging in the behaviour cheated others.

Perceived little risk of punishment or health for the behaviour

As the quote from Dr. Ferrari hinted above, those involved in professional cycling – including the team management and team physicians along with the cyclists – understood that no effective test existed for EPO use despite the drug's place on cycling's Prohibited List. The decision to ban EPO without a sufficient test followed from lessons learned after the use of blood transfusions at the 1984 Olympic Games (Gleaves, 2015). Prior to the 1984 Olympic Games, the International Olympic Committee (IOC) knew about the potential use of blood transfusions but concluded that without a test it could not credibly ban the procedure. This led some athletes to view blood transfusions as a permitted means to enhance performance. In response, the IOC and many international federations including the *Union Cycliste Internationale* (UCI) adopted the strategy to ban potential performance-enhancing substances even if no test existed.

Cyclists' perception of relative immunity persisted even after the UCI introduced efforts to detect EPO use. Still without a test, in 1997 the UCI introduced a 50% haematocrit rule as a limited step to enforce the ban on EPO (Waddington & Smith, 2009: 227). The haematocrit test left the door open for riders to boost their haematocrit up to 50% without serious risk of detection and then only punished a rider exceeding the limit with a two-week 'health suspension' if their blood values exceeded the 50% limit. Hence, cyclists continued to perceive relative immunity from detection of EPO use assuming their haematocrit levels remained under the threshold. After the first test for EPO appeared at the 2000 Olympic Games, cyclists further refined their EPO use by combining it with blood transfusions, micro-dosing, and avoidance of out-of-competition testing (CIRC et al., 2015: 32). Indeed, until the UCI introduced the Athletes' Biological Passport in 2008, careful athletes continued using EPO minimal risk of detection (USADA, 2012).

Even if the cyclists believed their risk of punishment was low, their belief that EPO presented little risk to their health contributed to the drug's widespread embrace. Riders dismissed press accounts of cyclists dying as a result of EPO – rumours that later remain unproven (López, 2011) – since most knew many riders using EPO but could point to few cyclists who had died or suffered harmful side-effects. Some cyclists of the EPO era, such as George Hincapie, recalled Ferrari's comments equivocating the health effects of EPO to orange juice (Hincapie, 2012: 4). Others saw it as a safer alternative to risker practices or substances. For example, Michael Barry, who admitted using EPO, explained, 'I had always deliberately avoided hGH because I thought it posed more health risks than EPO and testosterone' (Barry, 2012: 10). Peter Janssen, a team doctor for professional cycling teams from 1988–1992 explained later that he not only considered EPO harmless but that he would give the blood booster to his own son if his son was racing the Tour de France or the Giro d'Italia (Andrews, 2010). The perceptions of low, or at least lower health risks, made the choice to use EPO easier for professional cyclists, which, in turn, increased the number that eventually used the banned substance.

Received support from licenced medical professionals to engage in the behaviour

A second ingredient in the EPO era came the licenced medical professionals who facilitated the professional cyclists' EPO use. Not only did teams such as Gewiss-Ballan employ doctors like Michele Ferrari but riders also had access to an emerging cottage industry of medical doctors who specialised in helping elite athletes. These doctors existed on a spectrum with some providing ordinary treatments for illnesses and tests to support nutrition and training load. In the middle were doctors who evaluated physiological capacity such as VO2 capacity, body composition, and other biometric indicators of performance. And finally, there were the medical doctors using their legal power to prescribe controlled pharmaceutical substance to enhance athletes' capacities. Such prescriptions included anabolic steroids, cortisone, amphetamines, and eventually EPO (Brissonneau, 2015). Swiss professional cyclist Rolf Järmann explained that he got his EPO by asking doctors, who 'knew exactly what I wanted it for but they were happy to help' (Cyclingnews, 2000).

The success of Gewiss-Ballan's partnership with Michele Ferrari initiated a trend among top professional cycling teams to seek physicians willing to take a more proactive role enhancing performance. Now the job was not just to manage illnesses and injuries, but also procure and administer banned pharmaceutical substances. For example, begging in 1993 the German professional cycling team Telekom used Dr. Andreas Schmid and later Dr. Lothar Heinrich to procure EPO and determine dosages for riders (Schafer, Schanzer, & Schwabe, 2009). Numerous team doctors, including Eric Rijckaert, Eufemiano Fuentes, Luigi Cecchini, Pedro Celaya, and Luis Garcia del Moral, have admitted or been investigated for facilitating doping at their teams. Christian Vande Velde, who raced for US Postal Service and Liberty Seguros, claimed that both teams had organised doping programmes in which, 'team doctors were very involved in providing performance enhancing drugs' (Vande Velde, 2012: 20). When team doctors refused to support doping practices, such as Prentice Steffen at the US Postal Service team, team management brought in new staff (Hamilton & Coyle, 2012: 41).

Not only did doctors administer EPO to riders, but their status as medical doctors allowed them to convince riders to use despite their reluctance. For example, when cyclist Michael Barry asked the team doctor about injections, he reported the doctor 'would act offended and ask, "Don't you trust me?"' (Barry, 2012: 8). This provided the EPO use at least a veil of legal authority, since the doctors each had licences to acquire the substance and the technical knowledge to safely administer the injection. It also provided the practice with a degree of social capital since the riders were more likely to go along with a person who held the position of a medical doctor.

Believed refraining from the behaviour would not stop others from doing it

Even though many professional cyclists viewed EPO as low risk, they report feeling reluctant about doping. Their internal moral qualms about doping faded as they increasingly believed not only that many other cyclists used EPO but also that their individual abstinence made no difference. For example, British cyclist David Millar conceded that he did not think his commitment not to use EPO was going to change the sport. Before he started doping, Millar ultimately concluded that his decision not to dope had no effect on cycling's entrenched doping culture. Millar reported that such thinking influenced his eventual decision to use EPO (Millar, 2012).

Other professional cyclists of the EPO era echo the same thought process. Laurent Roux, a professional cyclist from 1994 to 2002 explained that, 'At the start, with the Castorama team, I didn't use drugs. But I was sidelined, so then I did what everybody did' (Abt, 1998). Frenchman Nicolas Aubier, who raced five seasons as a professional starting in 1992, explained in 1997 that 'The use of doping products has become so general that anybody not taking anything is regarded as abnormal' (Cyclingnews, 1997).

Logically, there was a period where EPO had not fully saturated professional cycling. However, even in the nascent days of EPO, riders faced the growing reality that their own choice to not use EPO made no difference to the riders around them. They could each see the changes in performance for some riders or some teams; they knew the risk was relatively low. Perhaps if they believed their decision would make a difference, more would have resisted and EPO would not have flourished.

Believed refraining from the behaviour placed one at a disadvantage

Faced with the growing feeling of powerlessness, riders also increasingly believed that refraining from EPO placed them at a disadvantage. EPO improves performance in cycling and the evidence was clear to riders. Many could see EPO boosting their teammates or opponents. Those who used EPO also noticed its benefit on their own performance. In fact, Tyler Hamilton points out that professional cycling developed a term for racing without EPO – one was racing *pan y agua*; on bread and water – to describe the disadvantage a rider faced (Hamilton & Coyle, 2012: 45). By 1997, Nicolas Aubier explained, 'Frankly, I can't imagine a rider belonging to the top 100 and not taking EPO, growth hormones or another product' (Cyclingnews, 1997).

As much as cyclists may have disliked doping, many found competing at a disadvantage even worse. Professional cyclist Jonathan Vaughters explained the exact dilemma riders faced, 'If you just said no when the anti-doping regulations weren't enforced, then you were deciding to end your dream, because you could not be competitive' (Vaughters, 2012: 9). Another professional cyclist from the EPO era, Michael Barry, explained that by the time he finally used EPO, 'I had already resigned myself to the fact that I would need to start doping in order to be competitive' (Barry, 2012: 10).

Professional cyclist Jörg Jaksche explained that the perception of disadvantage creates an inertia that drives behaviour: because everyone dopes, everyone has to dope. For Jaksche, 'The logic is you adjust your performance level to the rest, because everyone is doing it' (Woodland, 2007). Floyd Landis put it bluntly, 'There was no good scenario. It was either cheat or get cheated. And I'd rather not be the guy getting cheated' (Cyclingnews, 2011). Such assessments show cyclists believed not using EPO placed them at a competitive disadvantage in a profession where results were the ultimate measurement of success.

Did not believe engaging in the behaviour cheated others

While riders believed they would be at a disadvantage if they did not use EPO, they also reasoned that using EPO did not really cheat the riders they raced against because they considered most of the other riders also used EPO. In the rare case of a rider not using EPO, the cyclists believed that this constituted a personal choice for the rider who certainly had access to EPO, knew others were using EPO, and still decided not to use EPO. In either case, they did not see their decision as cheating other riders. It was not their fault EPO was widespread and if they used, it only leveled the playing field. For example, Richard Virenque explained in his confession, 'I live in a world where the rules are set up a long time in advance. I didn't cheat other riders' (BBC, 2000).

Had riders believed their actions placed others at a disadvantage, perhaps using EPO would have been harder to justify. For instance, Lance Armstrong confessed to Oprah Winfrey that, 'I kept hearing I'm a drug cheat… I went in and just looked up the definition of cheat and the definition of cheat is to gain an advantage on a rival or foe that they don't have. I didn't view it that way. I viewed it as a level playing field' (BBC, 2013). A teammate of Armstrong, Tyler Hamilton wrote in his book that, 'I've always said you could have hooked us up to the best lie detectors on the planet and asked us if we were cheating, and we'd have passed. Not because we were delusional – we knew we were breaking the rules – but because we didn't think of it as cheating. It felt fair to break the rules, because we knew others were too' (Hamilton & Coyle, 2012: 95).

What is obviously true is that each individual rider could not know with certainty that every single other rider really used EPO. In fact, previous quotes point out that many cyclists tried to race without EPO and knew other riders trying to do the same. It is also reasonable to assume many riders using EPO wished to drown out the voices of those who resisted the practice. Compounded with what riders saw and heard, many may have felt that *nearly* everyone was using EPO. Moreover, convincing themselves and their peers that *everyone* was doping meant that riders could still imagine themselves as ethical people and deserving of their success (see the chapter by Christiansen). So obviously some riders who followed the rules did not earn the results they deserved. But for the vast majority of those racing during the EPO era, they either did not or chose not to believe that they were depriving someone else of something. As it stood, riders often believed their own decision to use EPO did not cheat the people they were racing against, but they would themselves be disadvantaged if they did not.

Therapeutic use exemptions

Despite EPO use by some riders, including micro-doses, the era of widespread and unchecked EPO use in professional cycling appears to be in the past. More robust testing, less hypocrisy, and pressure from sponsors wanting to avoid tainting their brand eroded the team-supported doping programmes. However, a new issue seems to be looming on the horizon – the misuse of therapeutic use exemptions (TUE). Unlike the cyclists using prohibited EPO, therapeutic use exemptions (TUE) permit athletes to take medications that exist on the prohibited substance list for legitimate medical treatment. According to WADA's TUE Expert Group, the TUE 'enables athletes with genuine ill-health to compete in fair, equitable competition' (Gerrard, 2017: 370).

The risk, however, is that some athletes without legitimate medical needs might employ TUEs to use otherwise prohibited substances to boost their performance. Historically, cyclists employed false TUE's for cortisone. In fact, many of the above quoted cyclists who used EPO, including Lance Armstrong, Jörg Jaksche, Christian Vande Velde, and David Millar – all reported the TUE provided a large loophole for glucocorticoids that would easily register in drug tests.

These cases, however, occurred during the EPO era, but the misuse of TUEs appears to have continued. In fact, the Athletes' Biological Passport and increased testing for EPO and anabolic-androgenic steroids implemented in the 2000s may have unintentionally increased TUE misuse. Closing the door to these drugs made less powerful but medically plausible banned substances such as glucocorticoids more appealing. The UCI's Cycling Independent Reform Commission (CIRC) stated in 2015 that riders and team doctors 'reported that TUEs are systematically exploited by some teams and even used as part of performance enhancement programmes' (CIRC, 2015: 60). The CIRC also found reforms to the TUE policy before 2016 may have actually made TUE misuse easier since 'riders and team personnel find the current system for TUE application much easier to abuse than during the period when only a so-called "Declaration of Use" had been required' (CIRC et al., 2015: 61).

Reforms, including those suggested by the CIRC and to WADA's International Standard for Therapeutic Use Exemptions, (2016), do not appear to have solved these issues. Following a hack of WADA's TUE applications in 2016, which suggested that 2012 Tour de France winner Bradley Wiggins may have misused TUEs, Richard McLaren, a Canadian lawyer appointed by WADA to investigate Russian doping, acknowledged that in the current system, 'TUEs are open to abuse' (BBC, 2016). In an open letter to WADA, the *Mouvement Pour un Cyclisme Crédible* (MPCC) criticised WADA for failing to address glucocorticoids and tramadol, an opioid pain reliever (MPCC, 2017). A report by a committee in the United Kingdom's House of Commons concluded that Wiggins and his team, Team Sky, engaged in unconventional use of the asthma treatment triamcinolone, and concluded that the TUE system is 'open to abuse'. The report further stated that, 'drugs were being used by Team Sky, within the WADA rules, to enhance the performance of riders, and not just to treat medical need' (House of Commons & Digital, 2018: 32). British cyclist Chris Froome, multiple time winner of the Tour de France, drew further scrutiny following an adverse analytical finding for an asthma medication in September 2017 (Dreier, 2018).

Statically, evidence indicates cycling may have more athletes permissibly using banned substances than other sports. According to the WADA's *Anti-Doping Rule Violations Report* for 2013–2015, cycling has a higher percentage of its 'Adverse Analytical Findings' classified as permissible because of TUEs or authorised route of administration than the average for all other sports. Such statistics may point to cycling possibly having higher rates of misuse for certain substances. At the same time, other plausible explanations exist such as more

Table 8.1 Summary of WADA Anti-Doping Rule Violation Reports 2013–2015

		AAFs	*Medical reason*	*No case to answer for*	*Percentage dismissed (%)*
2015	All other sports	2278	254	157	18
	Cycling	244	46	21	27
2014	All other sports	2066	205	273	23
	Cycling	221	20	44	29
2013	All other sports	2262	196	295	22
	Cycling	278	27	52	28

testing of the same athletes or more athletes with sport-related conditions such as exercise-induced asthma. However, statistics about TUEs and the use of prescribed medications regulated in-competition or through route of administration for cycling are not publicly available so it is impossible to identify problematic trends.

Others seem to be simply exploring substances that do not require a TUE. One example involves thyroid medication. Rumours indicate cyclists, as well as runners, have used levothyroxine, medication intended for thyroid disorders, to help athletes lose weight and thus boost performance. In a 'Secret Pro' column, an anonymous professional cyclist described 'lots of chatter' about the misuse of thyroid medication to help cyclists misusing thyroid medication to help with weight loss and indicated in his opinion its 'prevalence among us elite athletes seems awfully high' (Secret Pro, 2017). Other prescription substances rumoured to be misused to boost performance include telmisartan (for hypertension) and tramadol (a pain reliever) (Hamilton, 2016). Since WADA has not included these substances in the banned substance list, no regulations govern their use in sport. This means that riders do not require a TUE (or even must report their use of the prescription) because it falls outside of WADA's regulations.

With the rumours and evidence of possible TUE misuse, parallels between the early days of EPO in cycling and TUEs do appear. But does it have the necessary ingredients listed above that fuelled the EPO era?

First, riders with TUEs face low risk for punishment (ingredient 1). In fact, their risk of punishment is even lower. When anti-doping tests could not detect EPO misuse, riders still had to avoid being caught using EPO. With a TUE, riders essentially have a 'free pass' should they run into any problems. Whether riders fear health risks also remains unclear. David Millar, who reported using cortisone with a TUE, called it a 'once-a-year drug' because of its negative side-effects (Millar, 2016). Yet most of the TUEs still fall within some standard for accepted medical practices so they do not appear to be present health risks more significant than EPO, which cyclists tolerated.

Second, support from licenced medical practitioners (ingredient 2) can make obtaining and employing a TUE for performance enhancement more feasible. The little bit known about TUE misuse suggests medical doctors may be finding ways around the TUE system through their diagnoses, reports, and coaching of symptoms. The British inquiry into Team Sky raised serious doubts about their team doctor, Dr. Richard Freeman's role in the TUEs and called for investigation by Britain's General Medical Council 'for [Dr. Freeman's] failings' (House of Commons & Digital, 2018: 31). This concern should be taken more seriously in light of the significant role doctors played in making EPO available to cyclists in the 1990s.

What remains to be seen is how cyclists will come to interpret the spate of stories about TUE misuse (ingredients 3, 4, and 5). The 1994 Flèche Wallonne convinced many that EPO was necessary if one was in professional cycling. Allegations linking Team Sky riders, their doctors, and TUEs mean five of the last six winners of the Tour de France raise some question whether a team has systematically exploited the TUE loophole. Team Sky's dominance might convince more cyclists that TUEs are necessary just as Gewiss-Ballan marked a turning point in attitudes about EPO. One thing the EPO era showed was that cyclists would not accept an unlevelled playing field. And if they do not see sporting officials enforcing the rules, they will begin trying to solve matters on their own. If the riders perceive that TUE misuse is widespread, the necessary ingredients that made possible the EPO era appear present in cycling to fuel a kind of grey-zone TUE era.

Potential reforms for a new era

On the other hand, cycling has the chance to employ lessons from its past to help better navigate the present. At the moment, publicly available evidence of TUE misuse in cycling does not show cycling has anything close to a 'TUE era'. While efforts to prevent TUE misuse are ongoing, a more worrying problem is the *perception* about TUEs in cycling. These perceptions can create their own inertia – as cyclists increasingly believe they need a TUE to be competitive, then more might look to exploit a loophole in the TUE system, which drives more cyclists to pursue TUEs because of their widespread use.

One reform should involve universal reporting and transparency regarding TUE information. As it stands now, athletes can apply for TUEs from their national anti-doping organisation (NADO) or their sports international federation. Since the UCI automatically recognises TUEs from certain NADOs, they may never know a rider has a TUE. According to Renee Anne Shirley, former head of the Jamaican Anti-Doping Commission, NADOs provide 'virtually no supervision'. Shirley also reports that David Howman claimed 'that around 50% of TUEs are not seen by WADA because they're not logged into their tracking system, ADAMS' (Benson, 2017). This appears to be the case with the UCI, as the organisation only reports to have granted a modest number of TUEs since 2010.

The number of TUEs granted by the UCI does not include all of the TUEs in cycling, however. The UCI offers 'Automatic Recognition' of TUE decisions

Table 8.2 Number of TUEs granted annually by the UCI

Year	*TUEs granted*
2009	239
2010	97
2011	55
2012	46
2013	31
2014	25
2015	13
2016	15
2017	20

Source: www.uci.ch/clean-sport/therapeutic-use-exemptions/.

made by 21 National Anti-Doping Organizations (NADO). According to the UCI, if a rider receives a TUE from one of these specified NADOs, which includes all of the major cycling countries, 'he/she does not need to apply to the UCI for recognition of that TUE', and that, 'The TUE is automatically recognised by the UCI, without further action required by the Rider' (UCI, 2018). So, the UCI might not ever know how many riders from France, Belgium, Italy, or Spain, for example, have TUEs since these are not reported to the UCI.

Compiling all of the TUEs, including the prescribing doctor's information, can help identify patterns of misuse. Publicly reporting certain anonymous TUE data, including the number of athletes using TUEs, the number denied, and the substances used, can alleviate concerns that riders have TUE misuse. Such information would combat perceptions that 'everyone is doing it'.

A second reform involves the medical doctors. Medical doctors played a significant role in the EPO era. It would be naïve to assume teams could not again conscript doctors to provide necessary diagnoses to support a TUE determination for an athlete. Since these doctors provide the documentation to the TUE Committees for their review, they can heavily shape diagnoses and reports to justify granting a TUE.

To the greatest extent possible, TUE should distance team physicians and personal doctors from the TUE process. Instead, the UCI should move towards more independent assessments, not just from the TUE Committee but also for the diagnosing and application. This would make applications for questionable maladies more difficult and reduce the number of athletes acquiring false TUEs. This presents certain challenges for some international federations, including logistics and costs, but perhaps not for cycling. Given professional cycling's stable pool of registered athletes, cycling could pursue such an approach, especially for TUE's for drugs more likely to be exploited.

The history of EPO's spread into cycling in the 1990s and cyclists' reactions showed how doping can become a nearly universal practice in a sport. In particular, five key ingredients permitted EPO to become nearly ubiquitous in the sport. However, these ingredients can and may be coalescing again to form a new TUE era. Drawing parallels from the lessons of cycling's EPO culture, the article concludes that these two TUE misuses have the potential to grow into a new 'TUE era', whereby TUE misuse undermines the credibility of sport through persistent rule violations and encourages unnecessary health risks. These two suggested reforms can help protect the intended purpose of TUE while preventing their widespread misuse. Without appropriate policy reforms to address TUE misuse, cycling may find itself in another era of moral equivocation where athletes justify violating the spirit, if not the letter, of anti-doping because they believe 'everyone is doing it'.

Note

1 Unless otherwise cited, evidence of these views draws upon and summarises views expressed in the many detailed interviews, biographies, and affidavits from individuals involved in doping during this era.

References

Abt, S. (1998, 11 October). CYCLING; Riders Are Still Critical of the French Police and Courts for Their Role in Drug Affair. *New York Times*.

Andrews, C. (2010, 10 May). Former Team Doctor Claims EPO is Not Harmful. *Velonation*. Retrieved from www.velonation.com/News/ID/4122/Former-team-doctor-claims-EPO-is-not-harmful.aspx

Barry, M. (2012). *Affidavit*. Retrieved from d3epuodzu3wuis.cloudfront.net/Barry%2c+Michael+Affidavit.pdf

BBC. (2000). Virenque Admits Taking Banned Drugs. *BBC Online*. Retrieved from http://news.bbc.co.uk/sport2/hi/other_sports/988095.stm

BBC. (2013, 18 January). Lance Armstrong & Oprah Winfrey: Interview Transcript. *BBC*. Retrieved from www.bbc.com/sport/cycling/21065539

BBC. (2016, 16 September). TUE System Can Be Abused by Athletes – Dr Richard McClaren. *BBC Sport*. Retrieved from www.bbc.com/sport/37382825

Benson, D. (2017, 21 November). Bradley Wiggins' TUE case highlights crisis facing anti-doping authorities. *Cyclingnews*. Retrieved from www.cyclingnews.com/features/bradley-wiggins-tue-case-highlights-crisis-facing-anti-doping-authorities/

Brissonneau, C. (2015). The 1998 Tour de France – Festina, from a scandal to an affair in cycling. In V. Møller, I. Waddington, & J. Hoberman (Eds), *Routledge Handbook of Drugs and Sport* (pp. 181–192). New York: Routledge.

CIRC, Marty, D., Nicholson, P., & Haas, U. (2015). *Report to the President of the Union Cycliste Interantionale*. Retrieved from www.uci.ch/mm/Document/News/CleanSport/16/87/99/CIRCReport2015_Neutral.pdf

Cyclingnews. (1997, 17 January). Doping widespread according to riders. *Cycling News*. Retrieved from http://autobus.cyclingnews.com/results/archives/jan97/doping.html

Cyclingnews. (2000, 8 September). Järmann admits EPO use *Cycling News*. Retrieved from http://autobus.cyclingnews.com/results/2000/sep00/sep8news.shtml

Cyclingnews. (2011, 31 January). Landis: It was either Cheat or get Cheated. *Cycling News*. Retrieved from www.cyclingnews.com/news/landis-it-was-either-cheat-or-get-cheated/

Dreier, F. (2018, 17 January). Commentary: The Simplest Explantion for Froome's Salbutamol Test. *Velonews*. Retrieved from www.velonews.com/2018/01/commentary/commentary-the-simplest-explanation-for-froomes-salbutamol-test_454985

Gerrard, D. (2017). The use and abuse of the therapeutic use exemptions process. *Current Sports Medicine Reports*, *16*(5), 370.

Gleaves, J. (2015). Manufactured dope: How the 1984 US Olympic Cycling Team rewrote the rules on drugs in sports. *International Journal for the History of Sport*. doi:10.1080/09523367.2014.958667

Hamilton, J. (2016, 10 August). Olympic Athletes Still Use Some RX drugs as a Path to 'Legal Doping'. *National Public Radio*. Retrieved from www.npr.org/sections/health-shots/2016/08/10/488862344/olympic-athletes-still-use-some-rx-drugs-as-a-path-to-legal-doping

Hamilton, T. & Coyle, D. (2012). *The Secret Race: Inside the Hidden World of the Tour de France: Doping, Cover-ups, and Winning at all Costs*. New York: Bantam Books.

Hincapie, G. (2012) Affidavit.

House of Commons, & Digital, C., Media, and Sport Committee. (2018). *Combatting Doping in Sport: Fourth Report of Series 2017–19*.

Lindsey, J. (2012, 5 December). From the Inside. *ESPN*. Retrieved from www.espn.com/espn/otl/story/_/id/8683670/jonathan-vaughters-lance-armstrong-ex-teammate-talks-doping-espn-magazine-interview-issue.

López, B. (2011). The invention of a 'drug of mass destruction': Deconstructing the EPO myth. *Sport in History*, *31*(1), 84–109.

Millar, D. (2012). *Racing Through the Dark: Crash. Burn. Coming Clean. Coming Back*. New York: Touchstone.

Millar, D. (2016, 14 October). How to Get Away with Doping. *New York Times*.

MPCC. (2017). Open Letter to Mr Olivier Niggli Director General World Anti-Doping Agency.

Rouet, J.-M. (1994, 22 April). Gewiss roule en Ferrari *L'Equipe*.

Schafer, H.J., Schanzer, W., & Schwabe, U. (2009). *Final Report of the Expert Commission Investigation of Doping Against Doctors in the Sports Medicine Department of the Freiburg Clinic*.

Secret Pro (2017, 9 November). Sketchy thyroids, confused commissaires, and more. *CyclingTips*. Retrieved from https://cyclingtips.com/2017/11/the-secret-pro-sketchy-thyroids-confused-commissaires-and-more/

UCI (2018). Theraputic Use Exemption. Retrieved from www.uci.ch/clean-sport/therapeutic-use-exemptions/

USADA (2012). *Reasoned Decision of the United States Anti-Doping Agency on Disqualification and Ineligibility* Retrieved from http://d3epuodzu3wuis.cloudfront.net/Reasoned-Decision.pdf

Vande Velde, C. (2012). Affidavit.

Vaughters, J. (2012, 11 August). How to Get Doping Out of Sports. *New York Times*.

Waddington, I. & Smith, A. (2009). *An Introduction to Drugs in Sport: Addicted to Winning?* New York: Routledge.

Woodland, L. (2007). Jakshe Admits Taking Banned Substances & Blood Doping. *Cycling News*.

World Anti-Doping Agency. (2016). ISTUE Therapeutic Use Exemption Guidelines.

Chapter 9

Cycling teams preventing doping

Can the fox guard the hen house?

Fabien Ohl

Doping is often perceived as part of cycling because cycling teams have been involved in doping for years. Moreover, for many people, there is no chance of teams ever preventing doping in cycling. Paraphrasing Travis Tygart, the head of the United States Anti-Doping Agency (USADA) describing the International Olympic Committee officials' role in anti-doping governance, requesting teams to prevent doping is akin to 'the fox guarding the hen house'.[1]

However, when Jean-Pierre Strebel, the UCI (*Union Cycliste Internationale*) general secretary, asked me in 2010 how I could help to improve anti-doping through prevention, my proposal was to better understand cycling culture and to change the culture of performance production, especially the organisation of cycling teams and their human resources. My first suggestion was to change the role of physicians, to exclude the staff previously sentenced for doping, to improve riders' follow-up and to analyse the precariousness of riders' careers. Most academics, critical journalists, anti-doping specialists, and even sports organisations' staff were doubtful in the face of such a preposterous proposal. Indeed, I was certainly slightly naïve and not totally aware of the difficulties. However, two main arguments motivated me to think that it is possible to rely on teams, at least some of them, to prevent doping.

The first argument is theoretical. How can academics analyse doping in cycling as a legacy of its cultural history and believe that it is impossible to change? Although culture may be reproduced, it may also evolve, especially in a changing environment. The second argument has to do with the concept of sociology. To me, sociology can be useful to feeding some of the social changes. Cycling is the sport that is mostly associated with doping (López, 2015), and it is stigmatised for cheating. Cycling is an easy target. It is certainly beneficial for other sports organisations, some journalists, and even some academics, to use cycling to denounce the misuse of the sport, its lack of ethics, etc. Although the role of an academic may not be the one of 'moral entrepreneur' (Becker, 1963) crusading to stop doping, because he views it as wrong, providing critical analysis that may be a resource to increase social actors' agency can be part of the job. There is no doubt that doping was a resource for some teams and riders to 'do their job'. However, in 2010, the doping legacy was already a burden for some of the riders, staff, the UCI, and organisers. Some of them already suffered from the negative image of cycling and from the stigmatisation of the riders. In addition, in my conception of sociology, I support the idea of being sometimes able to offer a humble contribution to social changes. My involvement also relies on previous observations showing that to prevent doping risks, teams are the key actors (Ohl, Fincoeur, Lentillon-Kaestner, Defrance, & Brissonneau, 2015). These factors explain why I agreed to work with the UCI. Moreover, instead of merely observing riders and teams' staff through a moral lens, we looked at them as workers (Aubel, Lefèvre, & Ohl, 2015; Aubel & Ohl, 2016). However, such an involvement in the changes may place us, as sociologists, in difficult and ambiguous positions because of the following:

- it is difficult to know how our work is going to be used by the protagonists;
- the question of confidence often influences our interactions; some riders and teams did not trust us and were sceptical of our work. Many riders do not clearly differentiate between sociologists and journalists. We are both asking for interviews, both are addressing 'boring questions on doping' and both may transform their purpose and feed the rather negative image of professional cycling. It has happened at least once that we were even lumped in with agents from the World Anti-Doping Agency (WADA);
- it is also very difficult to trust any of the informants, riders and staff, on doping issues without the feeling of being disrespectful of distance, as one of the basic methodological sociological rules;
- the main focus of the team's staff and riders is on performance. However, staff members must face many other important constraints: on their economic resources, to obtain and keep sponsors; on their organisation, especially logistics and planning the team's and riders' schedules; on riders' follow-up; on their precariousness, the economic pressure and the instability of their condition; on the constraints coming both from UCI and the race organisers; on doping as a threat to the entire team; and on their blurred professional identity. Thus, if you tell them that you want to understand cycling culture, teams and riders, you are not a priority on their agenda. Furthermore, teams' staff and riders do not always understand that our involvement is not part of a moral crusade against cheaters.

Performance-enhancing drug use as part of a culture

Obviously, for most people in 2018, including federations, the International Olympic Committee (IOC), riders and teams, doping is usually perceived as cheating. As a consequence, many people in sports and anti-doping equate the fight against doping with the identification and punishment of cheaters.

However, this widely disseminated representation is based on a narrow view that individualises doping and ignores that substance use can be part of a culture

(Smith & Waddington, 2009). That is why a short historical examination allows us to see how doping was constructed as a social norm and how what appears normal at one moment is later considered problematic; it helps us to understand how sports, sciences, historical events, media, politics, or even the economy interact in the process of forming and fixing norms of what is allowed to produce performances and, as a consequence, what is prohibited and considered as unfair. Doping is often analysed as a widespread practice that goes back centuries. This misconception relies on a confusion between substance use and doping. Ancient Greeks did indeed use various enhancing substances at the Olympic Games, but this practice was not truly condemned, nor considered doping. Neither was the use of various substances at the end of the nineteenth century. One cannot analyse these behaviours as cheating, or as a lack of ethics or character, since at the end of the nineteenth century, drug use was rather seen as an improvement technique or an experimentation vis-a-vis performance (Hoberman, 2002). Athletes from the first half of the twentieth century did experiment with all kinds of substances and techniques, but there were no rules, no norms that people agreed on to define doping. Therefore, in 1924, the Pélissier brothers, the cycling heroes of that era, could speak about their consumption of cocaine, chloroform, ointments, pills, and other enhancing techniques without risk of being disqualified from the Tour de France. Furthermore, a few years later, during the Cold War, sports organisations, federations, and countries were at the very heart of the organisation of doping (Hunt, 2011), which shows that seeing dopers only as individual cheaters is truly a narrow view.

The new definitions of doping, emerging in the 1960s (Dimeo, 2007), requalified many enhancing substance uses in sport as doping. However, definitions of doping in the 1960s are very different from the actual definition in the WADA code. Doping has been permanently reworked: it is a social norm that is contested, transgressed, redefined, and subject to controversies, even with the 2018 legal arsenal. For example, despite a 152-page WADA code manual, which includes a long list of prohibited substances, and debates over doping cases that involve lawyers, scientists, experts, arbitration courts, and a 98-page arbitral award,[2] the rider Alberto Contador still denies doping and claims that the banned substance had entered his body after he had eaten a contaminated steak.[3] Thus, to be consistent, it is more relevant to analyse doping in cycling as a social deviance rather than as merely cheating (Brissonneau et al., 2008).

The legacy of enhancing-drug use and the recurrence of cycling culture

Cycling culture has a legacy of performance-enhancing drug use going back to the nineteenth century (Dimeo, 2007; Hoberman, 2002). However, the meaning and acceptance of drugs has changed significantly over time. The culture of drugs was shared by a very large number of riders and was often a part of the job. Various external changes in the values and the uses of sports, from amateurism to the Cold War (Dimeo, 2007; Gleaves & Hunt, 2016), have combined with an increasing supply of enhancing drugs (Paoli & Donati, 2014) to alter the external perception of performance doping in sports. Consequently, the behaviour of teams' staff and riders failed to adapt to a new context, one in which people appear to be more concerned with doping issues. Scandals arise from this gap between the recurrence of doping culture and a new context characterised by new rules, norms, and organisations in charge of anti-doping. After 1998, riders and teams did not immediately understand why their ordinary professional doping 'skills', meaning their knowledge of how to use and hide performance-enhancing drugs, were no longer tolerated. Riders were not truly concerned with moral values. Often doping was not perceived as cheating but rather as a professional skill (Brissonneau, Aubel, & Ohl, 2008). Many teams shared this doping culture in solidarity: they exchanged drugs if necessary, circulated doping tactics, agreed in upholding the *omertà*, did not feel that doping was unfair, etc. In many cases, riders were under the influence of strong family or peer pressure in cycling. A win-at-all-costs mentality, including drugs, can be learned in clubs, with peers, staff, or even parents. The Rumsas family is an example of a family that continued to reproduce the culture of doping, despite the new cultural context of cycling. The father, Raimondas Rumsas, had a controversial career (sentenced for doping in 2003 at the Giro), the mother was arrested at the French border in 2002 with 37 different drugs in her car, and one of the sons, Raimondas Rumsas Junior, tested positive in September 2017 for growth hormone, just five months after his 21-year-old brother Linus, competing for the elite under 23, died. The role of family culture of doping in L. Rumsas's death is under investigation. However, when parents, who are experts in cycling, normalise a culture of doping to support training and competition, it is very likely that young riders may reproduce this culture. Of course, the recurrence of doping culture can also be supported by relatives, peers, team and staff members, even physicians. For example, when R. Rumsas was arrested for doping in Italy in June 2005, A. Taucius, the Lithuanian cycling federation's general secretary, declared himself willing to help Rumsas face this difficult situation.

Therefore, when Mario Zorzoli, the UCI Chief Medical Officer, asked me to find new and innovative ways to prevent doping, I translated this request into more sociological terms as the need to implement solutions that would help limit the recurrence of the doping culture. The mechanisms of recurrence have already been analysed by Pierre Bourdieu and Jean-Claude Passeron, but in the field of education. These authors underline the role of the interaction between educational institutions and agents' culture to analyse how the reproduction of social hierarchies work (Bourdieu & Passeron, 1990). For them, the successful education paths are explained by adapted social dispositions at school. Bourdieu also analyses the reproduction of culture while showing a correspondence between social agents' habitus, shaped through socialisations, and their specific positions in a field (Bourdieu, 1984). In cycling, to be professional, riders also require specific socialisations to fit with the *doxa* (the core values and what is taken for granted) of a field. They must accept to train hard, to suffer, to compete, to dedicate their whole mind and body to succeed in cycling. Without such a rider habitus, there is minimal chance for someone to succeed and even to remain in cycling. This means that, at least before 1998, most of the riders' habitus were matched with organisations completely focused on the production of performance. Although not all of the riders doped, doping was part of the *doxa* and there was no incentive to change anything within the teams, except something that might enhance performance. Many riders were socialised to the doping culture as a part of their training, mostly under the influence of 'insiders', specifically the staff and the more experienced riders (Brissonneau et al., 2008). Thus, the key issue is to identify what can change this reproduction of the 'traditional' cycling culture.

Method: to observe and understand cycling culture

Our seminal study was initially funded by WADA in 2006. It was focused on the socialisation of young riders in a comparative analysis between three countries (Ohl et al., 2015). A second set of studies was funded by the UCI, from 2011 to 2017. One of the first steps was to present and discuss our previous research and some results to three groups of sports directors. Our focus was on the working conditions of the entire 'cycling world', mainly the riders but also the staff, with attention to the organisation of work and to the external constraints teams must face when producing performances. Although some teams did not want to collaborate, UCI support allowed us to have access to ten professional teams in the first and second world divisions (UCI WorldTeams (WTT) and UCI Professional Continental Teams (PCT)). The research team conducted interviews (in most cases eight per team: usually two to three riders, the team manager, the trainer, sports directors, the physician, and the sponsor) and collected other information on staff, budgets, salaries, and communication within the team (a total of more than 100 interviews). The research team also compiled the UCI quantitative databases that included information on riders' careers, the results, sanctions, and employment of the riders and the team (Aubel & Ohl, 2015). Despite UCI support, the inquiries to teams were not always easy. Some cycling teams refused to cooperate; they did not trust us and denied us access to sensitive information. Some were afraid because, as sociologists, we want to publish papers and that was not well perceived. For many riders and staff, sociologists are similar to journalists, with whom they often have ambivalent relations. They require media for visibility but complain about journalists' quest for spectacular headlines that stigmatise teams and riders through misleading or exaggerated information on doping. The riders feel that their performances are belittled and their anti-doping efforts are discredited. Defiance increases because they feel that such a treatment is unfair, considering the investment of the teams and the UCI in anti-doping.

In 2016, we received a grant from the Swiss National Science Foundation (SNSF) that allows us to be independent from the UCI, but this increases the difficulties in obtaining access to the teams. However, a new set of interviews (approx. 60) and observations were conducted in another type of relation. We were only interacting on a voluntary basis, with no pressure for them to collaborate. Information became more difficult to collect, with no access to 'confidential' information such as the salaries or exchanges among the staff on riders' training and competitions. It was a less institutionalised relation, and riders and staff spoke to us more voluntarily. It was also an opportunity to increase the diversity of interviewees, with more younger riders from a broader diversity of cultural backgrounds and to attend training camps to gather interviews and some ethnographic observations. The data collected in these studies were not directly used in this chapter. We just relied on the publications derived from them (e.g. Aubel & Ohl, 2014; Aubel & Ohl, 2015; Fincoeur, Cunningham & Ohl, 2018; Ohl et al., 2015) to provide a comprehensive overview of the cycling culture and its changes.

Is anti-doping in cycling a great failure?

What do we know about the professional cycling culture today? If we rely on examples such as the Rumsas family, we know that the recurrence of doping culture in cycling is working very well. These spectacular cases feed claims by academics, journalists, and citizens that current anti-doping is a failure. The situation can also explain why some academics suggest legalising performance-enhancing drugs in sports, while others support a harm-reduction approach (Møller, Waddington, & Hoberman, 2015). The many anti-doping crises of recent years offer good arguments to support such critical positions, although statements are often broad and sweeping. On the one hand, the main changes in the organisation of anti-doping are minimised, while on the other, the actual cycling culture changes are neglected.

The new context of anti-doping in cycling

There is a gap between the exaggerated promises of the 1980–1990s, during which the IOC and sports organisations claimed that a new scientific anti-doping era would eradicate doping, and the numerous scandals that have occurred since then. However, this gap does not mean that nothing has changed. Since 1998, important changes can be observed at two levels: first, in the organisation of anti-doping, and second, in the social representation of anti-doping.

WADA was created in 1999, and the anti-doping rules were clarified thanks to a World Anti-Doping Code that is regularly updated. The Code's intention is to clarify the anti-doping norms, at least for professional riders and for athletes more broadly. The NADOs' (National Anti-Doping Organisations) work and networks were also improved. Some agencies are independent and completely dedicated to anti-doping, whereas others may still be tolerant or even support doping, as was the case for RUSADA (Russian Anti-Doping Agency) during the Sochi games in

2014. The laboratories also must follow strict compliance rules, have higher quality standards and more WADA controls. Although the Russian laboratory was at the core of the organisation of doping in connection with the support of the FSB (Federal Security Service of the Russian Federation), most laboratories provided reliable anti-doping testing. While some doping tests are not completely efficient, others, such as those on erythropoietin (EPO), have undergone considerable improvement (see Reid and Sottas's chapter).

Anti-doping changed in cycling with the creation of the Cycling Anti-Doping Foundation (CADF) in 2008 and its conquest of independence, when the UCI stepped down from the CADF foundation board in 2013. The development of the biological passport and the integration of intelligence specifically enhanced the fight against doping by the CADF. Approximately 80% of the CADF comes from teams, riders, and event organisers. Its budget is as high as 20% of the UCI budget (6.7 million Swiss francs (CHF), approx. 6.9 US$2018, in 2016 for CADF, UCI 2014 is 34 million CHF, approx. 35 US$2018, source: *CADF Business Report* 2016). This is a very high ratio compared to that of other international federations (e.g. FIFA's expenses for 2016 in medicine and sciences are only at a ratio of 0.25% of the budget (3.5 million US$ in a 1.4 billion budget per year: *Rapport financier 2016*, Bahreïn, May 2016, p. 72). The move from exclusive in-competition to more out-of-competition testing, undeniably improved the results of the fight against doping. The UCI also established the Legal Anti-Doping Services (LADS) in 2013. The LADS' key role is to manage anti-doping results. The legal management of doping cases was conducted inside UCI by the legal department before the creation of the LADS. It is now a unit separate from the UCI in order to increase its independence. Furthermore, UCI created its Anti-Doping Tribunal, in 2015, in charge of the disciplinary proceedings and to render decisions concerning violations of the anti-doping rules. These tasks were previously delegated to the National Federations. The Anti-Doping Tribunal may help to increase the level of expertise. Which can be a support for the coherence and the independence of decisions. And compared to the previous situation, in which National Federations were in charge of sanctioning the athletes, it eventually may reduce potential conflict of interests.

Parallel to the renewed organisation of anti-doping, the social representations of doping did change considerably. Audiences that were not very sensitive to doping issues became much more concerned. Governments, international organisations, consumers, sponsors, journalists, physicians, etc., built up doping as a threat to health and ethics, sometimes in a kind of moral panic (Critcher, 2014). Thus, the doping in cycling media coverage changed. Very few books and papers were published before the Festina case in 1998 (López, 2015), and a massive amount of the literature on doping and cycling spread thereafter. Not only was the cycling culture's tolerance to doping high, but the culture among the journalists who covered cycling also tolerated the practice. Some of the journalists were very close to the riders and even attended parties in which drugs were shared (Brissonneau et al., 2008). The journalists who had access to the background of cycling culture even respected the *omertà*. The strong association between cycling and doping (López, 2015) shaped a negative image of cycling. It increased the team's sponsorship pressure on the staff and the riders. The deterioration of riders' professional identity also changed riders' sensitivity to doping issues. Obviously, the sensitivity is completely different in 2018 compared to what it was in the 1990s. For example, riders were striking at the 12th stage of the 1998 Tour de France because they perceived French police inquiries on Festina and TVM teams as being unfair, despite the 235 EPOs, 120 amphetamines, 82 growth hormones, and 60 testosterone doses they found in the Festina soigneur's car, and the 88 illegal products on the TVM team.

In 2018, several riders now complain when other riders are in what seems to be the 'grey zone', such as in Froome's Adverse Analytical Finding (AAF) for salbutamol at the 18th stage of the 2017 Tour of Spain. Salbutamol is related to inhaled salbutamol, which is not forbidden if it is under 1600 micrograms per 24 hours (the presence in urine of salbutamol in excess of 1000 ng/mL is not consistent with therapeutic use of the substance and will be considered as an Adverse Analytical Finding (AAF)). Romain Bardet perceives this as a threat for cycling:

> It is never good news and it is not good news for cycling as a whole. We would prefer not to receive such news. No one is keen on such an issue. Everyone is more or less affected, the credibility of cycling [most of all].
>
> (R. Bardet, a professional rider ranked 2nd in the 2016 Tour de France and 3rd in 2017, AP and AFP, 17/12/17)[4]

In 1998, Laurent Jalabert (1st in the UCI ranking, leading a strike in 1998) vehemently demanded that journalists report on the race results instead of discussing judicial matters. Jalabert even told the Spanish sporting magazine *Marca* that the UCI controllers '*resembled 50 per cent Count Dracula and 50 per cent neo-Nazi*'.[5] There is a gap, at least in riders' public discourse, between the 1990s and 2018. Thus, there is no doubt that the discourse has completely changed, both for riders and journalists. Of course, that certainly does not guarantee that cycling is doping-free, but it clearly expresses a massive change in what the *doxa* and the dominant norms are.

Observing or supporting the changes in a cycling team's culture?

The social history of doping shows that enhancing-drug use, how doping is organised, and how anti-doping emerged and is structured, has substantially changed in recent years. However, cycling's doping culture did not change much, as for a long time using drugs was an ordinary way of producing performances. In the 1990s, doping was difficult to avoid for a young rider wishing to be successful in cycling. Experimented riders and staff shared the doping culture with young riders (Brissonneau et al., 2008) and, of course, this facilitated moral disengagement (Boardley & Kavussanu, 2011). Although the 1998 Festina affair caused a genuine clash, the autonomy of cycling may explain that despite Festina, the creation of the WADA and the new regulations, the culture did not change very much in the following years. Riders and teams adapted their practices and instead of competing without doping, they became more inventive in hiding it better. Armstrong's driver delivering the drugs, riders hiding uncontaminated urine from controls, adding salt or spitting in the urine to spoil the analysis: these are examples that show riders' and teams' ability for innovative tricks to escape anti-doping controls. Nevertheless, previous research (Fincoeur & Paoli, 2014) and our own observations from 2006 to 2018 suggest that the cycling culture has changed, moving from a team-organised doping to a more individualised doping. During the 1990s, as former rider Christian (a pseudonym) explained it: 'in cycling, we discuss three things. That's what I often say, that the top-level sport can be summarised to three tricks: the sex, the food and the dose (of drugs)' (Brissonneau et al., 2008). We also interviewed young riders in France, Belgium, and Switzerland in 2007 and 2008; at this time discussions on 'legal' drugs, as they told us, were a resource for learning how to perform (Ohl et al., 2015). This grey zone in legal pharmacology appears to have remained a problem. The prevalence of 'authorised' pharmacology uses seems still high, which means the persistence of a culture of pharmacology.[6] However, a general manager of a World Tour team, interviewed in 2017, told us that his team has forbidden the use of legal drugs since 2016. Nevertheless, it was a real issue for the team to convince some of the coaches and DS (*Directeurs Sportifs*) to avoid the risky grey zone of legal drugs. After internal discussions, this was accepted by the staff and seems to have been applied by the riders. Furthermore, compared to the young European riders interviewed in 2006, there is truly a large difference with the ones, not yet in top professional teams, that we interviewed in 2016–2018. Legal drug use is not a subject for most of them in most western-European countries. However, some young riders, from non-western-European countries, also told us that performance-enhancing drugs are widespread in their country and that they perceived anti-doping control in their country only as a great farce.

Excluding past dopers to avoid the recurrence of doping?

To respond to the UCI's demand to improve doping prevention, one key idea was a break with past culture. To limit the recurrence of the cycling culture, we suggested that people involved in doping in the past not be allowed to be hired by a professional team or have relations with riders. This coherent sociological idea, which may support a break with the past culture, is very difficult to implement because it is not easy to identify all the riders and staff that have been involved in doping in the past. Parts of the doping cases are well-known because some riders speak out, but other dopers simply deny that they doped. As we know, claiming a strong commitment to anti-doping does not mean being a 'clean' athlete, just as a bad reputation is not adequate to exclude someone from a professional team: real evidence of doping is required. Even athletes and coaches with a good reputation might have been involved in doping. Furthermore, such a decision may sanction people that speak out, while those that did not disclose their doping keep their jobs. Using such a criterion to exclude someone could be both unfair and counterproductive. In addition, it is difficult to legislate on exclusion from a cycling team. An employee of a team has a working contract, and even if he doped in the past, it may be illegal to exclude him from work, especially those individuals already sanctioned. As with other legal issues, one cannot be sanctioned twice for the same act of misconduct.

Teams that do not seem to be directly involved in doping

Additionally, it is naïve to believe that this radical change, mainly based on exclusion, could guarantee a new 'clean' culture of cycling without any change in the practical and structural aspects of cycling. Without more 'structural' changes, the 'new clean' riders and staff may also use doping as a strategy to face difficulties. Furthermore, the interviews and observations collected during our various studies also convince us to believe that the culture has changed. Doping is no longer included in a strong organisation that provides drugs for the whole team as part of the training process, which is a significant change. This change means that doping is no longer a shared culture among and between the teams, as was primarily the case. It is very unlikely today to find a soigneur supporting one of his colleagues from another team to provide drugs, as was the case previously. Of course, this does not mean that cycling is free of doping. However, when doping occurs, it is more individual and hidden. Doping may eventually be limited to a small sub-group within a team, but it is quite unlikely that the whole UCI, WTT, or PCT is involved in doping. Given the size of the team and the diversity of the staff – all the teams we had access to hired staff from other sports, physiologists, or coaches, some with no cycling background – it would be difficult and even impossible to keep such an organisation secret in a culture of cycling that no longer favours the *omertà*. The Armstrong case may have been a kind of turning point (Dimeo, 2014) in the professional cycling doxa providing a different ethos. In addition, today, many teams and riders sign contracts and charters to demonstrate that they will be completely committed to anti-doping. Such a pledge is often a requirement of sports organisations, and especially of sponsors who fear for their image. Claiming new values, a commitment to clean sport, a break with the past norms of doping: these often form the basis of anti-doping policies. Obviously, moreover, a weak staff commitment to 'clean' cycling can favour athletes' moral disengagement (Boardley & Kavussanu, 2011).

Cycling teams' new conditions and organisation of work

Although team commitment to 'clean' sport may limit moral disengagement, it is only a necessary condition, but not at all a sufficient one. Teaching riders the value of clean sport may not be sufficient to change their behaviours. Rather, we suggest that teams focus on addressing the day-to-day experiences of training and competing. This focus not only means changing words to do things differently (Austin, 1975), or simply shifting the discourse on clean sport; it also means doing things differently, and that can change how people think.

Team Sky and their general manager Dave Brailsford did comment profusely on the new generation of 'clean' teams and riders, but the controversies on Wiggins's TUE (Therapeutic Use Exemption) and on Froome AAF show that words were disconnected from the idealistic clean practices that were put on stage. In addition, this fact presents risks for the image of cycling. However, team influence on doping is certainly today more often indirect (Houlihan, 2002). Doping may not be organised by the teams, but it may appear as one of the options for individual riders to face professional constraints, to do their job, make money, gain prestige, or stay in the peloton. These reasons are why we focused on the organisation of work to support some changes in the actual culture (Ohl et al., 2015; Aubel & Ohl, 2014). We recommended that the UCI pay more attention to teams' organisation and support to the riders. As a consequence, this means focusing on their working and social conditions, observing how team staff organise the production of performance, and suggesting practical changes that may diminish indirect risks of doping. We focused especially on different topics that were sometimes already on teams' agenda, even if expressed differently. Our seminal work for the WADA (Brissonneau, Defrance, Fincoeur, Lentillon-Kaestner, & Ohl, 2009) suggests an emphasis on teams' values, organisation, and support for the rider. The culture of cycling was characterised by training, recovering, and managing the workload through doping. That situation is less the case in 2018 because most teams seem willing to escape the culture of doping. However, until recently, some teams still had a non-professional approach to organisation, a weak support of riders and a bad management of their workload and planning (Aubel, Lefèvre, & Ohl, 2015). Thus, the idea was to improve riders' working conditions to be sure that their workload is acceptable and that they have enough time to recover without doping. However, it is difficult to change a culture without trying to reduce precariousness, which is a structural aspect of the cycling culture. The results of our WADA grant (Brissonneau et al., 2009) underline the key role that team organisation can play. For example, a team's staff entirely dedicated to performance is a mistake, as physicians should only take care of riders' health, not try to improve their performance.

Attitudes to and experiences of work have also changed. Staff that experienced the post-Festina, after 1998, and remained involved in doping, had to hide doping, although some physicians find it exciting to develop skills relating to drug use (see Fincoeur's chapter), while others have no regrets about those years. Working as a physician was very stressful; it obliged them to hide, to take risks, to be coherent when cheating, etc. The new experience of work, in which they are not involved in doping, is judged more positively. However, being involved in anti-doping can also mean providing a better support to the riders. Some teams favour a mixing of cultures; some of the performance managers, physicians, or coaches had no cycling background when they joined a team. This aspect reduces cultural homogeneity and helps in not reproducing doping culture. Hiring highly skilled team staff, trainers, biomechanics, physiologists, and psychologists who do not share the past cycling culture, nor a doping culture, may help to change the norms, to improve riders' support and to make *omertà* unlikely. Sharing more information on riders' performances, profile, shape, difficulties, etc., may help to support riders but also to control them. Staff are also more careful when hiring riders in the teams. Some of them privilege countries, clubs, or farm-teams committed to fighting doping. One team's head of performance explained to us (during a training camp in 2018) that he always analyses the training data before any recruitment. For riders, having adequate qualitative support for a coherent follow-up is crucial. However, support may be ambivalent. Some riders also complain because of a perceived decrease in their autonomy. Highly scientific support appears to make riders feel that they are losing control of their work. Some interviewees (in 2018) were even worried about new social drug consumption, such as mixing alcohol with *Lexomil*, as the expression of negative working experiences and difficult transitions. However, taking *Lexomil* is not a new phenomenon, and the changes in its prevalence are very difficult to assess.

From our observations, it appears that a renewed and reinforced organisation of anti-doping, combined with some teams' efforts to change the way they produce performances, made the recurrence of drugs culture more difficult. Changes in how teams are working can be observed: instead of using drugs, some of them try to find alternative methods to preclude doping as a privileged means of producing performance. Other suggestions, such as developing riders' education, were less convincing for the teams and the UCI because they perceived it as difficult to manage. However, cycling as the only job option is risky, and supporting alternative careers, riders' education, distance learning, etc., would facilitate riders' transition if they lose their job. As explained by a WTT staff member who has previously doped, it was easier for his colleague, another staff member, not to dope because he did not depend on cycling; his studies gave him other options beyond cycling, and that made it easier to refuse doping.

Conclusion

The recurrence of doping culture has become increasingly difficult because of the abovementioned changes within cycling, anti-doping, and the broader environment. Not because of a sudden, more 'ethical', generation of teams and riders, this change occurred under external pressures, thanks to a better organisation of anti-doping and a decreasing tolerance of doping by a broader audience of journalists, consumers, governments, sponsors, etc. It is understandable that defiance is still expressed towards cycling teams, but it is clear that some team members are truly willing to prevent doping. Furthermore, many of the new riders joining the WTT and PCT in 2018 do not appear to share the previous culture of doping. Some were not even born in 1998, and with the changes in the culture and the organisations, it is less likely that they learned to ride with drugs. This fact means that no one knows the hen better than the fox, and that may help it guard the hen house – at least if it is closely monitored. However, this fox-and-hen metaphor is simplistic for sports and doping, because culture can change much faster than instincts can.

Lastly, saying that doping is no longer recurring does not mean that doping is no longer an issue in cycling. First, because we mainly had access to the teams willing to cooperate, this certainly gives an over-representation of the teams that are the most committed to changing the cycling culture. Other teams simply did not want to have sociologists observing how they work. Some of those teams had good reasons: because they are fed up with being under scrutiny by anti-doping agencies, journalists, and researchers judging their work. For other teams, at best, it is simply because they do not think that teams have a social responsibility in doping. A manager from a team that had to face doping charges told us that the rider who doped was just an idiot, and that is all! He and his team did not want to take any responsibility, notwithstanding the absence of any appropriate support for and follow-up of the riders that may help to prevent doping, and despite the damage it could have on his team and on cycling generally. Other managers simply did not want us to have access to their team's 'professional secrets' or to their back-stage, including the 'grey-zone' of 'authorised' pharmacology uses. As suggested by other observers 'It's not blatant doping as it was in the early days, but there certainly seems to be anecdotal evidence that there's a lot of marginal stuff going on'.[7] However, there are also good reasons for such a resistance. As sociologists, we are observing their culture, and the publication of our results may have consequence on their image. Some of the teams' staff, the riders, and even people at the UCI, suffer from the legacy of doping and the systematic association between cycling and doping. In addition, telling them that a sociological understanding of the cycling culture may provide tools to inflect it is not always sufficient to convince them.

Notes

1 www.reuters.com/article/us-sport-doping-wada-tygart-idUSKBN16K1LV 13 March 2017, 'US anti-doping chief says WADA is the "fox guarding hen house"', Karolos Grohmann.

2 See CAS 2011/A/2384 UCI v. Alberto Contador Velasco & RFEC CAS 2011/A/2386 WADA v. Alberto Contador Velasco & RFEC, ARBITRAL AWARD delivered by the COURT OF ARBITRATION FOR SPORT in Lausanne, 6 February 2012.

3 See Henry Robertshaw, 'One of the biggest injustices in sport': Alberto Contador still angry at doping ban and loss of Grand Tour titles, *Cycling Weekly*, www.cyclingweekly.com/author/henryrobertshaw, 26 September 2017.
4 Source: *VeloNews.com*, published 14 December 2017, www.velonews.com/2017/12/news/tony-martin-froome-case-scandal-double-standard_453365
5 Source: http://autobus.cyclingnews.com/results/1998/sep98/sep10.shtml
6 See, The 2017 WADA MONITORING PROGRAM (In Competition Monitoring: Mitragynine, Tramadol, Codeine In and Out of Competition Monitoring: Telmisartan, Glucocorticoids and Beta-2 Agonists), shows that the prevalence of Tramadol, Glucocorticoids and Codeine is still high in cycling.
7 Robin Parisotto, quoted in 'Casting a critical eye on corruption in sport: Q&A with anti-doping expert Robin Parisotto', by Shane Stokes, *Cyclingtips*, 15 June 2018. https://cyclingtips.com/2018/06/casting-a-critical-eye-on-corruption-in-sport-qa-with-anti-doping-expert-robin-parisotto/

References

Aubel, O., Lefèvre, B., & Ohl, F. (2015). Les équipes cyclistes « professionnelles » face aux nouvelles injonctions au professionnalisme. *Sociologie du Travail*, *57*(4), 470–495.

Aubel, O. & Ohl, F. (2014). An alternative approach to the prevention of doping in cycling. *International Journal of Drug Policy*, *25*(6), 1094–1102.

Aubel, O. & Ohl, F. (2015). De la précarité des coureurs cyclistes professionnels aux pratiques de dopage: L'économie des coproducteurs du WorldTour. *Actes de la recherche en sciences sociales*, *209*(4), 28–41.

Aubel, O., & Ohl, F. (2016). Le sportif en travailleur face à la lutte anti-dopage. Éléments de critique et propositions. *Science & Motricité*, 9(2), 33–43.

Austin, J.L. (1975). *How to do Things with Words*. Oxford: Oxford University Press.

Becker, H.S. (1963). *Outsiders. Studies in the Sociology of Deviance*. New York: The Free Press.

Boardley, I.D. & Kavussanu, M. (2011). Moral disengagement in sport. *International Review of Sport and Exercise Psychology*, 4(2), 93–108.

Bourdieu, P. (1984). *Distinction: A Social Critique of the Judgement of Taste*. Cambridge: Harvard University Press.

Bourdieu, P. & Passeron, J.C. (1990). *Reproduction in Education, Society, and Culture*. London: Sage.

Brissonneau, C., Aubel, O., & Ohl, F. (2008). *L'épreuve du Dopage : Sociologie du Cyclisme Professionnel*. Paris: Presses Universitaires de France.

Brissonneau, C., Defrance, J., Fincoeur, B., Lentillon-Kaestner, V., & Ohl, F. (2009). Carrière sportive et socialisation secondaire en cyclisme sur route: les cas de la Belgique, la France et la Suisse. *Rapport de Fin de Recherche Financée Par l'Agence Mondiale Antidopage (AMA). Lausanne*.

Critcher, C. (2014). New perspectives on anti-doping policy: from moral panic to moral regulation. *International Journal of Sport Policy and Politics*, 6(2), 153–169.

Dimeo, P. (2007). *A History of Drug Use in Sport: 1876–1976: Beyond Good and Evil*. London: Routledge.

Dimeo, P. (2014). Why Lance Armstrong? Historical context and key turning points in the 'cleaning up' of professional cycling. *The International Journal of the History of Sport*, *31*(8), 951–968.

Fincoeur, B., & Paoli, L. (2014). Des pratiques communautaires au marché du dopage. *Déviance et Société*, 38(1), 3–27.

Fincoeur, B., Cunningham, R., & Ohl, F. (2018). I'm a poor lonesome rider. Help! I could dope. *Performance Enhancement & Health*, 1–6.

Gleaves, J. & Hunt, T. (2016). *A Global History of Doping in Sport: Drugs, Policy, and Politics*. London: Routledge.

Hoberman, J. (2002). *Mortal Engines: The Science of Performance and Dehumanization of Sport*. New Jersey: The Blackburn Press.

Houlihan, B. (2002). *Dying to Win: Doping in Sport and the Development of Anti-Doping Policy*. Strasbourg: Council of Europe Pub.

Hunt, T. (2011). *Drug Games: The International Olympic Committee and the Politics of Doping, 1960–2008*. Austin: University of Texas Press.

López, B. (2015). Drug use in cycling. In V. Møller, I. Waddington, & J. Hoberman (Eds), *Routledge Handbook of Drugs and Sport* (pp. 89–102). London: Routledge.

Møller, V., Waddington, I., & Hoberman, J. (2015). *Routledge Handbook of Drugs and Sport*. London: Routledge.

Ohl, F., Fincoeur, B., Lentillon-Kaestner, V., Defrance, J., & Brissonneau, C. (2015). The socialization of young cyclists and the culture of doping. *International Review for the Sociology of Sport*, 50(7), 865–882.

Paoli, L. & Donati, A. (2014). *The Sports Doping Market: Understanding Supply and Demand, and the Challenges of their Control*. New York: Springer.

Smith, A. & Waddington, I. (2009). *An Introduction to Drugs in Sport: Addicted to Winning?* London: Routledge.

Chapter 10

Blowing the whistle on doping in cycling

Kelsey Erickson

The public perception that wrongdoing is prevalent in organisations worldwide is increasing (Gundlach, Martinko, & Douglas, 2008), and sport organisations are certainly not exempt. Indeed, global media headlines have been littered with examples of sport corruption (e.g. sexual abuse, bribery, match-fixing) across numerous national borders (e.g. USA, England, Australia) and sports (e.g. soccer, gymnastics, cricket). Growing recognition for the magnitude of corruption in international sport has prompted significant interest in exposing and eradicating wrongdoing in sport and individuals are being increasingly encouraged – and expected – to play an active role in this pursuit. It has therefore become necessary to determine the most effective means for facilitating this and one avenue that has proven particularly effective for exposing both individual and systemic corruption in sport is *whistleblowing*.

Given sport's growing interest in the concept of whistleblowing, the aim of this chapter is to: (1) familiarise the reader with the issue of whistleblowing, (2) review whistleblowing behaviour specifically in the sporting context and (3) consider the (potential) role of whistleblowing for exposing and deterring doping in the sport of cycling. To begin, an overview of the existing whistleblowing literature is offered.

Whistleblowing

The concept of whistleblowing has been widely researched within the public sectors for decades and is commonly defined as, '… the disclosure by organisation members (former or current) of illegal, immoral, or illegitimate practices under the control of their employers, to persons or organisations that may be able to affect action' (Near & Miceli, 1985: 4). As such, it is a prosocial behaviour that is considered useful for preventing, remedying against, and/or exposing fraud, corruption (Vandekerckhove, 2006), and wrongdoing (Miceli, Near, & Schwenk, 1991). The latter – wrongdoing – refers to conduct falling along a spectrum of behaviour ranging from unprofessional and improper to illegal behaviour within an organisation (Teo & Caspersz, 2011). The concept of whistleblowing is therefore relevant to varied organisations (e.g. business, government, education) and has the potential to expose a broad range of unethical behaviours.

Whistleblowing was originally considered a one-off event, but scholars are increasingly viewing it as a process that oftentimes involves multiple (progressive) attempts at reporting wrongdoing (e.g. Vandekerckhove & Phillips, 2017; Richardson & McGlynn, 2015). This evolution in the whistleblowing literature reflects the complexity of the behaviour. When deciding what to do in a possible whistleblowing situation, individuals are confronted with a serious dilemma stemming from *the morality of loyalty* and *the morality of principle* (Uys & Senekal, 2008). *Morality of loyalty* refers to an obligation to people, organisations, or groups within a particular context. Within this, 'organisational loyalty' suggests that an individual should act in good faith for the best interests of all involved in an organisation, constantly seeking to protect its reputation. Meanwhile, the *morality of principle* suggests that individuals should adhere to certain abstract principles irrespective of those involved in the situation. Consequently, while whistleblowing is often considered the right and easy option when viewed as an abstract; in reality, norms favouring obedience to authority and group loyalty make it more difficult than often acknowledged (Dungan, Waytz, & Young, 2015). Individuals are ultimately condemned to failure if/when they become aware of wrongdoing because regardless of which choice they make (whistleblow or stay silent), they are doing something wrong and/or hurting someone (Geva, 2006).

Given the complexity of whistleblowing, it is not surprising that exploring the factors that make someone more or less likely to report wrongdoing (i.e. determinants) has attracted significant interest from researchers. Generally speaking, the determinants can be categorised as: individual, situational, and environmental. Commonly identified *individual* determinants include: whether whistleblowing is considered integral to one's role responsibility (Miceli & Near, 2002); job performance, education level, whether or not one holds a supervisory position (Mesmer-Magnus & Viswesvaran, 2005; Miceli & Near, 1988); whether or not one endorses fairness over loyalty (Dungan et al., 2015); if an individual is extroverted (Bjørkelo, Einarsen, & Matthiesen, 2010); subjective norms about whistleblowing (Vadera, Aguilera, & Caza, 2009); and one's level of whistleblowing education (Caillier, 2017). *Situational* factors influencing whistleblowing behaviour include: perceived support (for whistleblowing) from management (Keenan, 2000); whether the organisational climate/culture supports whistleblowing (Miceli & Near, 1985, 1988; Berry, 2004); the severity of wrongdoing (Miceli & Near, 1992); and the (non-)relationship between the observer and the whistleblower (Mesmer-Magnus & Viswesvaran, 2005). It is worth noting that individual determinants are generally inconsistent across research studies whereas situational determinants tend to be more stable (Culiberg & Mihelic, 2017). Finally, *environmental* factors related to country and culture are thought to further influence whistleblowing behaviour (Culiberg & Mihelic, 2017). Within this, religion and historical factors have been deemed significant (O'Sullivan & Ngau, 2014) and experts therefore advise against generalising whistleblowing findings across cultural contexts (Miceli, Near, & Dworkin, 2009).

Importantly, the fear of retribution (e.g. job loss, negative labels) constitutes the dominant deterrent to whistleblowing and its deterrent effect is enhanced when an organisation lacks clear whistleblowing policies that protect whistleblowers (Rennie & Crosby, 2002). The reality is that whistleblowing regularly involves significant social and economic costs for the whistleblower and can be a psychologically harrowing experience (Fotaki, Kenny, & Scriver, 2015; Hermandorfer, 2015). Consequences for whistleblowers are commonplace regardless of the specific context in which the behaviour occurs. Research has consistently identified retaliation towards whistleblowers in the form of: (1) being bullied, shunned, negatively labelled, and discredited by others (Dasgupta & Kesharwani, 2010; Teo & Caspersz, 2011); (2) having one's reputation, job and livelihood seriously jeopardised (Baron, 2013); and (3) being victimised by employers with lawsuits, job loss, defamation, and disgrace (Rennie & Crosby, 2002; Uys & Senekal, 2008). The mere *possibility* that whistleblowing might result in an individual facing one or more of these reactions is oftentimes enough to deter someone from engaging in the behaviour (De Maria, 2006).

As demonstrated, there is a substantial body of empirical research that has explored whistleblowing in the public sectors. But, is the same true within the sporting context? This will be revealed in the next section.

Whistleblowing in sport

Following high-profile cases of whistleblowing in sport (e.g. Yuliya and Vitaly Stepanov regarding Russian Athletics), the concept of reporting wrongdoing in sport has garnered increasing interest from researchers (Erickson, Backhouse, & Carless, 2017; Whitaker, Backhouse, & Long, 2014), the media and anti-doping organisations worldwide. To encourage whistleblowing, significant resources have been (and are) directed towards 'Report Doping' platforms, including the World Anti-Doping Agency's (WADA) Speak Up! Platform (2017) and accompanying Whistleblowing Program (2016), which outlines the rights afforded to whistleblowers. As the introduction of these resources illustrates, an emphasis on intelligence-driven approaches to anti-doping has emerged and the WADA are compelling those with information on doping to come forward. Reinforcing this, the WADA Code (WADC; Article 10.6.1; WADA, 2015) now includes the possibility for individuals to have the length of their sanctions reduced (and/or removed entirely) for providing substantial assistance leading to an anti-doping rule violation (ADRV). Thus, providing a new incentive for individuals to engage in whistleblowing on doping.

Yet, research on whistleblowing in sport has not kept pace with these developments in anti-doping policy and practice. Unlike the public sectors, whistleblowing literature specific to the sporting context is in its infancy. Nonetheless, there is already an indication that whistleblowing in sport is similar – but different – to whistleblowing in traditional industries (Richardson & McGlynn, 2015). That is, (potential) whistleblowers in sport are faced with further challenges not relevant to the broader industries. These include: (a) an absence of evidence-based whistleblowing policies, (b) a 'win at all costs' mentality (Richardson & McGlynn, 2015), and (c) the threat of retaliation from a range of stakeholders (e.g. fans, sponsors, media) who are not directly attached to the individual/organisation against whom they are reporting (Richardson & McGlynn, 2011, 2015). Complicating matters further, prospective *doping* whistleblowers are met with: (d) (the perception that) athletes who report doping are treated more harshly than doping athletes (Whitaker et al., 2014), (e) the existence of a 'code of silence' and 'omerta' in sport (Shipley, 2013; Whitaker et al., 2014; Kimmage, 2017), (f) a lack of knowledge and education related to whistleblowing (Whitaker et al., 2014), and (g) being faced with a true moral dilemma (Erickson et al., 2017). Collectively, there are a number of potential barriers to blowing the whistle in sport, especially in relation to doping behaviours.

Considering the mounting calls for whistleblowing within the global anti-doping community, it is concerning that there are only two published papers exploring the issue (i.e. Erickson et al., 2017; Whitaker et al., 2014). Whitaker and colleagues (2014) noted a difference in the way individual (track and field) versus team-sport (rugby) national level British athletes approached the issue of blowing the whistle on doping, with rugby athletes demonstrating more hesitation at the thought of whistleblowing in comparison to their counterparts. The authors therefore suggest that endorsing a code of silence may cause team-sport athletes to refrain from reporting a fellow teammate for doping despite disagreeing with their behaviour. Additionally, the authors underline the significance of contextual factors in determining how individuals in sport approach the issue of whistleblowing. Building on the preliminary research, Erickson and colleagues (2017) identified for the first time that in situations of reporting doping, individuals are faced with a 'true moral dilemma' – two equally valid and demanding moral options (Uys & Senekal, 2008). As a result, individuals must choose between (1) reporting the doping athlete to protect the rights of athletes at large to compete in 'clean sport' (i.e. doping-free) or (2) staying quiet to protect the doping athlete's athletic career, reputation, and wellbeing given the social consequences associated with being labelled a 'doper' (Georgiadis & Papazoglou, 2014). Notably, someone gets harmed regardless of the final choice. Ensuing from the true moral dilemma, US and UK university track and field student-athletes were hesitant to blow the whistle on doping despite being personally opposed to engaging with doping substances and/or methods. Student-athletes instead suggested they would be willing to personally confront the doping athlete(s). The authors therefore propose that whistleblowing is not the *only* avenue for addressing doping in sport and suggest that engaging the wider sporting community in the pursuit of clean sport may require providing individuals with additional means for actively addressing/deterring the behaviour. An approach of this nature would acknowledge the importance of relationships in determining how individuals address doping situations.

The dearth of literature exploring the issue of whistleblowing on doping leaves us with a limited understanding of the behaviour. In particular, what the experience is like, determinants of the behaviour and current attitudes towards whistleblowing in sport (i.e. whistleblowing culture). That said, while empirical evidence is lacking, media stories have provided critical insights regarding sport-specific forms of whistleblower retaliation. For example, Yuliya and Vitaly Stepanov – the Russian couple who first blew the whistle on systemic doping in Russia – were forced to take their infant son and flee Russia without the prospect of returning (James, 2014). Yuliya has subsequently been referred to by such names as a 'traitor' and 'Judas' (Ash, 2016; Tsvetkova & Strohecker, 2015). Moreover, following fears that hackers had determined the family's location in the US, Yuliya warned, 'if something happens to us, all of you should know it was not an accident' (Axon, 2016a). By 'something', Yuliya was implying *death*. Offering further insights, Grigory Rodchenkov – the former Moscow Lab Director and central actor in the Russian doping programme (Harris, 2017) – fled Russia before corroborating the Stepanovs' story due to fear for his safety and is currently under witness protection in the US (Stokes, 2017). Fear for his safety is reasonable considering two former Russian doping officials died under mysterious circumstances in 2016 (Kramer, 2016) and Grigory himself has received multiple death threats (Walker, 2017). As a consequence of blowing the whistle, Grigory will forever have to look over his shoulder and he also fears potential retaliation directed towards his family, whom he had to leave behind in Russia (Waldron, 2017). As seen, the lives of both sets of whistleblowers, and their families, have been forever altered by whistleblowing on doping.

Importantly, in response to public concerns for the safety of these global whistleblowers, the International Olympic Committee (IOC) formally denied responsibility (Grohmann, 2016). The reaction sparked worry that whistleblowers will now be further deterred from coming forward (Axon, 2016b); yet, without established whistleblowing policies in place, the response from the IOC is ultimately justified. As it stands, there is no clear indication of who (e.g. WADA, IOC) is responsible and accountable for protecting and compensating doping whistleblowers, nor when/how to facilitate such provisions.[1] Thus, revealing a critical gap in existing sport policy and provision that is currently hindering the potential for whistleblowing to serve as an effective means for exposing and, ideally, reducing doping behaviour in sport.

On the whole, it appears that there is much work to be done if global sport wants to encourage and facilitate whistleblowing as an effective means for exposing and deterring doping. But, is the same true for the sport of cycling? In response to this question, the following section outlines anti-doping developments in the sport of cycling before offering suggestions for (further) encouraging and facilitating whistleblowing on doping in the sport.

Whistleblowing in cycling

It is no secret that cycling has had a turbulent past with doping. High-profile doping scandals in the late 1990s (e.g. Festina affair) and 2000s (e.g. Lance Armstrong) brought to the public's attention the doping problem permeating the sport. The fact that 36 of the 45 Tour de France podium finishers during the time period of 1996 to 2010 were tainted by doping was certainly testimony to this (USADA, 2012). Another important revelation during this time period was the potential collusion of the world governing body for the sport of cycling – the *Union Cycliste Internationale* (UCI). The report produced by the US Anti-Doping Agency (USADA) that exposed Lance Armstrong's doping included evidence suggesting that the UCI had potentially been aware of Lance's doping and, at best, turned a blind eye or, at worst, helped conceal it (USADA, 2012; CIRC, 2015). The UCI was eventually forced to acknowledge that doping was taking place in cycling and that the anti-doping measures they had in place at the time were not sufficient for deterring the behaviour.

Signalling a turning point in the UCI's approach towards doping, stricter anti-doping rules have since been introduced (UCI, 2015a, 2015b). A central component of these updated rules is an explicit expectation (i.e. incentive) for individuals to blow the whistle on doping in cycling. Indeed, riders and support personnel are now required to report (i.e. whistleblow) potential ADRVs to their respective anti-doping organisations (Articles 21.1.7 & 21.2.7; UCI, 2015b) and failure to do this can result in punishment. It is worth emphasising the novelty of this rule. As previously mentioned, the updated WADC includes the substantial assistance provision which offers an incentive for individuals to assume the role of a whistleblower in order to reduce their own (impending) sanctions (Article 10.6.1; WADA, 2015). However, a significant limitation of this incentive is that it only applies to individuals facing a sanction. Thus, it does not provide an incentive for the vast majority of athletes and support personnel. Conversely, *all* individuals in the sport of cycling have an incentive to whistleblow since it is clearly outlined as their responsibility and there are consequences for not satisfying the expectation. Further, individuals are more likely to whistleblow if they feel it is integral to their role within an organisation (Miceli & Near, 2002). Thus, it seems the UCI has taken a strong step towards facilitating whistleblowing on doping with the introduction of these rules (i.e. Articles 21.1.7 & 21.2.7). Importantly, they are bolstered by the addition of *team* sanctions. Specifically, for UCI-registered teams, if two individuals contracted (i.e. rider and/or rider support personnel) by the team receive an ADRV within a 12-month period, the whole team can be suspended between 15–45 days (Article 7.12.1) or up to 12 months in the case that three or more associated individuals receive ADRVs (Article 7.12.3). On top of this, UCI World Teams and Professional Continental Teams face the further consequence of a financial fine whereby the team will be required to pay the UCI 5% of their annual budget if two associated individuals receive ADRVs in a 12-month period (Article 11.3) and the same applies in situations where three or more individuals are sanctioned (Article 11.4). The prospect of team-wide sanctions based on the doping behaviours of individuals within those teams provides an incentive for individuals to expose the doping behaviours of fellow team members (athletes and support personnel) in an attempt to avoid being punished alongside them.

Taken together, the UCI has implemented valuable incentives for blowing the whistle on doping that do not currently exist within the majority of international sport federations.

There is one further distinction that warrants attention though, and that is the creation of the Cycling Anti-Doping Foundation (CADF) – cycling's independent anti-doping organisation. The CADF was established in 2008 and became truly independent from the UCI in 2013. Its mandate is to run the UCI's anti-doping programme in compliance with the WADC and UCI Anti-Doping Rules. The CADF is also responsible for encouraging and facilitating whistleblowing on doping and has introduced two primary avenues for engaging with the behaviour. Specifically, the CADF hosts an online platform that allows individuals to complete an encrypted online form which is then sent directly to appropriate members of the CADF. Alternatively, whistleblowers can send an email directly to the CADF (CADF, 2017), who guarantee complete confidentiality and protection for sources (i.e. whistleblowers) regardless of the approach adopted.

Following the creation of the CADF, the UCI commissioned the 'Cycling Independent Reform Committee' (CIRC) in 2014 with a mandate to review doping practices in cycling during the 1990s and 2000s (O'Shea, 2014). The review process culminated in a report presented to the UCI President that offered insights into past and current doping attitudes and behaviours in the sport, together with recommendations for moving the sport forward (CIRC, 2015). Among the many important insights presented, it was suggested that the attitude towards whistleblowers needs to evolve towards recognising the positive role they (can) play in cleaning up cycling. Yet, the same Report identified that a culture of omerta in cycling has existed and, critically, still exists (to an extent). This omerta culture included such things as keeping quiet about doping (individually and collectively), not exposing those who have/are engaged with it, and shunning cyclists who do not take part in the behaviour (CIRC, 2015). Essentially, doping secrets were shared by professional cyclists, yet hidden from the public (Lentillon-Kaestner, Hagger, & Hardcastle, 2011). The implications of this enduring culture cannot be overlooked.

The mafia-like omerta culture in cycling (Laser, 2015) can deter individuals from whistleblowing on doping since speaking up or acting in a way that contradicts the norm is considered risky behaviour (Baron, 2013). Moreover, the likelihood of whistleblowing can be socially influenced (Gundlach, Douglas, & Martinko, 2003) and jeopardising the trust of a teammate or fellow athlete may be considered significantly more damaging than an ADRV (Taunton, 2011).

Meanwhile, it has been suggested that finding a team after accepting an ADRV is easier than finding a team after whistleblowing on doping in cycling (CIRC, 2015). Further, research with student-athletes (Erickson et al., 2017) and national level athletes (Whitaker et al., 2014) highlight the concern for relationships, reputation, and not knowing how to whistleblow, as representing significant deterrents to whistleblowing on doping. Yet, it does appear that the omerta culture is beginning to shift. Indeed, cyclists have indicated that doping now contradicts the social norms within the sport (e.g. Ohl, Fincoeur, Lentillon-Kaestner, Defrance, & Brissonneau, 2015) and it is no longer assumed that banned substances are a necessity within the sport (Lentillon-Kaestner et al., 2011). Many cycling teams have openly adopted a zero-tolerance approach to doping and take active steps towards deterring the behaviour (e.g. additional doping tests; Fincoeur, Van de Ven, & Mulrooney, 2014). Thus, choosing not to dope no longer equates to being excluded from the sport (Lentillon-Kaestner et al., 2011).

While cycling does indeed appear to be moving towards creating a culture of intolerance towards doping, actively encouraging and facilitating whistleblowing on doping can boost this effort. The following section therefore draws upon existing whistleblowing literature to provide an outline of possible avenues for creating a positive whistleblowing culture in cycling. Ultimately, the goal is to create a culture that not only *tolerates* whistleblowers but *celebrates* them.

Creating a culture of whistleblowing in cycling

Immediate changes

Whistleblowing policy and whistleblower protection

Whistleblowing policies have the potential to: (1) reduce the negative stigma attached to the label 'whistleblower' (e.g. snitch, tattletale), (2) deter athletes who may be considering doping from engaging with substances as they will no longer feel confident that their behaviour will be kept secret, and (3) create a truly open environment. Thus, offering a safe haven that allows individuals to report wrongdoing without the fear of retribution (Winneker, 2016). Despite known benefits, with the exception of the WADA's Whistleblowing Program (WADA, 2016), established whistleblowing policies in sport are rare. This gap in provision is particularly noticeable within the context of reporting doping. Designing and implementing an evidence-based whistleblowing policy that clearly outlines the rights afforded to whistleblowers is one way that the UCI could send the message that they are serious about breaking the cycling omerta. Such protections are designed to insulate whistleblowers against threats of and/or actual acts of reprisal that result from reporting wrongdoing within a particular context (Hermandorfer, 2015).

Whistleblower support

Whistleblowers can benefit from receiving independent advice (i.e. removed from the UCI and CADF) on the whistleblowing process. For example, through gathering information related to what can be expected during the whistleblowing process and being familiarised with available resources (Lewis & Vandekerckhove, 2015). One way this could be facilitated within sport would be by means of appointing a whistleblower ombudsman (King & Hermodson, 2000; Richardson & McGlynn, 2011). The ombudsman would provide a point of call for individuals who may not feel comfortable disclosing their information to someone directly within the organisation (King & Hermodson, 2000); thus, enabling them to take action despite existing reservations.

Whistleblowing education

Even the most sophisticated whistleblowing policies and procedures are ultimately futile if those expected to engage with them are not aware of and equipped to utilise them. Whistleblower education is therefore necessary and has been shown to increase engagement with whistleblowing (see Caillier, 2017). Offering whistleblowing education signals that an organisation cares about and values whistleblowing (Cho & Song, 2015). Such provisions are standard practice within government agencies, and effective whistleblowing education should include: (a) providing information on available whistleblowing channels (including the pros/cons of each route), (b) information regarding how to utilise them effectively (and when), and (c) familiarising individuals with whistleblower rights (i.e. relevant whistleblower policy) (Berry, 2004; Caillier, 2017).

Long-term changes

Ethical culture

A strong ethical culture in an organisation – one that encourages, celebrates, and supports whistleblowing – plays a central role in stimulating individuals to whistleblow on wrongdoing (Berry, 2004; King III & Hermodson, 2000; Miceli & Near, 1988). 'Ethical culture' can be defined as the elements of the perceived organisational climate that condone unethical behaviour and promote ethical behaviour (Trevino & Weaver, 2003). In its absence, individuals are less likely to whistleblow due to concerns that they will be negatively impacted by it (Whitaker et al., 2014). A critical step towards establishing an ethical culture is for organisations to shift the focus from the *messenger* to the *message* in incidences of whistleblowing (Uys, 2008; Uys & Senekal, 2008). In other words, rather than seeing whistleblowers as the *cause* of the problem, they should be viewed as initiators of *problem-solving* (Richardson & McGlynn, 2011) and as change agents (Near & Miceli, 1995). Leaders and management play an important role in this context by serving as role-models who can reinforce the importance of ethics (Kaptein, 2011). It is therefore essential that they are held accountable if/when they fail to achieve this.

Conclusion

Blowing the whistle on wrongdoing is an increasingly important and effective means for exposing and deterring corrupt behaviour. While the public sectors have a longstanding history of engaging with whistleblowing research, the sport context is lacking in this area and, consequently, provisions for encouraging and facilitating whistleblowing are limited. This is particularly true within the specific anti-doping context and raises concerns for whether individuals will be willing to come forward with doping information. Although there has been an increase in the number of resources available for reporting suspected doping behaviours, information regarding how, when, and why to engage with them is rarely provided. Moreover, there is a lack of established whistleblowing policies and procedures in place within sport; thus, placing would-be whistleblowers at heightened risk for receiving negative backlash as a result of their choice to come forward.

The sport of cycling has been implicated by doping scandals for decades, which has resulted in updates being made to its anti-doping policies and practices. However, while multiple whistleblowing platforms have been introduced by the CADF, limited attention has been afforded towards establishing and implementing robust whistleblowing policies and practices alongside these. Establishing robust policies would demonstrate that the UCI is serious about breaking cycling's omerta culture and committed to supporting and facilitating whistleblowing on doping. In turn, this would likely increase individuals' willingness to report suspected doping in the sport and, eventually, create a truly transparent cycling culture. Critically, the significance of the wider cycling community cannot be overlooked in this context. Cyclists are only one of many key actors (e.g. coaches, trainers, managers, sponsors, etc.) that collectively constitute the 'cycling community'. Therefore, in order for cycling to truly move beyond its doping past, a concerted effort from all relevant stakeholders will be required. The UCI is therefore tasked with designing and disseminating whistleblowing education and resources to all relevant parties in the cycling community and helping them recognise and accept their personal responsibility to contribute towards this change. That said, changing a culture takes time, especially when it is a well-established culture involving many agents of influence, as is the case in cycling. It will not happen overnight but, hopefully the insights provided in this chapter can serve as a catalyst towards experiencing this evolution in the sport of cycling.

Note

1 The WADA's Speak Up! platform (WADA, 2017) and Whistleblower Program (WADA, 2016) now outline WADA's policy and procedures for addressing whistleblowing cases *specifically* reported to them.

References

Ash, L. (2016, 30 December). Yuliya Stepanova: What do Russians think of doping whistleblower? Retrieved from www.bbc.com/news/magazine-38406627

Axon, R. (2016a, 15 August). Russian whistleblower fears for her safety after account hacked. *USA Today*. Retrieved from www.usatoday.com/story/sports/olympics/rio-2016/2016/08/15/russian-whistleblower-yuliya-stepanova-email-hacked-fears-for-her-safety/88772528/

Axon, R. (2016b, 26 July). IOC decision on Russian whistleblower baffling. *USA Today*. Retrieved from www.usatoday.com/story/sports/olympics/rio-2016/2016/07/26/ioc-decision-russian-whistleblower-/87566562/

Baron, S.J.F. (2013). Inaction speaks louder than words: The problems of passivity. *Business Horizons*, 56(3), 301–311.

Berry, B. (2004). Organizational culture: A framework and strategies for facilitating employee whistle-blowing. *Employee Responsibilities and Rights Journal*, 16(1), 1–11.

Bjørkelo, B., Einarsen, S., & Matthiesen, S.B. (2010). Predicting proactive behaviour at work: exploring the role of personality as an antecedent of whistleblowing behaviour. *Journal of Occupational & Organizational Psychology*, 83(2), 371–394.

CADF. (2017). Report Doping. Retrieved from www.cadf.ch/intelligence/

Caillier, J.G. (2017). An examination of the role whistle-blowing education plays in the whistle-blowing process. *The Social Science Journal*, 54(1), 4–12.

Cho, Y.J. & Song, H.J. (2015). Determinants of whistleblowing within government agencies. *Public Personnel Management*, 44(4), 450–472.

CIRC. (2015). *Cycling Independent Reform Commission: Report to the president of the union cycliste internationale*. Retrieved from www.uci.ch/mm/Document/News/CleanSport/16/87/99/CIRCReport2015_Neutral.pdf

Culiberg, B. & Mihelic, K.K. (2017). The evolution of whistelblowing studies: A critical review and research agenda. *Journal of Business Ethics*, 146(4), 787–803.

Dasgupta, S. & Kesharwani, A. (2010). Whistleblowing: a survey of literature. *The IUP Journal of Corporate Governance*, IX(4).

De Maria, W. (2006). Brother secret, sister silence: Sibling conspiracies against managerial integrity. *Journal of Business Ethics*, 65, 219–234.

Dungan, J., Waytz, A., & Young, L. (2015). The psychology of whistleblowing. *Current Opinion in Psychology*, 6, 129–133.

Erickson, K., Backhouse, S.H., & Carless, D. (2017). 'I don't know if I would report them': Student-athletes' thoughts, feelings and anticipated behaviours on blowing the whistle on doping in sport. *Psychology of Sport and Exercise*, 30, 45–54.

Fincoeur, B., Van de Ven, K., & Mulrooney, K. (2014). The symbiotic evolution of anti-doping and supply chains of doping substances: How criminal networks may benefit from anti-doping policy. *Trends in Organized Crime*, 17, 1–22.

Fotaki, M., Kenny, K., & Scriver, S. (2015). Whistleblowing and mental health: A new weapon for retaliation? In D. Lewis & W. Vandekerckhove (Eds), *Developments in*

Whistleblowing Research 2015. London: International Whistleblowing Research Network.

Georgiadis, E. & Papazoglou, I. (2014). The experience of competition ban following a positive doping sample of elite athletes. *Journal of Clinical Sport Psychology*, 8(1), 57–74.

Geva, A. (2006). A typology of moral problems in business: A framework for ethical management. *Journal of Business Ethics*, 69(2), 133–147.

Grohmann, K. (2016, 20 August). Any dangers to whisleblower Stepanova not an IOC issue. *Reuters*. Retrieved from www.reuters.com/article/us-olympics-rio-stepanova-idUSKCN10V0Q4

Gundlach, M.J., Douglas, S.C., & Martinko, M.J. (2003). The decision to blow the whistle: A social information processing framework. *Academy of Management Review*, *28*(1), 107–123.

Gundlach, M.J., Martinko, M.J., & Douglas, S.C. (2008). A new approach to examining whistle-blowing: The influence of cognitions and anger. *SAM Advanced Management Journal*, 40–50.

Harris, N. (2017, 14 January). Grigory Rodchenkov is the man at the centre of Russia's state-sponsored doping plot who could this week become Putin's Public Enemy No 1. *Daily Mail*. Retrieved from www.dailymail.co.uk/sport/othersports/article-4120694/Grigory-Rodchenkov-man-centre-Russia-s-state-sponsored-doping-plot-week-Putin-s-Public-Enemy-No-1.html

Hermandorfer, W.D. (2015). Blown coverage: Tackling the law's failure to protect athlete-whistleblowers. *Virginia Sports & Entertainment Law Journal*, *14*(2), 250–276.

James, R. (2014, 17 December). Russian doping whistleblowers 'have more proof'. *Agence France Presse*. Retrieved from http://sports.yahoo.com/news/russian-doping-whistleblowers-more-proof-205417947-spt.html

Kaptein, M. (2011). From inaction to external whistleblowing: The influence of the ethical culture of organizations on employee responses to observed wrongdoing. *Journal of Business Ethics*, 98(3), 513–530.

Keenan, J.P. (2000). Blowing the whistle on less serious forms of fraud: A study of executives and managers. *Employee Responsibilities and Rights Journal*, *12*(4), 199–217.

Kimmage, P. (2017, 22 December). Half a century on from Simpson's death, cycling's omerta still rules in the peloton. *Ireland Independent*. Retrieved from www.independent.ie/sport/other-sports/cycling/paul-kimmage-half-a-century-on-from-simpsons-death-cyclings-omerta-still-rules-in-the-peloton-35957750.html

King, G. & Hermodson, A. (2000). Peer reporting of coworker wrongdoing: A qualitative analysis of observer attitudes in the decision to report versus not report unethical behavior. *Journal of Applied Communication Research*, *28*(4), 309–329.

Kramer, A. (2016, 15 February). Nikita Kamayeu, Ex-Head of Russian Antidoping Agency, Dies. *New York Times*. Retrieved from www.nytimes.com/2016/02/16/world/europe/nikita-kamayev-ex-head-of-russian-antidoping-agency-dies.html

Laser, T. (2015). Doping in cycling: Incentivizing the reporting of UCI anti-doping rules violations through organizational oversight and accountability. *John Marshall Law Review*, 49(2).

Lentillon-Kaestner, V., Hagger, M., & Hardcastle, S. (2011). Health and doping in elite-level cycling. *Scandinavian Journal of Medicine and Science in Sports*, *22*(5), 596–606.

Lewis, D. & Vandekerckhove, W. (2015). *Developments in Whistleblowing Research 2015*. London: International Whistleblowing Research Network.

McGlynn, J. & Richardson, B.K. (2014). Private support, public alienation: Whistle-blowers and the paradox of social support. *Western Journal of Communication*, *78*(2), 213–237.

Mesmer-Magnus, J.R. & Viswesvaran, C. (2005). Whistleblowing in organizations: An examination of correlates of whistleblowing intentions, actions and retaliation. *Journal of Business Ethics*, *62*(3), 277–297.

Miceli, M.P. & Near, J.P. (1985). Characteristics of organizational climate and perceived wrongdoing associated with whistle-blowing decisions. *Personnel Psychology*, *38*(3), 525–544.

Miceli, M.P. & Near, J.P. (1988). Individual and situational correlates of whistle-blowing. *Personnel Psychology*, *41*, 267–281.

Miceli, M.P. & Near, J.I. (1992). *Blowing the Whistle: The Organizational and Legal Implications for Companies and Employees*. New York: Lexington Books.

Miceli, M.P., Near, J.P., & Dworkin, T.M. (2009). A word to the wise: How managers and policy-makers can encourage employees to report wrongdoing. *Journal of Business Ethics*, *86*(3), 379–396.

Miceli, M.P., Near, J.I., & Schwenk, C. (1991). Who blows the whistle and why? *Industrial and Labor Relations Review*, *45*(1), 113–130.

Near, J.P. & Miceli, M. (1985). Organizational dissidence: The case of whistle-blowing. *Journal of Business Ethics*, *4*(1), 1–16.

Near, J.I. & Miceli, M. (1995). Effective whistle-blowing. *Academy of Management Review*, *20*(3), 679–708.

Ohl, F., Fincoeur, B., Lentillon-Kaestner, V., Defrance, J. & Brissonneau, C. (2015). The socialization of young cyclists and the culture of doping. *International Review for the Sociology of Sport*, *50*(7), 865–882.

O'Shea, S. (2014, 8 January). UCI announces Cycling Independent Reform Commission. *Cycling News*. Retrieved from www.cyclingnews.com/about/

O'Sullivan, P. & Ngau, O. (2014). Whistleblowing: a critical philosophical analysis of the component moral decisions of the act and some new perspectives on its moral significance. *Business Ethics: A European Review*, *23*(4), 401–415.

Rennie, S.C. & Crosby, J.R. (2002). Ethics. Students' perceptions of whistle blowing: implications for self-regulation. A questionnaire and focus group survey. *Medical Education*, *36*(2), 173–179.

Richardson, B.K. & McGlynn, J. (2011). Rabid fans, death threats, and dysfunctional stakeholders: The influence of organizational and industry contexts on whistle-blowing cases. *Management Communication Quarterly*, *25*(1), 121–150.

Richardson, B.K. & McGlynn, J. (2015). Blowing the whistle off the field of play: An empirical model of whistle-blower experiences in the intercollegiate sport industry. *Communication & Sport*. doi:10.1177/2167479513517490

Shipley, A. (2013, 6 April). Baseball Starts Playing Hardball in South Florida Doping Probe. *Sun Sentinel*. Retrieved from http://articles.sun-sentinel.com/2013-04-06/news/fl-mlb-drug-probe-20130407_1_usada-lance-armstrong-u-s-anti-doping-agency

Stokes, D. (2017, 30 November). Doping whistleblower Grigory Rodchenkov urges Russia to come clean. *CNN*. Retrieved from www.cnn.com/2017/11/29/sport/russia-doping-whistleblower-grigory-rodchenkov-winter-olympics-ioc/index.html

Taunton, J. (2011). *PEDs Pose Significant Health Risk for Athletes, Children and Youth Final Report of the Task Force on the Use of Performance Enhancing Drugs in Football*. Report to the Canadian Centre for Ethics in Sport. Retrieved from http://cces.ca/sites/default/files/content/docs/pdf/cces-taskforcefootballfinalreport-e-web.pdf

Teo, H. & Caspersz, D. (2011). Dissenting discourse: Exploring alternatives to the whistleblowing/silence dichotomy. *Journal of Business Ethics*, *104*, 237–249.

Trevino, L.K. & Weaver, G.R. (2003). *Managing Ethics in Business Organizations: Social Scientific Perspectives*. Stanford: Stanford University Press.

Tsvetkova, M. & Strohecker, K. (2015, 20 November). Branded a traitor, Russian sports whistleblower hides abroad. *Reuters*. Retrieved from www.reuters.com/article/us-athletics-corruption-whistleblower/branded-a-traitor-russian-sports-whistleblower-hides-abroad-idUSKCN0T91PL20151120

UCI (2015a). New UCI Anti-Doping Rules introduced to reflect 2015 World Anti-Doping Code and further strengthen cycling's anti-doping procedures [Press release]. Retrieved from www.uci.ch/pressreleases/new-uci-anti-doping-rules-introduced-reflect-2015-world-anti-doping-code-and-further-strengthen-cycling-anti-doping-procedures/

UCI (2015b). Anti-Doping Rules. Retrieved from www.uci.ch/mm/Document/News/Rulesandregulation/16/85/60/20161216UCIADRPart14-FINALversionenligne2016.12.16_English.pdf

USADA (2012). *Report on the Proceedings Under the World Anti-Doping Code and the USADA Protocol*. Retrieved from https://d3epuodzu3wuis.cloudfront.net/ReasonedDecision.pdf

Uys, T. (2008). Rational loyalty and whistleblowing: The South African context. *Current Sociology*, *56*(6), 904–921.

Uys, T. & Senekal, A. (2008). Morality of principle versus morality of loyalty: The case of whistleblowing. *African Journal of Business Ethics*, *3*(1), 38–44.

Vadera, A.K., Aguilera, R.V., & Caza, B.B. (2009). Making sense of whistle-blowing's antecedents: Learning from research on identity and ethics programs. *Business Ethics Quarterly*, *19*(4), 553–583.

Vandekerckhove, W. (2006). *Whistleblowing and Organizational Social Responsibility: A Global Assessment*: Ashgate.

Vandekerckhove, W. & Phillips, A. (2017). Whistleblowing as a protracted process. A study of UK whistleblower journeys. *Journal of Business Ethics*, 1–19.

WADA (2015). World Anti-Doping Code. Retrieved from www.wada-ama.org/sites/default/files/resources/files/wada-2015-world-anti-doping-code.pdf

WADA (2016). Whistleblowing Program. Retrieved from www.wada-ama.org/sites/default/files/whistleblowingprogram_policy_procedure_en.pdf

WADA (2017). Speak Up! Retrieved from https://speakup.wada-ama.org/WebPages/Public/FrontPages/Default.aspx

Waldron, T. (2017, 15 December). Russian Olympic Doping Whistleblower Fears Putin Will Retaliate Against His Family. *Huffington Post*. Retrieved from www.huffingtonpost.com/entry/grigory-rodchenkov-russia-doping-putin_us_5a27193ee4b0c2117626922d

Walker, S. (2017, 17 November). Russian Olympic official says doping whistleblower should be executed. *Guardian*. Retrieved from www.theguardian.com/sport/2017/nov/17/russian-olympic-official-says-doping-whistleblower-should-be-executed

Whitaker, L., Backhouse, S.H., & Long, J. (2014). Reporting doping in sport: National level athletes' perceptions of their role in doping prevention. *Scandinavian Journal of Medicine & Science in Sports*, *24*, 515–521.

Winneker, J. (2016). It's time to blow the whistle on performance enhancing drugs in sport. *Lewis & Clark Law Review*, *20*(1), 55–90.

Chapter 11

Performance data to improve cycling's credibility?

Raphaël Faiss and Martial Saugy

Athletes fight for glory and produce a spectacle that experts are eager to dissect. While true performance is often a result of hard work to overcome one self, doping beyond any accepted ergogenic aid represents a common shortcut (Fitch, 2012; Wagner, 1991). Performance production is dense like never before with many very close competitors; sometimes disappointing spectators expecting dramatic failures. In that context, cheaters try to be stronger, reach higher, and be faster by all possible means.

In the current globalised digital world, where seemingly every step is accounted for, monitoring (race or training) performance helps objectifying successes and failures (Jobson, Passfield, Atkinson, Barton, & Scarf, 2009; Passfield, Hopker, Jobson, Friel & Zabala, 2017). Experts and scientists have gathered performance data for decades to better understand the mechanisms underlying performance production (Borresen & Lambert, 2009; Faria, Parker & Faria, 2005a; Sweeting, Cormack, Morgan & Aughey, 2017). Still, the best indicator of performance capacity is performance itself, especially when monitoring instruments can display ones' physical performance as it occurs. Such information may help athletes maintain a better health, but also allow abnormal performances to be flagged. Athletes who misuse doping substances often seek physiological changes that improve their performance (Morente-Sanchez & Zabala, 2013).

The Athlete's Biological Passport (ABP) was invented to thwart athletes using prohibited substances identical to those naturally produced by the human body (Sottas, Robinson, Rabin, & Saugy, 2011). Since its progressive implementation with the longitudinal and personalised assessment of biomarkers of doping, the APB has become a strong tool for the indirect detection of doping (in blood) (Saugy, Lundby, & Robinson, 2014; Zorzoli, Pipe, Garnier, Vouillamoz, & Dvorak, 2014).

While doping alters biomarkers measured in the ABP, exercise training is also known to influence these same parameters (Bouchard, 2015). Conversely, variation in biomarkers observed in the ABP may coincide with improving (or declining) athletic performance. Numerous studies have associated variations in biological parameters to performance alterations as either explaining variables or confounding factors. For example, endurance sports rely essentially on aerobic energy production (i.e. with oxygen). At the same time, maximal oxygen consumption is highly related to the athlete's total haemoglobin mass. Indeed, several analytical approaches allow modelling of performance capacity precisely from work capacity for certain sports (Busso, 2003; Calvert, Banister, Savage, & Bach, 1976; Mujika, Padilla, Pyne, & Busso, 2004).

To our knowledge, the ABP has been subject of more than 90 studies to date published in peer-reviewed scientific publications. From its emergence through a pilot project with the International Cycling Union (UCI) in 2008 (Zorzoli & Rossi, 2010), the ABP includes a haematological module introduced officially in December 2009 aiming to identify enhancement of oxygen transport and any form of blood transfusion or manipulation (Schumacher, Saugy, Pottgiesser, & Robinson, 2012). A steroidal module was additionally introduced in January 2014 aiming to identify endogenous anabolic androgenic steroids when administered exogenously and other anabolic agents (Sottas, Saugy, & Saudan, 2010). Besides, experts recently created a working group to implement the 2015 World Anti-Doping Code that clearly includes the ABP and confounding factors in the strategy of its implementation (Dvorak et al., 2014). It is thus noteworthy to underline the current widespread acceptance of the ABP as a valuable tool for the indirect detection of doping.

Very interestingly, from the official 2015 ABP guidelines, the term passport refers indeed not only to a longitudinal profile of the athlete's haematological markers but also 'includes all other relevant information also comprising training and competition results' (Vernec, 2014). The inclusion of performance models (including competition results and training contents) to support the ABP are hence formally fulfilled. In other words, the ABP is not limited to the longitudinal analysis of multiparametric biomarkers present in biological samples but should also include its confounding factors and other parameters like performance. However, the implementation of performance data to complement the ABP still represents a challenge (Hopker et al., 2018; Iljukov & Schumacher, 2017; Menaspa & Abbiss, 2017).

Nevertheless, the inclusion of performance in the ABP opens the door for what can be called a 'performance passport', which can complement the ABP approach.

To date, a thorough analysis of training content or athletes' performance has never been done specifically for this purpose. Such an analysis presents challenges, including identifying relevant variables and gathering sufficient data for a properly valid analysis. It is thus a first priority to define the kind of performance that should be monitored and evaluated in such a 'performance passport'.

For instance, many studies have investigated performance determinants and variations related to training content, especially in endurance sports. In addition, several attempts to develop mathematical models describing human performance and its physiology have been made with some interesting achievements for running (McLaughlin, Howley, Bassett, Thompson, & Fitzhugh, 2010; Peronnet & Thibault, 1989; Tokmakidis, Leger, Mercier, Peronnet, & Thibault, 1987; Ward-Smith, 1985; Ward-Smith & Mobey, 1995).

Historically, even though physiological mechanisms underlying athletic performance have been described earlier, the pioneer contribution of Monod and Scherrer defined a linear relationship between the time to exhaustion and total work performed (Monod & Scherrer, 1965) to introduce a concept of critical power (CP). The asymptotic inversely proportional relationship between time to exhaustion and work rate was then inceptively introduced in 1973 at the Second International Symposium on Biochemistry of Exercise (Magglingen, Switzerland) (Howald & Poortmans, 1975). A further milestone was then set with the mathematical modelling of world records in running by Perronet and Thibault to investigate athletic performance towards a reference value (Peronnet & Thibault, 1989; Peronnet, Thibault, Rhodes, & Mckenzie, 1987). The latter finally led Grappe and Pinot to allow the computation of an objective measure of performance in cycling (i.e. mechanical power) to assess performance in cyclists with a 'record power profile' (Pinot & Grappe, 2011, 2015).

For instance, the record power profile is now often integrated in the monitoring of elite cyclists (Pinot & Grappe, 2015). However, the longitudinal utilisation of cycling power data cannot be simplified with a unique reference measurement of performance (Jobson, Passfield, Atkinson, Barton, & Scarf, 2009; Menaspa & Abbiss, 2017; Passfield, Hopker, Jobson, Friel, & Zabala, 2017). Still, a record power profile may yield interesting data complementary to assessments of critical power or maximal mean power (Menaspa & Abbiss, 2017).

Relevant models have also been proposed to determine the relationship between training and performance in endurance athletes (Busso, 2003; Millet et al., 2002). Exercise training is definitely the common way to improve performance capacity. Doping may then obviously influence either performance directly or training capacity. The application of the ABP as a strategy to indirectly detect doping highlights the association between performance and biological markers that may in turn also be influenced (in a certain physiological range) by training (Figure 11.1).

Interestingly, in cycling, physiological variables in connection with training and factors affecting performance have been widely described both for endurance (Faria et al., 2005a; Faria, Parker & Faria, 2005b) and resistance training (Yamamoto et al., 2010). Moreover, studies have been able to describe determinants of cycling performance in major competitions by means of cycling power output analysis (Vogt et al., 2006; Vogt et al., 2007, 2007b). The physiological demands in cycling can also be described in different racing situations and at different competitive levels (Abbiss, Menaspa, Villerius, & Martin, 2013; Menaspa, Abbiss, & Martin, 2013; Menaspa, Quod, Martin, Peiffer, & Abbiss, 2015). Cycling power meters have undeniably emerged as an almost necessary tool for cyclists in training and racing during the past decade.

Interestingly, the whole conception of a longitudinal monitoring of performance in cycling relies on the validity of the objective measurement of the athlete's mechanical power produced in the field. In cycling, power reflects the

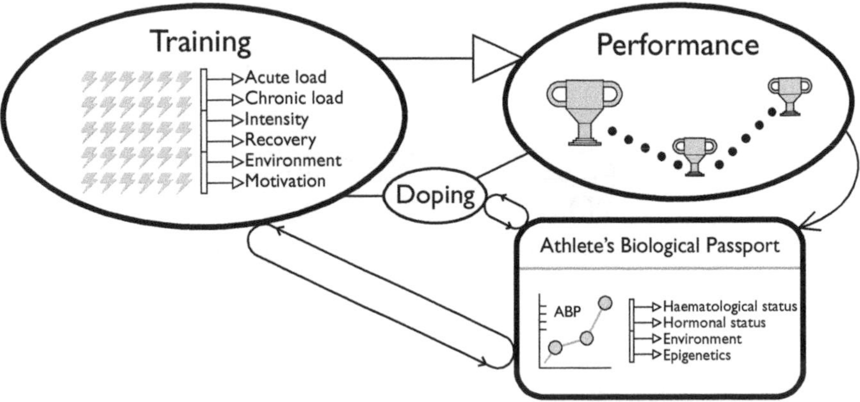

Figure 11.1 Relationship between training and performance (potentially altered by doping) with an unknown yet probable association of variables measured during training and biomarkers of the Athlete's Biological Passport.

force applied at the pedals to overcome resistive forces opposed to forward motion. Mechanical power is currently measured most accurately with computation of torque being applied on the cranks (measured with strain gauges) and angular velocity. From its original development with the patent for the first 'spider-based' power meter submitted by Ulrich Schoberer in 1986 (SRM, Schoberer Rad-Messtechnik, Jülich, Germany), devices allowing mechanical power to be recored have been subject to rapid and continuous development in the last decade. In parallel to the further development of the SRM, several other power meters have gone through a (not necessarily successful) scientific validation process (Bertucci, Duc, Villerius, Pernin, & Grappe, 2005; Duc, Villerius, Bertucci, & Grappe, 2007; Gordon, Franklin, Davies, & Baker, 2007; Granier, Hausswirth, Dorel, & Yann, 2017; Hurst & Atkins, 2006; Nimmerichter, Schnitzer, Prinz, Simon, & Wirth, 2017; Sparks, Dove, Bridge, Midgely, & McNaughton, 2015). The rapid market expansion to recreational cyclist has seen the emergence of a multitude of different systems measuring cycling power output. Depending on device brand, mechanical power is mostly measured by strain gauges at the crankset, crank, chain ring, pedal, or cog level thus reflecting the intensity of the effort produced by the cyclist while pedalling. For instance, eight different devices were used in UCI World Tour Teams (Figure 11.2), illustrating the current variety of sources to record mechanical power in professional cyclists.

While one can question the accuracy of the measurement with manufacturers often claiming a measurement error below 2%, athletes' and trainers' feedback support a fair reliability of the devices. The SRM was considered as a Gold Standard for a long time (especially in its 'science' version with most strain

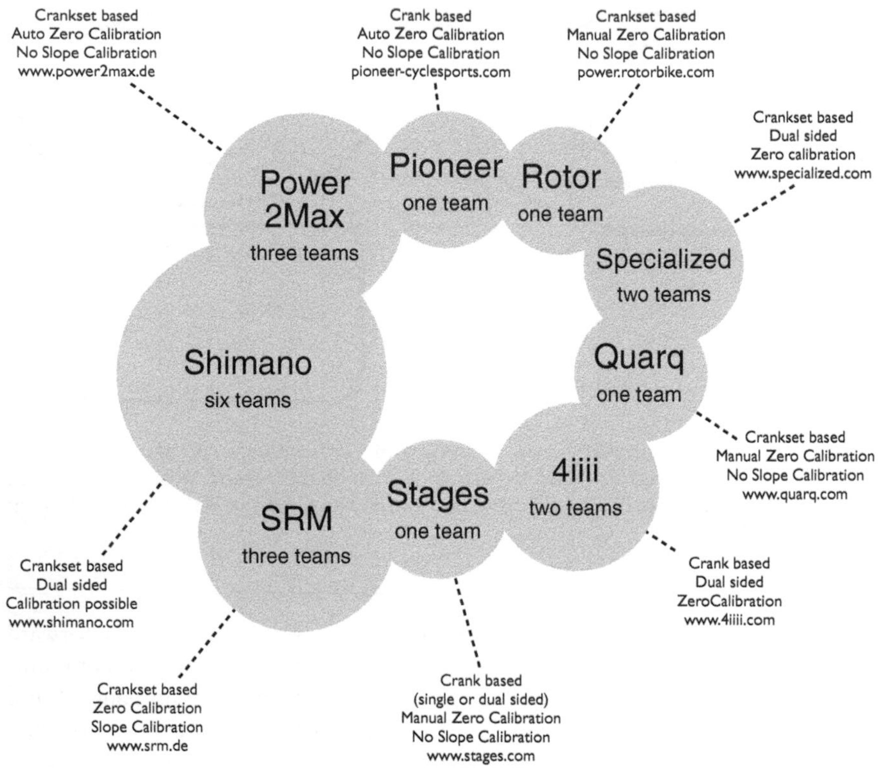

Figure 11.2 **Illustration of different power meter brands in use by first division professional cycling teams in 2018 with principal characteristics.**

gauges). One important factor is certainly the ability to calibrate properly each single mobile power meter (or sometimes even called ergometre) to ensure simultaneously a high accuracy (is the recorded value the 'true' power?), high precision (is the recorded value reproducible with the exact same conditions applied?). In addition, the concept of bias refers to the difference between the mean of the measurements and true or reference value (Walther & Moore, 2005).

In this context, a scientific evaluation and comparison of power meters (54 from nine different brands) in use by professional and elite cyclists allowed a valuable analysis of their accuracy and precision (Maier, Schmid, Muller, Steiner, & Wehrlin, 2017). While mean deviation ('trueness') was in average less than 1%, coefficients of variation of the power meters were 1.2% with >10% of the devices deviating by more than 5%. Maier et al. (2017) conclude that 'current power meters used by elite and recreational cyclists vary considerably in their trueness; precision is generally high but differs between manufacturers'.

The importance of a proper calibration procedure is underlined with both a proper 'zero calibration' (when no torque is being applied) and 'slope calibration' (increment of torque effectively measured when more forces are being applied to the cranks).

The latter highlights the impossibility to directly use standalone data for a thorough interpretation of when data are recorded without knowledge of the accuracy and precision of each single device mounted on each single bicycle. Broadcasting live power outputs of riders during races originating from uncalibrated sensors is hence questionable, also because such values require sufficient knowledge for a proper interpretation by commentators. Nevertheless, the widespread use of such power meters offers a great opportunity to gather training and racing data for further analyses because such devices become more reliable with time. At this stage, gathering properly standardised and accurate data remains a complicated challenge. Then, identifying if certain data reflects maximal effort capacity is the next obstacle (Abbiss et al., 2013). Do we imagine the blackboard official at the Tour de France showing Borg scales to the riders on his motorcycle to record their perceived exertion?

Instead, many markers measured in the ABP (e.g. haematocrit, haemoglobin, cortisol, testosterone, insulin, interleukins, among others) have been shown to be altered by exercise (Hill et al., 2008; Leal et al., 2006; Novosadova, 1977) (and not only by doping). If training can thus be precisely monitored with properly recorded power output data, it would be of particular interest to test any influence of training content (and thus performance profile) on selected markers from the ABP to determine putative concomitant variations.

These variations may be linked with differences in performance levels seen during training or races. Since power meters seem to record mechanical power with a consistent reproducibility, variations in power output values would yield a satisfactory interpretation of performance variations computed from precise (while maybe biased) sensors. Then doping behaviours could be better targeted from specifically selected biomarkers in connection with performance variations. However, to date, there is no conclusive evidence highlighting associations between variations in the ABP and performance changes in competitive athletes. An evolution of the ABP with new biomarkers that can be related to performance would thus represent an attractive strategy for indirect detection of the use of doping substances or methods (Menaspa & Abbiss, 2017).

With the emergence of new research fields in human biology (i.e. 'omics' approaches), a personalised longitudinal assessment of each athlete's system biology is feasible where systemic performance would yield as an additional confounding variable (Kuster, Merkus, van der Velden, Verhoeven, & Duncker, 2011).

In conclusion, understanding performance in cycling is very complex, and targeting abnormal performance even more. The prestige of the monuments of cycling or the visibility of the Grand Tour races entice many athletes to work hard to reach an optimal fitness level. Because pain is temporary but glory forever, doping behaviours represent a recurrent shortcut. The introduction of the ABP in cycling certainly helped deter blood doping practices while cheaters may have adjusted their doping practices meanwhile to avoid being flagged due to abnormal haematological values. Exercise physiologists have in parallel constantly contributed to improve the understanding of performance production in cycling with regards to exercise training and modelling of mechanical power distribution during efforts, for example. The progress of the ABP with the addition of new biomarkers (e.g. from 'omics' technologies) could help defining links with performance variations. Proper acquisition and standardisation of performance data with adequate modelling may finally help experts in their longitudinal concomitant interpretation of cyclists' haematological, biological, and performance profiles.

Finally, systematic scientific approaches could help tightening the net for counterfeiters. Real winners never cheat and cheaters never really win ...

References

Abbiss, C.R., Menaspa, P., Villerius, V., & Martin, D.T. (2013). Distribution of power output when establishing a breakaway in cycling. *Int. J. Sports Physiol. Perform.*, *8*(4), 452–455.

Bertucci, W., Duc, S., Villerius, V., Pernin, J.N., & Grappe, F. (2005). Validity and reliability of the PowerTap mobile cycling powermeter when compared with the SRM Device. *Int. J. Sports Med.*, *26*(10), 868–873.

Borresen, J. & Lambert, M.I. (2009). The quantification of training load, the training response and the effect on performance. *Sports Med.*, 39(9), 779–795.

Bouchard, C. (2015). Adaptation to acute and regular exercise: From reductionist approaches to integrative biology. *Prog. Mol. Biol. Transl. Sci.*, *135*, 1–15.

Busso, T. (2003). Variable dose-response relationship between exercise training and performance. *Med. Sci. Sports Exerc.*, *35*(7), 1188–1195.

Calvert, T., Banister, E.W., Savage, M.V., & Bach, T. (1976). A systems model of the effects of training on physical performance. *IEEE Transactions on Systems, Man, and Cybernetics*, SMC-6(2), 94–102.

Duc, S., Villerius, V., Bertucci, W., & Grappe, F. (2007). Validity and reproducibility of the ErgomoPro power meter compared with the SRM and Powertap power meters. *Int. J. Sports Physiol. Perform.*, *2*(3), 270–281.

Dvorak, J., Baume, N., Botre, F., Broseus, J., Budgett, R., Frey, W.O., ... Zorzoli, M. (2014). Time for change: a roadmap to guide the implementation of the World Anti-Doping Code 2015. *Br. J. Sports Med.*, *48*(10), 801–806.

Faria, E.W., Parker, D.L., & Faria, I.E. (2005a). The science of cycling: factors affecting performance – part 2. *Sports Med.*, *35*(4), 313–337.

Faria, E.W., Parker, D.L., & Faria, I.E. (2005b). The science of cycling: physiology and training – part 1. *Sports Med.*, *35*(4), 285–312.

Fitch, K. (2012). Proscribed drugs at the Olympic Games: permitted use and misuse (doping) by athletes. *Clin. Med. (Lond)*, *12*(3), 257–260.

Gordon, R.S., Franklin, K.L., Davies, B., & Baker, J.S. (2007). Further mechanical considerations between polar and SRM mobile ergometer systems during laboratory-based high-intensity, intermittent cycling activity. *Res. Sports Med.*, *15*(4), 241–247.

Granier, C., Hausswirth, C., Dorel, S., & Yann, L.M. (2017). Validity and reliability of the stages cycling power meter. *J. Strength Cond. Res.* doi:10.1519/JSC.0000000000002189

Hill, E.E., Zack, E., Battaglini, C., Viru, M., Viru, A., & Hackney, A.C. (2008). Exercise and circulating cortisol levels: the intensity threshold effect. *J. Endocrinol. Invest.*, *31*(7), 587–591.

Hopker, J., Schumacher, Y.O., Fedoruk, M., Mørkeberg, J., Bermon, S., Iljukov, S., ... Sottas, P.E. (2018). Athlete performance monitoring in anti-doping. *Front Physiol.*, in press. doi:10.3389/fphys.2018.00232

Howald, H., & Poortmans, J.R. (1975). *Metabolic Adaptation to Prolonged Physical Exercise* (Springer Basel AG ed.). Basel: Birkhäuser.

Hurst, H.T., & Atkins, S. (2006). Agreement between polar and SRM mobile ergometer systems during laboratory-based high-intensity, intermittent cycling activity. *J. Sports Sci.*, *24*(8), 863–868.

Iljukov, S. & Schumacher, Y.O. (2017). Performance profiling-perspectives for anti-doping and beyond. *Front Physiol.*, 8, 1102.

Jobson, S.A., Passfield, L., Atkinson, G., Barton, G., & Scarf, P. (2009). The analysis and utilization of cycling training data. *Sports Medicine*, 39(10), 833–844.

Kuster, D.W., Merkus, D., van der Velden, J., Verhoeven, A.J., & Duncker, D.J. (2011). 'Integrative Physiology 2.0': integration of systems biology into physiology and its application to cardiovascular homeostasis. *J. Physiol.*, 589(Pt 5), 1037–1045.

Leal, L.K., Costa, M.F., Pitombeira, M., Barroso, V.M., Silveira, E.R., Canuto, K.M., & Viana, G.S. (2006). Mechanisms underlying the relaxation induced by isokaempferide from Amburana cearensis in the guinea-pig isolated trachea. *Life Sci.*, *79*(1), 98–104.

Maier, T., Schmid, L., Muller, B., Steiner, T., & Wehrlin, J.P. (2017). Accuracy of cycling power meters against a mathematical model of treadmill cycling. *Int. J. Sports Med.*, *38*(6), 456–461.

McLaughlin, J.E., Howley, E.T., Bassett, D.R., Jr., Thompson, D.L., & Fitzhugh, E.C. (2010). Test of the classic model for predicting endurance running performance. *Med. Sci. Sports Exerc.*, *42*(5), 991–997.

Menaspa, P. & Abbiss, C.R. (2017). Considerations on the assessment and use of cycling performance metrics and their integration in the Athlete's Biological Passport. *Front Physiol.*, 8, 912.

Menaspa, P., Abbiss, C.R., & Martin, D.T. (2013). Performance analysis of a world-class sprinter during cycling grand tours. *Int. J. Sports Physiol. Perform.*, 8(3), 336–340.

Menaspa, P., Quod, M., Martin, D.T., Peiffer, J.J., & Abbiss, C.R. (2015). Physical demands of sprinting in professional road cycling. *Int. J. Sports Med.*, *36*(13), 1058–1062.

Millet, G.P., Candau, R.B., Barbier, B., Busso, T., Rouillon, J.D., & Chatard, J.C. (2002). Modelling the transfers of training effects on performance in elite triathletes. *Int. J. Sports Med.*, *23*(1), 55–63.

Monod, H. & Scherrer, J. (1965). The work capacity of a synergic muscular group. *Ergonomics*, 8(1–4), 329–338.

Morente-Sanchez, J. & Zabala, M. (2013). Doping in sport: A review of elite athletes' attitudes, beliefs, and knowledge. *Sports Medicine*, *43*(6), 395–411.

Mujika, I., Padilla, S., Pyne, D., & Busso, T. (2004). Physiological changes associated with the pre-event taper in athletes. *Sports Med.*, *34*(13), 891–927.

Nimmerichter, A., Schnitzer, L., Prinz, B., Simon, D., & Wirth, K. (2017). Validity and reliability of the Garmin vector power meter in laboratory and field cycling. *Int. J. Sports Med.*, *38*(6), 439–446.

Novosadova, J. (1977). The changes in hematocrit, hemoglobin, plasma volume and proteins during and after different types of exercise. *Eur. J. Appl. Physiol. Occup. Physiol.*, *36*(3), 223–230.

Passfield, L., Hopker, J. G., Jobson, S., Friel, D., & Zabala, M. (2017). Knowledge is power: Issues of measuring training and performance in cycling. *J. Sports Sci.*, *35*(14), 1426–1434.

Peronnet, F. & Thibault, G. (1989). Mathematical analysis of running performance and world running records. *J. Appl. Physiol. (1985)*, *67*(1), 453–465.

Peronnet, F., Thibault, G., Rhodes, E.C., & Mckenzie, D.C. (1987). Correlation between ventilatory threshold and endurance capability in marathon runners. *Medicine and Science in Sports and Exercise*, *19*(6), 610–615.

Pinot, J. & Grappe, F. (2011). The record power profile to assess performance in elite cyclists. *Int. J. Sports Med.*, *32*(11), 839–844.

Pinot, J. & Grappe, F. (2015). A six-year monitoring case study of a top-10 cycling Grand Tour finisher. *J. Sports Sci.*, *33*(9), 907–914.

Saugy, M., Lundby, C., & Robinson, N. (2014). Monitoring of biological markers indicative of doping: the athlete biological passport. *Br. J. Sports Med.*, *48*(10), 827-U127.

Schumacher, Y.O., Saugy, M., Pottgiesser, T., & Robinson, N. (2012). Detection of EPO doping and blood doping: the haematological module of the Athlete Biological Passport. *Drug Test Anal.*, *4*(11), 846–853.

Sottas, P.E., Robinson, N., Rabin, O., & Saugy, M. (2011). The athlete biological passport. *Clin. Chem.*, *57*(7), 969–976.

Sottas, P.E., Saugy, M., & Saudan, C. (2010). Endogenous steroid profiling in the athlete biological passport. *Endocrinol. Metab. Clin. North Am.*, *39*(1), 59–73, viii–ix.

Sparks, S.A., Dove, B., Bridge, C.A., Midgely, A.W., & McNaughton, L.R. (2015). Validity and reliability of the look Keo power pedal system for measuring power output during incremental and repeated sprint cycling. *Int. J. Sports Physiol. Perform.*, *10*(1), 39–45.

Sweeting, A.J., Cormack, S.J., Morgan, S., & Aughey, R.J. (2017). When is a sprint a sprint? A review of the analysis of team-sport athlete activity profile. *Front Physiol*, *8*.

Tokmakidis, S.P., Leger, L., Mercier, D., Peronnet, F., & Thibault, G. (1987). New approaches to predict VO2max and endurance from running performances. *J. Sports Med. Phys. Fitness*, *27*(4), 401–409.

Vernec, A.R. (2014). The Athlete Biological Passport: an integral element of innovative strategies in antidoping. *Br. J. Sports Med.*, *48*(10), 817–819.

Vogt, S., Heinrich, L., Schumacher, Y.O., Blum, A., Roecker, K., Dickhuth, H.H., & Schmid, A. (2006). Power output during stage racing in professional road cycling. *Med. Sci. Sports Exerc.*, *38*(1), 147–151.

Vogt, S., Schumacher, Y.O., Blum, A., Roecker, K., Dickhuth, H.H., Schmid, A., & Heinrich, L. (2007a). Cycling power output produced during flat and mountain stages in the Giro d'Italia: a case study. *J. Sports Sci.*, *25*(12), 1299–1305.

Vogt, S., Schumacher, Y.O., Roecker, K., Dickhuth, H.H., Schoberer, U., Schmid, A., & Heinrich, L. (2007b). Power output during the Tour de France. *Int. J. Sports Med.*, *28*(9), 756–761.

Wagner, J.C. (1991). Enhancement of athletic performance with drugs. An overview. *Sports Med.*, *12*(4), 250–265.

Walther, B.A. & Moore, J.L. (2005). The concepts of bias, precision and accuracy, and their use in testing the performance of species richness estimators, with a literature review of estimator performance. *Ecography*, *28*(6), 815–829.

Ward-Smith, A.J. (1985). A mathematical theory of running, based on the first law of thermodynamics, and its application to the performance of world-class athletes. *J. Biomech.*, *18*(5), 337–349.

Ward-Smith, A.J. & Mobey, A.C. (1995). Determination of physiological data from a mathematical analysis of the running performance of elite female athletes. *J. Sports Sci.*, *13*(4), 321–328.

Yamamoto, L.M., Klau, J.F., Casa, D.J., Kraemer, W.J., Armstrong, L.E., & Maresh, C.M. (2010). The effects of resistance training on road cycling performance among highly trained cyclists: a systematic review. *J. Strength Cond. Res.*, *24*(2), 560–566.

Zorzoli, M., Pipe, A., Garnier, P.Y., Vouillamoz, M., & Dvorak, J. (2014). Practical experience with the implementation of an athlete's biological profile in athletics, cycling, football and swimming. *Br. J. Sports Med.*, *48*(10), 862–866.

Zorzoli, M. & Rossi, F. (2010). Implementation of the biological passport: the experience of the International Cycling Union. *Drug Test Anal.*, *2*(11–12), 542–547.

Chapter 12

What might a partially relaxed anti-doping regime in professional cycling look like?

Bengt Kayser

The affair(s) of cycling with doping

The combination of the words cycling and doping resonates strongly. Cycling arguably was the sport most in the spotlight when anti-doping started to pick up momentum at the turn of the twentieth century. Contrary to popular belief at that time, this was not necessarily because it was the sport most concerned. Already the Canadian Dubin inquiry after the 'Ben Johnson affair' at the 1988 Seoul Olympics, but also the more recent 'scandals' around athletics and the presumably pervasive state-sanctioned doping in Russia would attest to that; cycling was, and is not alone (Dimeo & Møller, 2018).

Cycling played an important triggering role in the globalisation of anti-doping. The advent of the World Anti-Doping Association (WADA) in 1999 and its agenda of harmonisation and globalisation of anti-doping took place in the aftermath of the 'Festina affair', when during the 1998 *Tour de France* team-organised doping was discovered. After doping substances were found in the car of a Festina team member, the French minister of sport Marie-George Buffet ordered a strong-armed intervention, presumably because she considered the cyclists as vulnerable, manipulated and exploited workers that had to be protected from their employers and the (commercial) *Tour* organiser (Mignon, 2003). Team cars and hotel rooms were searched; riders and personnel were arrested. At one stage the riders stepped off their bikes and sat down asking 'to be left alone so that they could do their job'. Several teams were excluded; other teams and individual riders left the *Tour* on their own. This '*Tour of Shame*' led to high levels of visibility of doping in cycling with much echo in the media and strong calls for change, which eventually led to WADA's inception (Hanstad, Smith & Waddington, 2008; Hunt, 2017).

It was not the first time that the doping-in-cycling theme drew attention. The deaths of cyclists Knud Enemark Jensen at the 1960 Rome Olympics and Tom Simpson on the Mont Ventoux during the 1967 *Tour*, both likely from heat stroke, but allegedly also from amphetamines, had already triggered some moral outrage, but no serious anti-doping action (Kayser & Møller, 2018; Møller, 2005).

In cycling the use of substances seemingly always was more or less part of the game. Early last century the brothers Henri and Francis Pélissier did not make it a secret how they affronted the hardship of participating in the *Tour*. In the article 'The Slaves of the Road' in *Le Petit Parisien*, a journalist described the riders' dealings with their suffering. The brothers showed him cocaine and chloroform containing pills and phials and exclaimed: 'In short, we are running on dynamite!' (Mignon, 2003). Numerous are the accounts of cyclists such as Jacques Anquetil[1] who made it clear that such behaviour was part and parcel of the trade, even though in those times it had more to do with constraints on workers' freedoms and the *Tour*'s organiser's authoritarianism than with doping (Mignon, 2003). Over the second half of last century, in parallel with the increasing disapproval of doping in sport, however, the behaviour was progressively pushed into hiding. Even though it was a public secret that doping was quite prevalent, a system of 'omerta' made it difficult to circumscribe.

It follows from the above cursory history of doping in cycling,[2] what is today called 'clean' cycling, i.e. competing without the use of forbidden substances or methods, is something that is rather new to cycling. In a way a new sport is being invented, cycling without doping. I do not negate that there were, and are many cyclists who did/do not want to use doping, but I make the point that for a long time doping was part of cycling, and for much of its existence the *Tour*'s podium was occupied by cyclists we now know doped (de Mondenard, 2011).

There are arguments to be made in favour of changing the way professional cycling is organised. Even though there are many public cycling clubs, national cycling associations, and an overarching UCI,[3] major professional cycling competitions are largely for-profit private enterprises. The *Tour*, arguably the biggest cycling event in terms of visibility, has always been in the hands of private enterprise. It is organised by the *Société du Tour de France*, a subsidiary of the Amaury press group, with a multi-million Euro budget (Mignon, 2003). The winner receives several hundreds of thousands of Euros in prize money, while many of the cyclists ('domestiques') in the peloton only have one-season contracts and meager base salaries. The above mentioned Pélissier brothers thus have their heirs among today's cyclists, who can be considered workers under great pressure to perform. Sociologists Ohl, Aubel, and Brissoneau (2015) described the specific culture of professional cycling, illustrating how it plays an important role in how cyclists see and realise their profession (see also Ivan Waddington's chapter in this book). Continuing this strand of work, Aubel, Lefèvre, Le Goff, & Taverna (2018) did a quantitative analysis of ten years of data (2005–2016) of cyclists in the first three world divisions and looked at predictors for an ADRV.[4] Even though ADRVs likely represent only a fraction of the 'real' doping population (de Hon, Kuipers, & van Bottenburg, 2015; Elbe & Pitsch, 2018; Pielke, 2017) it does shed interesting light on who gets caught. Aubel et al. (2018) found that the riders caught were those with more precarious career paths, i.e. those who were vulnerable at some point in their career. There further was some indication that those who had started their career before

2005 were more likely to have an ADRV than those who started after 2008, suggesting some effect of the anti-doping measures introduced in the cycling world during that period (Aubel et al., 2018).

Doping practice in cycling today

If at the time of the 'Festina affair' doping was more or less organised at team-level, the increasing surveillance and testing density progressively forced it into hiding, and nowadays doping has become more a matter of the individual (Fincoeur, Frenger, & Pitsch, 2013) (see also Bertrand Fincoeur's chapter in this book). Even though it would seem certain that the type of doping behaviour has changed,[5] the prevalence of doping in cycling is unknown, because it is impossible to quantify reliably. No actively doping athlete will admit to doping when asked. Surveillance and testing are limited by control density (how often a cyclist is tested) and by what is being looked for (not all compounds are tested for and there are limits to what tests can find). Official WADA data suggest a 1–2% ADRV rate. Actual doping prevalence is likely much higher, depending on sport and country (de Hon et al., 2015; de Hon, 2016; Elbe & Pitsch, 2018; Pielke, 2017; Pitsch & Emrich, 2011; Striegel, Ulrich, & Simon, 2010) (see also Werner Pitsch's chapter in this book).

It therefore is plausible that the peloton is made up of cyclists who play the game keeping to the official anti-doping rule as well as cyclists who trick the system by using adapted methods of doping or 'borderline-doping' in order to remain under the radar of detection.

For example, one way to circumvent anti-doping regulations is by asking for a therapeutic use exemption (TUE), which is a medically justified use of some substance for an ailment. TUE's are notoriously abused. Similarly to reports from Denmark (Overbye & Wagner, 2013), a survey among French speaking athletes revealed that about half had low trust in TUE management, 47% suspected abuse by fellow athletes and 46% had refrained from medically justified treatment, illustrating the ambiguity of the TUE rule (Bourdon, Schoch, Broers, & Kayser, 2015). The recent admission of the retired Dutch cyclist Lieuwe Westra of his use of cortisone with a TUE for non-existent knee problems and his statement of the rifeness of this practice among his fellow cyclists[6] illustrates the difficulty of separating medical treatment from doping and confirms the suspicion formulated by the athletes who participated in the Bourdon et al. (2015) and Overby & Wagner (2013) studies (for discussion of TUEs see also Andrew Bloodworth's and John Gleaves's chapters in this book).

Overall it would seem that the efficacy of today's anti-doping policy is highly questionable (de Hon, 2016; Dimeo & Møller, 2018; Moston & Engelberg, 2017). Given the likely ongoing undiscovered doping among some of the athletes on the podium, ranking close to (and above!) athletes who do not dope, and the frequent problem of most likely innocent athletes being sanctioned (de Hon, 2016; Dimeo & Møller, 2018), today's anti-doping arguably has immoral side-effects (Kayser, 2018). Thus, current anti-doping policy, in its quest to attain its goal of celebrating 'clean' champions, misses its target, while it uses means that come with non-negligible costs. These costs are not just monetary but include (mostly unintended but important) side-effects. It follows that current anti-doping policy may be potentially introducing problems of greater impact than are solved (Kayser, 2018), a situation dubbed a major crisis by Dimeo and Møller (2018).

Time for a rethink?

Given the above description of a highly non-satisfactory state of current anti-doping it would seem justified to discuss alternative strategies for the incessant calls for more surveillance density and punitive measures based on a 'zero-tolerance' stance whose promise of eradication of doping would seem illusory. Already recognising this in the runup towards the 2008 Olympic games, the prime scientific journal *Nature* published an intriguing editorial called 'A Sporting Chance'. It first made the point that as long as the anti-doping rule is in place one should keep to it. It then followed with:

> 'But this does not preclude the idea that it may, in time, be necessary to readdress the rules themselves. As more is learned about how our bodies work, more options become available for altering those workings. To date, most of this alteration has sought to restore function to some sort of baseline. But it is also possible to enhance various functions into the supernormal realm, and the options for this are set to grow ever greater. The fact that such endeavors will carry risks should not be trivialised. But adults should be allowed to take risks, and experience suggests that they will do so when the benefits on offer are enticing enough. By the end of this century the unenhanced body or mind may well be vanishingly rare. As this change takes place, we will have to re-examine what we expect of athletes. If spectators are seeking to reset their body mass index through pharmacology, or taking pills that enhance their memory, is it really reasonable that athletes should make do with bodies that have not seen such benefits? The more the public comes to live with the mixed and risk-related benefits of enhancement, the more it will appreciate that allowing such changes need not rob sport of its drama, nor athletes of their need for skill, training, character and dedication. [...] The first sport to change its rules to allow players to use performance-enhancing drugs will be attacked as a freak show or worse. [...] Perhaps the Tour de France could show the way ahead here. In terms of public respect, endurance cycling has the least to lose and perhaps the most to gain. To be sure, a change in the rules would lead to the claim that 'the cheats have won'. But as no one can convincingly claim that cheats are not winning now, or have not been winning in the past, that claim is not quite the showstopper it might seem to be. A leadership ready to ride

> out the outrage might be better for the sport in the long run. If some viewers and advertisers were lost along the way, the Tour could console itself with the thought that it got by with far less commercial interest in days gone by – and that it is more likely to re-establish itself through excellence and honesty than in the penumbra of doubt and cynicism that surrounds it now'.
>
> (Editorial, 2007)

Even though this quote may seem startling to some, the line of reasoning was not new. At the time of the 'Festina affair' in 1998, even Juan Antonio Samaranch, president of the International Olympic Committee (IOC), already seemed to prefer a more practical approach,[7] but his voice was rapidly silenced in favour of a more principled one. WADA was then launched and the publication of the first version of its World Anti-Doping Code in 2003 triggered academic interest. Several scholars critiqued the direction taken by WADA and developed reasoning in favour of a relaxation of the anti-doping rule (e.g. Kayser, Mauron, & Miah, 2005; Kirkwood, 2009; Savulescu, Foddy, & Clayton, 2004). Together with colleagues I have contributed to the development of a framework for a change to anti-doping policy using a harm minimisation approach (Kayser, 2018). Tolleneer and I (Kayser & Tolleneer, 2017) analysed the arguments for and against the introduction of a partial relaxation of the anti-doping rule and the introduction of harm minimisation measures at the level of the athletes themselves, the opponents in competition, the sport at stake, the spectators, and humanity. The result was that such a change in policy can be ethically defended. This justifies discussion on alternative anti-doping policies moving away from today's harsh regime based on a 'zero-tolerance' principle (Kayser, 2018). The question is how to operationalise such a proposal starting from the situation as of today. In the following sections I sketch the outlines of what such a policy change might look like.

Reconsidering doping in professional cycling

What I and colleagues have in mind is a framework where: (1) The anti-doping rule is relaxed within boundaries of acceptable health risks; (2) The athlete's health is monitored; (3) Some urine and blood testing subsists using pragmatic evidence-based cut-off levels to control risk. For this to be possible, among the three WADA criteria for the inclusion of methods and substances on the List (WADA, 2015), the health risk argument is retained, while the spirit of sport and the performance-enhancing criteria are dropped.[8] These conditions being met it then follows that instead of today's continuous yearly inclusion of more and more methods and substances on the List, WADA can also do the opposite, i.e. progressively take methods and substances off the List, one by one, while monitoring the outcomes. To satisfy those who are sceptical about this proposal, the Prohibited List and anti-doping controls would initially be maintained unchanged (Kayser, 2018). At the start nothing would practically change, but the underlying reasoning for the on-going anti-doping efforts would be fundamentally different. The change would be accompanied by the message that performance enhancement is not bad behaviour per se, but instead that performance enhancement is the crux of athletic endeavour.[9] The main message would be that for reasons of unreasonable health risk some techniques would remain or become forbidden, and therefore controls would still be necessary.

Such a change begs the question what are acceptable health risks and what is optimal athlete's health, which would need to be defined. Today the decisions on what is on the List are taken behind closed WADA-doors, without transparent communication of the reasons for putting something on the List. But secrecy is not necessarily a good housekeeper for good governance. I propose that WADA introduces a transparency with regard to the work of its various panels, such as the one deciding what to put on the List, as well as that it publishes its technical documents on doping sample analysis and interpretation. I also propose to introduce more democratic principles into anti-doping governance with a larger and elected athlete representation in order to better hear their voices (Kayser, 2018).

Shortening the Prohibited List

Hereunder I present four substances that can serve as examples for the proposed changes. I list them according to the presence vs. absence of performance-enhancing effects and of health risks.

No known performance enhancement, no known or little health risk

This category concerns compounds that were added to the List for reasons other than documented performance enhancing and/or health risks. WADA uses an all-inclusive terminology by stating that it is enough to suspect that something might have the potential for a performance-enhancing effect or potentially comes with a health risk. In January 2016, the drug meldonium was added to the List after being monitored since 2015. WADA stated that 'Meldonium was added [to the Prohibited List] because of evidence of its use by athletes with the intention of enhancing performance'.[10] Meldonium was developed in Latvia and is used in eastern Europe, mainly by patients with cardiovascular disease. In April 2016, WADA reported that more than 170 mostly Russian athletes had tested positive for meldonium. Since there is no evidence for any performance-enhancing effects of meldonium and because of its mild if any side-effects (Greenblatt & Greenblatt, 2016; Schobersberger, Dünnwald, Gmeiner, & Blank, 2017), it can be removed from the List. It would join the many other compounds used by athletes with the intention to enhance performance. Given the present lack of evidence for any relevant performance-enhancing effect WADA's decision to add meldonium is akin to putting a placebo on the List.

Performance enhancement, health risk

More complicated, because needing some tweaking with cut-offs, is for example erythropoietin (EPO), a popular means to increase the oxygen carrying capacity of blood used by endurance athletes in the nineties. The evidence suggests performance-enhancing effects, especially for endurance, even though not all research is univocal (Hardeman et al., 2014; Lundby & Olsen, 2011; Sgrò, Sansone, Sansone, Romanelli, & Di Luigi, 2018). In healthy athletes excessive use of EPO could theoretically lead to increased cardiovascular risk. That is reason to be prudent with its use, even though the so-called epidemic of EPO deaths during the EPO years was debunked as a myth (López, 2011). Nevertheless, it would seem reasonable to put some safety margin in place, which is actually what the UCI did during the EPO heydays in cycling. The fraction of red cells in circulating blood was not to exceed 50%, above which there was a no-start policy. Of course, there would be means to cheat somewhat around that cut-off level, e.g. by dilution, but that would be part of the game.

No known performance enhancement, health risk

I propose to begin by taking cannabis derivates off the List. It is argued that it might lower the threshold for taking risks in some high-risk sports such as snowboarding. The evidence base for that contention is nil, while there is ample evidence for an ergolytic effect. The potential health risks of cannabis use are acknowledged, but these are not different between the general population and athletes, causing one to question the ban for athletes only (Waddington, Christiansen, & Gleaves, 2013). Taking cannabis off the List would lead to a sizeable drop in ADRVs given the frequency of their detection and would allow athletes to be treated on a par with the general population.

Performance-enhancing effect, no or limited health risk

For this category there is a precedent. Caffeine was forbidden in 1984 at a urine threshold of 15 $\mu g{\cdot}mL^{-1}$, reduced to 12 $\mu g{\cdot}mL^{-1}$ in 1985. Since this urinary threshold cannot distinguish between social use and abuse of caffeine in sports, WADA removed caffeine from the List in 2004, which led to an increase in caffeine use (Del Coso, Muñoz, & Muñoz-Guerra, 2011). Both for endurance and explosive type activities, the evidence favours performance enhancement (for recent reviews see Grgic, Trexler, Lazinica, & Pedisic, 2018; Southward, Rutherfurd-Markwick, & Ali, 2018). In usual doses caffeine comes with limited health risk, but at higher dosage it exemplifies the maxim that the poison is in the dose (Jabbar & Hanly, 2013). Even though the overall evidence for performance enhancement is strong, the individual response varies. Genetic polymorphisms, epigenetic effects, and environmental factors are important determinants of the effects of caffeine (Pickering & Kiely, 2018). Just as genetic polymorphisms, epigenetic effects, and environmental factors are major (even though undeserved) determinants of athletic talent, the response to pharmacology also varies. This nullifies the argument that allowing doping would lead to a uniform increase in performance at an increased health cost. Because of the varying effects to identical stimuli between athletes, the outcome does not level out, but instead introduces further variance of performance. If the anti-doping rule would be relaxed, it would then be expected that the playing field would remain at least as dynamic as of today, opening the way towards valuing the exploitation of baseline talent by all means (Kayser, 2018).

These four examples could make up the start of a general reappraisal of what is on WADA's Prohibited List. The List would be updated yearly, mentioning not only what remains forbidden, what any threshold values are, but also what is permitted, with mention on proper use.

Harm minimisation

The above proposed relaxation of the anti-doping rule would imply an increase in the use of permitted technology, with potential harm. Harm minimisation, or harm reduction, concerns interventions that reduce negative health and other outcomes of drug use without necessarily reducing the use. The here proposed framework should therefore be accompanied by the following: (1) keeping to documented health risk for maintaining the List and reappraise regularly according to new evidence and epidemiology; (2) continuing controls for doping technology considered too dangerous; (3) evidence-based education and information on doping and anti-doping for athletes, athlete personnel, and the general public; (4) obligation of health checks of athletes by certified and regularly accredited doctors; and (5) low threshold medical counselling service to inquire about the use of any substance while minimising its health risk. The implementation of these points would take place in parallel to the discussion on what remains, is taken off, or put on the List. The fleshing out of the particularities and practicalities would, as for the List, be organised in a transparent and democratic fashion with a large voice for the athletes themselves.

Conclusion

I have sketched a change in doping policy in keeping with the practical constraints of reality. Given the impossibility of current anti-doping policy to reach its goal and its increasingly worrying side-effects, the proposed partial relaxation of the anti-doping rule in combination with a harm minimisation approach within a framework recognising that performance enhancement is the crux of elite athletic endeavour would seem a worthwhile pursuit. Like any proposal it has its weaknesses such as the unknowns of its promise, potential tendencies for runaway effects, the likely continuation of some cheating, a potential health cost, and the difficulty of shielding minors from undue practices. It also has strengths, including its resonance with the human enhancement debate in wider society, its practicality, its malleability, and its foundation on democratic principles and transparency.

Notes

1 See www.cyclisme-dopage.com/aveux.htm for a list (in French) of quotes from cyclists admitting their use of doping (visited July 2018).
2 For more in depth historical aspects of doping in cycling and in general see e.g. (de Mondenard, 2011; Dimeo, 2008; Dimeo & Møller, 2018; Gleaves, 2014; Hoberman, 2006; Hunt, 2011; Laure, 2004; López, 2013).
3 Union Cycliste Internationale: www.uci.org (visited July 2018).
4 ADRV: anti-doping rule violation, as defined in WADC: www.wada-ama.org/en/what-we-do/the-code (visited July 2018).
5 Because of surveillance and testing technology 'old-fashioned' doping e.g. with erythropoietin (EPO) injections is unlikely to go undetected. Instead other techniques like nightly intra-venous micro-injections are probably being used, to stay under the radar.
6 See www.nrc.nl/nieuws/2018/04/28/voormalig-wielrenner-westra-geeft-dopinggebruik-toe-a1601183, visited July 2018.
7

> Calling the 'Festina affair' a 'tough blow for all sports,' Juan Antonio Samaranch, the president of the International Olympic Committee, wants to reduce the list of drugs that athletes cannot use. 'The ones to blame are not the athletes but those around them', Samaranch was quoted as saying in the newspaper El Mundo today. 'Doping demands an exact definition – and I have been asking for it for years.' Samaranch said that while the I.O.C. would not consider legalising doping, the list of banned products 'must be reduced drastically.' 'Doping is everything that, firstly, is harmful to an athlete's health and, secondly, artificially augments his performance,' Samaranch said. 'If it's just the second case, for me, that's not doping. If it's the first case, it is.'
>
> (NYT, July 27 1998, www.nytimes.com/1998/07/27/sports/cycling-a-call-for-doping-changes.html, accessed July 2018)

8 The reader is referred to Kayser (2018) for a more detailed discussion on reasons for dropping these two criteria.
9 This would allow a move away from the strong tendency for doping to be increasingly seen as a *malum in se* (wrong or evil in itself), instead of *malum prohibitum* (wrong because it is prohibited).
10 www.wada-ama.org/en/media/news/2016-03/wada-statement-regarding-maria-sharapova-case (accessed July 2018).

References

Aubel, O., Lefèvre, B., Le Goff, J.M., & Taverna, N. (2018). Doping risk and career turning points in male elite road cycling (2005–2016). *Journal of Science and Medicine in Sport*. http://doi.org/10.1016/j.jsams.2018.03.003

Bourdon, F., Schoch, L., Broers, B., & Kayser, B. (2015). French speaking athletes' experience and perception regarding the whereabouts reporting system and therapeutic use exemptions. *Performance Enhancement & Health*, 3(3/4), 153–158.

de Hon, O. (2016, 18 November). *Striking the Right Balance: Effectiveness of Anti-Doping Policies*. Utrecht University.

de Hon, O., Kuipers, H., & van Bottenburg, M. (2015). Prevalence of doping use in elite sports: a review of numbers and methods. *Sports Medicine*, *45*(1), 57–69.

de Mondenard, J.P. (2011). *Tour de France, 33 vainqueurs face au dopage, entre 1947 et 2010*. Paris: Hugo et Compagnie.

Del Coso, J., Muñoz, G., & Muñoz-Guerra, J. (2011). Prevalence of caffeine use in elite athletes following its removal from the World Anti-Doping Agency list of banned substances. *Applied Physiology, Nutrition, and Metabolism*, *36*(4), 555–561.

Dimeo, P. (2008). *A History of Drug Use in Sport: 1876–1976*. London: Routledge.

Dimeo, P. & Møller, V. (2018). *The Anti-Doping Crisis in Sport*. London: Routledge.

Editorial. (2007). A sporting chance. *Nature*, *448*(7153), 512.

Elbe, A.M. & Pitsch, W. (2018). Doping prevalence among Danish elite athletes. *Performance Enhancement & Health*, 6(1), 28–32.

Fincoeur, B., Frenger, M., & Pitsch, W. (2013). Does one play with the athletes' health in the name of ethics? *Performance Enhancement & Health*, *2*(4), 182–193.

Gleaves, J. (2014). A global history of doping in sport: Drugs, nationalism and politics. *The International Journal of the History of Sport*, *31*(8), 815–819.

Greenblatt, H.K. & Greenblatt, D.J. (2016). Meldonium (Mildronate): A performance-enhancing drug? *Clinical Pharmacology in Drug Development*, 5(3), 167–169.

Grgic, J., Trexler, E.T., Lazinica, B., & Pedisic, Z. (2018). Effects of caffeine intake on muscle strength and power: a systematic review and meta-analysis. *Journal of the International Society of Sports Nutrition*, *15*(1), 11.

Hanstad, D.V., Smith, A., & Waddington, I. (2008). The establishment of the World Anti-Doping Agency A study of the management of organizational change and unplanned outcomes. *International Review for the Sociology of Sport*, *43*(3), 227–249.

Hardeman, M., Alexy, T., Brouwer, B., Connes, P., Jung, F., Kuipers, H., & Baskurt, O.K. (2014). EPO or PlacEPO? Science versus practical experience: panel discussion on efficacy of erythropoetin in improving performance. *Biorheology*, *51*(2–3), 83–90.

Hoberman, J. (2006). *Testosterone Dreams*. University of California Press.

Hunt, T.M. (2011). *Drug Games*. Austin: University of Texas Press.

Hunt, T.M. (2017). WADA and Doping in World Sport. In R. Edelman & W. Wilson (Eds), *The Oxford Handbook of Sports History* (pp. 1–13). Oxford: Oxford University Press.

Jabbar, S.B., & Hanly, M.G. (2013). Fatal caffeine overdose. *The American Journal of Forensic Medicine and Pathology*, *34*(4), 321–324.

Kayser, B. (2018). *Ethical Aspects of Doping and Anti-Doping: In Search of an Alternative Policy*. KU Leuven: Doctoral thesis.

Kayser, B., Mauron, A., & Miah, A. (2005). Viewpoint: Legalisation of performance-enhancing drugs. *Lancet*, *366*, *Suppl 1*, S21.

Kayser, B. & Møller, V. (2018, forthcoming). The anti-doping industry coming of age: in search of new markets. In K. Van de Ven & J. McVeigh (Eds), *Human Enhancement Drugs*. London: Routledge.

Kayser, B. & Tolleneer, J. (2017). Ethics of a relaxed antidoping rule accompanied by harm-reduction measures. *Journal of Medical Ethics*, *43*(5), medethics–2015–102659–286. http://doi.org/10.1136/medethics-2015-102659

Kirkwood, K. (2009). Considering harm reduction as the future of doping control policy in international sport. *Quest*, *61*(2), 180–190.

Laure, P. (2004). *Histoire du dopage et des conduites dopantes*. Paris: Vuibert.

López, B. (2011). The invention of a 'drug of mass destruction': Deconstructing the EPO myth. *Sport in History*, *31*(1), 84–109.

López, B. (2013). Creating fear: the 'doping deaths,' risk communication and the anti-doping campaign. *International Journal of Sport Policy and Politics*, 1–13.

Lundby, C. & Olsen, N.V. (2011). Effects of recombinant human erythropoietin in normal humans. *The Journal of Physiology*, 589(6), 1265–1271.

Mignon, P. (2003). The Tour de France and the doping issue. *The International Journal of the History of Sport*, 20(2), 227–245.

Moston, S. & Engelberg, T. (2017). *Detecting Doping in Sport*. London: Routledge.

Møller, V. (2005). Knud Enemark Jensen's death during the 1960 Rome Olympics: A search for truth? *Sport in History*, 25(3), 452–471.

Ohl, F., Aubel, O., & Brissoneau, C. (2015). *L'épreuve du Dopage*. Paris: Presses Universitaires de France.

Overbye, M. & Wagner, U. (2013). Between medical treatment and performance enhancement: An investigation of how elite athletes experience therapeutic use exemptions. *International Journal of Drug Policy*, 24(6), 579–588.

Pickering, C. & Kiely, J. (2018). Are the current guidelines on caffeine use in sport optimal for everyone? Inter-individual variation in caffeine ergogenicity, and a move towards personalised sports nutrition. *Sports Medicine*, 48(1), 7–16.

Pielke, R. (2017). Assessing doping prevalence is possible. So what are we waiting for? *Sports Medicine*, 48(1), 207–209.

Pitsch, W. & Emrich, E. (2011). The frequency of doping in elite sport: Results of a replication study. *International Review for the Sociology of Sport*, 47(5), 559–580.

Savulescu, J., Foddy, B., & Clayton, M. (2004). Why we should allow performance enhancing drugs in sport. *British Journal of Sports Medicine*, 38(6), 666–670.

Schobersberger, W., Dünnwald, T., Gmeiner, G., & Blank, C. (2017). Story behind meldonium – from pharmacology to performance enhancement: a narrative review. *British Journal of Sports Medicine*, 51(1), 22–25.

Sgrò, P., Sansone, M., Sansone, A., Romanelli, F., & Di Luigi, L. (2018). Effects of erythropoietin abuse on exercise performance. *The Physician and Sports medicine*, 46(1), 105–115.

Southward, K., Rutherfurd-Markwick, K.J., & Ali, A. (2018). The effect of acute caffeine ingestion on endurance performance: A systematic review and meta–analysis. *Sports Medicine*, 48(8), 1913–1928.

Striegel, H., Ulrich, R., & Simon, P. (2010). Randomized response estimates for doping and illicit drug use in elite athletes. *Drug and Alcohol Dependence*, 106(2–3), 230–232.

WADA. (2015). *World Anti-Doping Code*.

Waddington, I., Christiansen, A.V., & Gleaves, J. (2013). Recreational drug use and sport: Time for a WADA rethink? *Performance Enhancement & Health*, 2(2), 41–47.

Part III

Issues, controversies, and stakes

Chapter 13

The decline of trust in British sport since the London Olympics

Team Sky's fall from grace

Paul Dimeo and April Henning

Trust is a concept that is intangible, hard to measure, often used but rarely defined, and accepted by all political groups to be worth having. Nonetheless, recent discourses on fake news and political corruption mean that there are many recent examples whereby citizens' trust in leaders is abused and undermined in political negotiations, diplomacy, public relations, and commercial enterprise. The same can be said about sport. Sport has been idealised as a cultural context in which trust should be central to the ethical fabric; indeed, sport has been valorised as distinct to politics and business in that fair play and respect for one's opponents should be prioritised, sometimes (but not always) in favour of winning. At the same time, trust is central to sport if sport is going to have any meaning. A unique feature of sport is that the outcome is determined by the unscripted performances of athletes competing against each other in full view of the public. If fans cannot believe the results reflect honest competition, if they suspect matches are rigged, or that unseen forces have intentionally disrupted the playing field, not only will they cease watching sport but sport will cease to have any meaning.

Professional cycling knows these challenges all too well. The persistent denials by professional cyclists doping with EPO throughout the 1990s turned out to be lies. As revelations about doping poured out during the 2000s, the public who believed the lies, realised they had been duped. Moreover, cycling's governing body, the *Union Cycliste Internationale* (UCI) and anti-doping efforts, had proven themselves unreliable custodians of the sport. Into this integrity vacuum stepped Team Sky. Emerging from Britain's lottery funded and immensely successful track cycling programme, Team Sky promised its British fans to be different, to be 'clean'.

In this chapter, we argue that the high-profile debate over the use of drugs in British professional cycling can be understood as symptomatic of a wider malaise affecting British sport, which in turn can be contextualised, explained, and seen as part of a broader shift in scepticism regarding political leaders and media organisations. The British professional cycling team, Team Sky, represents both microcosm and protagonist in these wider social and cultural developments.

Lottery funding and British cycling

Team Sky's status as a microcosm for broader British scepticism stems from decisions made almost two decades before Britain would win the Tour de France. In 1993, British Prime Minister John Major proposed a national lottery, with funds allocated to 'good causes'. Major ensured sports would remain a major beneficiary of the National Lottery along with arts and culture. In 1998, Major justified this demand in front of the British Parliament because of 'the impact that sport can make on the twin priorities of health and education'. (Major, 1998). Despite this, 74% of British citizens in a 2000 poll indicated that lottery funding should be used to support the UK's National Health Service (Hall, 2000). The lottery funding for elite sport worked. UK sport spending was around £5 million per year before the 1996 Summer Olympics, but that increased to £54 million by the 2000 Summer Games and then to £264 million by 2012. This infusion of cash was intended to revitalise Olympic sport in the UK, fund high performance sport advances, and develop athletes into medal winners. The results of this renewed focus were clear, as the upsurge in spending was matched by the UK's climb up the medals table from 36th in 1996 to 3rd by 2012 (for a fuller discussion of British sports policy in this time period see Green, 2009).

London bid

The fusion of sport, public funds, and national benefit increased in 2003 when London prepared its bid for the 2012 Summer Olympic Games, supported by Prime Minister Tony Blair. Before the success of the lottery programme was fully realised, the UK Government emphasised the links between funding for high performance sport and the social benefits stemming from grassroots sport. Tessa Jowell, the culture secretary, claimed the bid would keep social interests as a central concern and aim to address issues including 'health, social inclusion, educational motivation and fighting crime' (Jowell, 2003). These social benefits accompanied the central argument for committing £17 million just to bid for the Games, and eventually around £11 billion to host the event: that being awarded the Olympics would galvanise elite sport to perform better than ever and have long lasting social and sporting legacies (Thornley, 2012).

A central beneficiary of these commitments to high performance sport was British Cycling, where Dave Brailsford and a number of future Team Sky staff and athletes first joined forces. Under the direction of coach Peter Keen, lottery funding was allocated to cycling and funnelled into track cycling from the mid-1990s, seeing the approach as a way to pick up Olympic medals. The 2000 Games supported his thesis as the UK took medals on the track, including a bronze by Bradley Wiggins. Track success continued through subsequent Games, but by the mid-2000s British Cycling was headed by Brailsford, who turned attention back to the roads and the Grand Tours (Moore, 2011). Sky became a national team sponsor before the 2008 Games before committing to fund the pro team that became Team Sky (Fotheringham, 2012).

Winning the Grand Tours

Though Team Sky maintains an international roster of talented cyclists, it has provided the main pipeline for developing cyclists from Britain. There are some exceptions to this: the sprinter Mark Cavendish was only in the team for one season; David Millar's early career peaked before Team Sky was created, and his post-ban return was with other teams. However, the most successful riders have been part of the team, notably Bradley Wiggins and Chris Froome, both of whom are highly decorated after having won several Grand Tours, as well as the 2018 Tour de France winner Geraint Thomas. The success of British cycling on the track inspired the creation of a professional road cycling team aiming to become the first British team to 'conquer' the Grand Tours. Founded in 2009, the climate in professional road cycling meant that Team Sky considered a strict anti-doping policy necessary to maintain trust. In some ways, Team Sky's internal anti-doping policy went beyond the usual requirements imposed by the UCI and WADA: for example, the Performance Director, David Brailsford, regularly made public statements that all the team members should not be suspected of doping and that no individual with a previous doping-related sanction would be hired.

Brailsford also spoke openly during this period to distance Team Sky from doping, and highlighting management and leadership practices as key to their success. To protect his riders from cycling's notorious doping past, Brailsford promised in 2009 that, 'We won't appoint foreign doctors. We've only appointed British doctors who have not worked in pro cycling before. We want to minimise risk' (Birnie, 2018). As an alternative narrative, he credited his team's success with the concepts of 'marginal gains' and 'growth mindset' in collaboration with the former table tennis player turned management psychology guru Matthew Syed, and the highly renowned psychologist Steve Peters.

In retrospect, 2011 was an important year. There was some success, though after Wiggins crashed in the Tour de France the team only managed two stage wins and 24th in the general classification. It was the winter between the 2010 and 2011, however, that Team Sky hired the former Rabobank team doctor Geert Leinders on a temporary basis. Leinders had been part of a doping programme which included Michael Rasmussen and Levi Leipheimer, and was banned for life in 2012 as part of the USADA investigation into blood doping and the use of performance enhancing drugs such as EPO. Team Sky's involvement with Leinders did not become public until July 2012, where it would erupt into controversy (Cycling News, 2012). During the 2011 season, it would later emerge, the medical support of riders, where their training and recovery was managed with medical professionals instead of just cycling specialists, was becoming more common. Corticosteroids were used, as did the infamous incident of the Jiffy Bag with unknown contents that was delivered for Wiggins just before the Criterium du Dauphine.

Nonetheless, the public image of Team Sky was based on a sense of trustworthiness, and 2012 became a season of remarkable success as Wiggins won the Tour de France and became the most decorated British Olympian with seven gold medals. Yet the image was secured and further enhanced by the numerous accolades and awards granted to members of the team: Bradley Wiggins was knighted in the Queen's New Years' Honours List of 2013 alongside Brailsford, who had also been given an MBE in 2005 and CBE in 2009 (these are among the most important and prestigious honours to be granted to a British citizen for public services: Member of the Most Excellent Order of the British Empire and Commander of the Most Excellent Order of the British Empire). British sport as a whole was brimming with confident pride after a position of 3rd in the London Olympics, a successful experience as hosts, and a programme of funding for community sports and elite talent in order to support the Olympic legacy.

The unravelling of trust

While Team Sky basked in the glories of its 2012 Grand Tour victory, behind the scenes all was not all rosy. One anonymous whistleblower claimed in 2017 that,

> In 2012 the team was under extreme pressure to perform. Dave B[railsford] and Shane Sutton put a great deal of pressure on the medical team in particular Richard Freeman to provide more proactive medical support. Using TUEs was openly discussed in hushed voices as a means of supporting health and wellbeing.
>
> (DCMS, 2018)

Leinders had been dismissed with the news from the USADA investigation, and an internal investigation in 2012 led the senior management to release three more coaching staff: Bobby Julich, Steven de Jongh, and Sean Yates (Gallagher, 2012).

The case of Jonathan Tiernan-Locke exposed another crack in the façade. Tiernan-Locke had only been part of the team for nine months when notified of an adverse analytical finding emerging from a biological passport test taken in September 2012 while he was a member of another team (Endura). Team Sky terminated his contract in July 2014 when the decision was made to ban him for two years and strip him of the world championship title and Tour of Britain win from 2012. While this case did not hit the headlines in the same way that later revelations of Wiggins' use of medicines and Froome's salbutamol test would, there is no doubt that Tiernan-Locke's situation cast a shadow over Team Sky's reputation. If he had used a banned drug in either 2012 or 2013 that led to a high reading in his ABP scores, then Sky had accidently employed a doper who could have spread news among the other riders about how to dope. However, Tiernan-Locke always protested his innocence, claiming instead that the high score was result of dehydration after a day of binge drinking. If this is so, then Team Sky employed a cyclist who did not follow guidelines on healthy lifestyles and professional conduct. Curiously, UK Anti-Doping accepted that he had been over-indulging in alcohol two days before the test, but that would not have led to the dehydration cause for an anomalous reading. Tiernan-Locke would later reveal that the controversial painkiller tramadol was being widely distributed to cyclists during the 2012 season (BBC, 2016a).

By 2013, Team Sky had appeared to weather the controversy. Brailsford's decisive actions with coaching staff associated with doping had supported his reputation for doing things 'the right way'. Brailsford had famously asserted to the press that,

> Sky started as a clean team and we will continue to be a clean team. It is the guiding principle to what we do. A British winner of the Tour de France is worthless unless he is a clean rider. People must continue to be able to believe in us.

Accepting this narrative, the *Telegraph* promised its readers that 'Sky can claim to be delivering on their vow to build a scandal-free team' (Gallagher, 2012).

Entering their third season, Team Sky appeared to also deliver on its promise to dominate cycling's Grand Tours. They had transformed from a fledgling British squad to a powerful presence at all of professional cycling's stage races. Chris Froome replaced Bradley Wiggins as Team Sky's leader at the Tour de France and won the first of his Tour de France titles in 2013. A subsequent victory would occur in 2015, when the team also won the World Championships. For some, this period of success – after demonstrably cutting ties with riders and staff associated with doping – proved their credibility and trustworthiness at a period when cycling appeared to be recovering from the USADA investigation of 2012. Team Sky, with 'marginal gains' as their mantra, epitomised a new era by winning numerous titles seemingly without the need for illicit performance enhancement.

At the same time, Team Sky's riders, including Wiggins and Froome, continued to face veiled accusations of doping. Froome's dominance at the 2013 Tour de France garnered unfavourable comparisons to Lance Armstrong (Fotheringham, 2013). Team Sky released Froome's power data from 2011 to 2013 in an effort to defend their rider's performances from doping allegations. Such steps presented Team Sky as an outfit with nothing to hide. Still, the allegations and questions implying doping certainly shaded the squeaky-clean image.

The situation within British sport was changing and, as a British cycling team, Team Sky could not avoid these changes. The legacy of the 2012 London Olympics, where Wiggins had won gold in the Time Trial and where British Cycling collectively took home 12 medals, became increasingly scrutinised.

Critics noted that there was no sign of the much-vaunted Government promise that national participation rates in sport, exercise, and physical activity would increase. The future of the new Olympic Stadium remained uncertain (it was eventually given to West Ham United on a low-cost lease arrangement). However, when Glasgow hosted the 2014 Commonwealth Games, there was an over-riding sense that it had been successful, if on a much smaller scale. Ironically, David Millar was allowed to captain the Scottish cycling team at those 2014 Games. While there were no major cycling scandals, two Welsh athletes had been disqualified after testing positive for a banned substance found in nutritional supplements. Nonetheless, the climatic build-up to hosting two major international multi-sport events within two years of each other left an aftermath of uncertainty as to the value of elite sport. Having dominated the cycling events with a great deal of money devoted to the sport, Britain faced the inevitable question wondering 'so what was that for' at a time when health issues such as obesity, ageing populations, and substance abuse remained prominent sources of anxiety for which organised sport had not provided any remedies (Weed et al., 2015).

Doping, bullying, and TUEs

Towards the end of 2014, the German media company ARD and their leading investigative reporter, Hajo Seppelt, broadcast evidence of widespread doping in Russian sport. This signalled the beginning of a process which would lead to unprecedented investigations, first by Dick Pound and then by Richard McLaren, that would see Russian athletes banned from international events including the Olympics. The initial coverage by ARD focused on new information provided by whistleblowers, and created the unavoidable impression that one of the largest and most successful sporting countries had developed a systematic approach to doping and corruption.

Though the Russian doping allegations implicated some cyclists, the details paled in comparison to another major report. In February 2015, a detailed report by the Cycling Independent Reform Commission (CIRC), led by a group of experts and based upon a range of sources including in-depth interviews, detailed the doping practices that had recently occurred in professional cycling. While the report was heavily focused on the problems of the 1990s to mid-2000s, and there was evidence that the situation had improved, this key section from the Executive Summary served to highlight the complex and subtle nature of contemporary doping problems:

> The general view is that at the elite level the situation has improved, but that doping is still taking place. It was commented that doping is either less prevalent today or the nature of doping practices has changed such that the performance gains are smaller. The CIRC considers that a culture of doping in cycling continues to exist, albeit attitudes have started to change. The

> biggest concern today is that following the introduction of the athlete biological passport, dopers have moved on to micro-dosing in a controlled manner that keeps their blood parameters constant and enables them to avoid detection. In contrast to the findings in previous investigations, which identified systematic doping organised by teams, at the elite level riders who dope now organise their own doping programmes with the help of third parties who are primarily outside the cycling team. At the elite level, doping programmes are generally sophisticated and therefore doctors play a key role in devising programmes that provide performance enhancement whilst minimising the risk of getting caught.
>
> (CIRC, 2015: 12)

In June 2015, a BBC documentary called 'Catch Me If You Can' saw investigative journalist Mark Daly experiment with EPO and demonstrate that testing methods do not always detect micro-dosing. In the same programme, the American coach Alberto Salazar was criticised for providing his athletes with performance-enhancing drugs and misusing the TUE system. For the British sport context, it highlighted that the hugely popular and successful runner Mo Farah was coached by Salazar and won both the 5,000m and 10,000m in the London Olympics. He was subsequently given a CBE in the 2013 New Years Honours. It was not directly alleged that he had received any banned substances. However, Farah had missed two anti-doping tests in 2015, including one just before the Olympics for which he claimed to have not heard the doping control officer ring his doorbell (Rumsby, 2015).

Similarly, in June 2015, Froome was interviewed in the media regarding two missed tests. The first had been in 2010 and the second in early 2015, when he claims that staff in the hotel he was staying in with his wife had refused to give his room information to the doping control officer.

The apparent scale of doping in world athletics and the Olympics was exposed in August 2015. Information about tests conducted between 2001 and 2010 was leaked to ARD and the Sunday Times (2015). Although the Athlete Biological Passport had not been fully implemented until 2009, the IAAF had collected over 12,000 samples from around 5000 athletes from 208 countries. When shown to experts, it was claimed that blood doping and the use of blood-related products such as EPO was rife in athletes. Major events like World Championships, the Olympics, and major Marathons had been won by athletes with suspicious blood count values. The scale of suspicious blood values was claimed to be: more than 1400 'abnormal' tests from over 800 athletes in 94 countries. This shone a critical light on British sport in three ways. First, Lord Sebastian Coe, who became President of the IAAF in 2015 after being a Vice President since 2007 and who was Chairman of the London Olympics Organizing Committee, said that this media coverage was a 'declaration of war' on his sport and organisation. This prompted much criticism, even within a Parliamentary Inquiry (see below). Second, major British events such as the London

Marathon and the 2012 Olympics were undermined, signalling a lack of certainty in the integrity of the medal allocations. Third, it was reported that leading British runner, Paula Radcliffe, an outspoken critic of doping athletes, had been identified in the leaked documents as having had three tests with suspicious readings. She was keen to deny that she had been doping. In September, the Conservative MP Jesse Norman said that British marathon winners were under suspicion, but he blamed the media for misrepresenting his comments and issued an apology to Radcliffe in January 2016 (Wilkinson, 2016).

These dark fears seemed confirmed in November 2015 when WADA's Independent Commission recommended that Russia's anti-doping agency, RUSADA, be found non-compliant with the WADA Code, its Moscow lab's accreditation revoked, its director removed, and that there were 'systemic failures' that undermined anti-doping efforts in athletics (Pound, McLaren, & Younger, 2015: 9). This report directly impacted the legacy of the 2012 London Games, saying the Games were sabotaged by the failure to act against athletes deemed suspicious. There were also questions about Coe's role in the IAAF-Russia doping scandal, including questions related to misleading answers to Parliament about when he became aware of the Russia allegations and corruption within the IAAF. Investigative reporting in June 2016 showed Coe had received information months before he claimed to have been made aware via the ARD documentary. There were further allegations that Coe's election as IAAF President was helped along by Papa Massata Diack, a former IAAF consultant and son of Coe's predecessor Lamine Diack, who was banned for life for his role in the Russia cover-up. In April 2016, further damage was done to British sport and specifically to the credibility of Team Sky when one of their key riders, Jess Varnish, made public claims about bullying, harassment, and sexism directed at her by one of the coaches, Shane Sutton (*Guardian*, 2016).

All of this was prelude to the series of events in the summer of 2016 leading up to the Rio Games. An Independent Report by Richard McLaren laid out the details of Russia's scheme to circumvent anti-doping, including at the 2012 London Games (McLaren, 2016). This led to a battle between WADA and the IOC over whether or not to bar the Russian team completely as WADA wanted, or to allow individual Russian athletes to demonstrate their eligibility, as the IOC eventually chose to do. While this crisis was on-going, news of British cyclist Lizzie Armistead's three missed anti-doping tests surfaced. Armistead avoided a sanction by demonstrating she was not at fault for the first missed test (Hattenstone, 2017). Despite this, fellow athletes, including Wiggins, criticised her and questions lingered against the backdrop of the Russian doping revelations. For his part, Wiggins was put in the centre of the story in September after the hacking group Fancy Bears leaked Wiggins' TUE information. The TUE information clearly contradicted Wiggins' claims in his autobiography that, 'I've never had an injection, apart from I've had my vaccinations, and on occasion I've been put on a drip'. Yet, during the 2011, 2012, and 2013 seasons he had been given injections of triamcinolone to treat his asthma (Bowden, 2016). He subsequently justified this, and the use of the powerful anti-inflammatory drug triamcinolone for allergies and respiratory problems, by saying that the drugs put him back on a 'level playing field'. What made his situation more controversial was that often these were administered just ahead of major races (BBC, 2016b). There were also still lingering questions around the infamous Jiffy Bag that was delivered for him in 2011, the contents of which still have never been explained.

All of this together had an erosive effect on public trust in sport institutions. A 2017 survey of British public found that one third of respondents reported losing faith in sport since 2016 (Kelner, 2017). Athletes, too, were faced with questions of confidence in sport as failures in duty of care to athletes resulted in reports of bullying, sexism, racism, sexual abuse, doping, and corruption. A 2017 Independent Report to the UK government reviewing duty of care for athletes found that sport bodies had not done enough to prevent athletes from various harms and recommended that the Government put in place a sport ombudsman. This failure showed the gap between national sporting success and athlete welfare (Grey-Thompson, 2017).

In March 2018, the Digital, Culture, Media and Sport (DCMS) select committee issued a report on doping in sport. It was scathing in its assessment of both Coe's misleading statements to Parliament and of British Cycling. The report stopped just short of accusing Wiggins and Brailsford of cheating, instead indicating they and Team Sky had crossed ethical lines – including those self-imposed by Brailsford – in its use of medications and other enhancing substances, possible abuse of TUEs, and others in pursuit of victories.

Most recently the focus has been on Froome's 2017 adverse analytical finding of salbutamol (an asthma drug for which he did not have a TUE) at twice the allowed level following his double victories at the Tour de France and Vuelta a Espana. Froome and Sky denied wrongdoing, maintaining that Froome did not exceed his allowed usage. Sky declined to suspend Froome until his case was resolved. Resolution would not come quickly, but Froome was allowed to continue racing in the interim. Froome and Sky continued to fight a competition ban, arguing that WADA's measure for salbutamol was flawed for not accounting for dehydration or drug retention over several days of competition. Following his Giro d'Italia win, the Tour de France organiser ASO said they would block Froome from competing if there was no ruling on his case. Days before the start of the Tour, UCI announced that Froome had been cleared and that it was ending its investigation. The case split the cycling world. This was exacerbated by UCI's decision not to release a reasoned decision on Froome, leaving many to guess at the science, reasoning, or pressure that informed the decision (Stokes, 2018). Froome rode the Tour de France but ended up third behind his own Sky teammate Geraint Thomas.

Discussion

The chronological narrative above presents a litany of controversies that collectively undermine much of the 'feel good factor' integral to British sport when hosting the 2012 Olympics and the 2014 Commonwealth Games. A number of overlapping issues help to explain the apparent erosion of trust.

First, hosting major sports events usually entails a cultural acceptance of the value of sport in order help promote the success of the host country, what some scholars refer to a 'boosterism', and which we might also align with the notion of 'manufactured consent'. That is to say, the media come to play an active role in emphasising good news stories while down-playing potential criticism. Politicians are keen to be associated with the success of such events, despite the significant investment required. At the same time, local communities and volunteers are engaged in the overall self-presentation of a unified nation getting behind the event. With the various successes, including in cycling, the Olympics looked like a highly positive experience. When Glasgow hosted the 2014 Commonwealth Games there was similar political and media support for the event, as it helped promote the image of the city overseas and had a tourism economic benefit. Once these events had finished, there was almost immediately reduced political interest in sport, and more investigative journalism emerged focusing on critical issues. Thus, as much as there has been a 'fall' in public trust, the 'rise' of positive stories and consensus around the benefits of hosting major events created a hype from which there was an inevitable anti-climax or hangover.

Second, the context in which Team Sky was operating arguably necessitated a shift towards both unremitting ambition and blurred ethical lines. Regarding the former, any professional cycling team is in a precarious position due to funding. Prize money is good for those who win races, but very modest for those further down the General Classification. It is an expensive sport, so the investment required for continued success can be over-whelming. The relationship with team sponsors can become challenging if there is a lack of success or if there are reputational issues. So, when Brailsford broke away from the relatively cloistered world of track cycling, and the security of Lottery funding, perhaps it was inevitable that new tensions would emerge. However, it is the blurred ethical lines that concern the argument of this chapter. Professional cycling has been fraught with doping for decades: it seemed highly optimistic that a completely new team could arrive on the scene with an uncompromising attitude to any coach, doctor, or rider tainted by doping and become immediately successful.

Third, Team Sky have made a singular contribution to this overall decline in trust by not being transparent and not explaining specific situations adequately. The Jiffy Bag contents, the allergies and illnesses apparently suffered by Wiggins and Froome, the delivery of testosterone patches to the Manchester Velodrome, the obvious refusal to directly answer questions at the Parliamentary Inquiry, the hiring and dismissal of key staff, and the occasional disorganisation with regards to medical records: these do not fit with the initial vision of a 'clean' team, nor with basic standards of accountability and clarity. They have left us with a distinct air of confusion as to the specific circumstances of 'medicalisation' and a sense that what is publicly known may only be the tip of the iceberg.

In sum, the ethical reputation of certain sports leaders and famous athletes in Britain is dramatically altered since the heady days of the London Olympics and Glasgow Commonwealth Games. This has been evident in numerous sports, and the overall culture of distrust also influenced by global events. Nonetheless, the recent history of professional cycling in Britain is replete with troubling issues that impact upon the reputation of the sport and the experiences of athletes whose welfare should be at the heart of elite sports culture and values.

References

BBC (2016a). UK Anti-Doping investigating Tiernan-Locke and Team Sky allegations, 7 October, www.bbc.co.uk/sport/cycling/37589241, accessed 5 August 2018.

BBC (2016b). Sir Bradley Wiggins: No unfair advantage from drug, 25 September, www.bbc.co.uk/news/uk-37462540, accessed 12 August 2018.

Birnie, L. (2018). Commentary: Eight years spent covering Team Sky. *VeloNews*, 7 March, www.velonews.com/2018/03/news/commentary-eight-years-spent-covering-team-sky_458885, accessed 1 August 2018.

Bowden, A. (2016). Wiggins clarifies 'no needles' claim following leak of medical records. *Road.cc*, 17 September, https://road.cc/content/news/204956-wiggins-clarifies-'no-needles'-claim-following-leak-medical-records, accessed 15 August 2018.

Cycling Independent Reform Commission (CIRC) (2015). *Report to the President of the UCI*, www.uci.ch/mm/Document/News/CleanSport/16/87/99/CIRCReport2015_Neutral.pdf, accessed 14 August 2018.

Cycling News (2012). Sky investigating team doctor Leinders but sees 'no risk': Brailsford defends hiring of controversial Belgian doctor, 12 July, www.cyclingnews.com/news/sky-investigating-team-doctor-leinders-but-sees-no-risk/, accessed 14 August 2018.

Digital, Culture, Media and Sport Committee (DCMS) (2018). *Combatting Doping in Sport Report*. London: House of Commons.

Fotheringham, W. (2012). How Britain became a cycling nation. *Guardian*, 14 July, www.theguardian.com/sport/2012/jul/14/british-cycling-world-beaters, accessed 6 August 2018.

Fotheringham, W. (2013) Tour de France 2013: Chris Froome furious over doping accusations – 'Lance Armstrong cheated. I'm not cheating. End of story. *Independent*, 16 July, www.independent.co.uk/sport/cycling/tour-de-france-2013-chris-froome-furious-over-doping-accusations-lance-armstrong-cheated-i-m-not-8709487.html, accessed 10 August 2018.

Gallagher, B. (2012). Sean Yates' fate proves Team Sky will show no mercy in doping cull. *Telegraph*, 27 October, www.telegraph.co.uk/sport/othersports/cycling/9638457/Sean-Yates-fate-proves-Team-Sky-will-show-no-mercy-in-doping-cull.html, accessed 30 July 2018.

Green, M. (2009). Podium or participation? Analysing policy priorities under changing modes of sport governance in the United Kingdom. *International Journal for Sports Policy and Politics*, *1*(2), 121–144.

Grey-Thompson, T. (2017). *Duty of Care in Sport: Independent Report to Government*, https://assets.publishing.service.gov.uk/government/uploads/system/uploads/attachment_data/file/610130/Duty_of_Care_Review_-_April_2017__2.pdf

Guardian (2016). Cyclist Jess Varnish says Shane Sutton told her to 'go and have a baby'. 23 April, www.theguardian.com/sport/2016/apr/23/jess-varnish-british-cyling-shane-sutton-go-and-have-a-baby, accessed 15 August 2018.

Hall, C. (2000). Use lottery money to fund NHS, says public. *Telegraph*, 7 August, www.telegraph.co.uk/news/uknews/1351737/Use-lottery-money-to-fund-NHS-says-public.html, accessed 8 August 2018.

Hattenstone, S. (2017). Cyclist Lizzie Armitstead: 'I could kick myself and kick myself'. *Guardian*, 1 April, www.theguardian.com/sport/2017/apr/01/lizzie-armitstead-cycling-missed-drugs-tests-sexism-in-sport-simon-hattenstone, accessed 14 August 2018.

Jowell, T. (2003). Speech to the Houses of Commons, cited in the *Guardian*, 'Full text of Tessa Jowell's statement to the Commons on the government's backing for London's Olympic bid', 15 May, www.theguardian.com/uk/2003/may/15/olympicgames.london, accessed 5 August 2018.

Kelner, M. (2017). General public is losing faith in scandal-ridden sports, survey claims. *Guardian*, 5 July, www.theguardian.com/sport/2017/jul/05/public-faith-sport-low-corruption-doping-scandals-survey, accessed 1 August 2018.

Major, J. (1998). Debate on National Lottery. House of Commons, 7 April 1998, cited in '1997 Onwards – Mr Major's Contribution to the National Lottery Debate', www.johnmajor.co.uk, accessed 9 August 2018.

McLaren, R. (2016). WADA Investigation of Sochi Allegations. www.wada-ama.org/sites/default/files/resources/files/20160718_ip_report_newfinal.pdf

Moore, R. (2011). *Sky's the Limit: British Cycling's Quest to Conquer the Tour de France*. London: Harper Collins.

Pound, D., McLaren, R., & Younger, G. (2015) *Independent Commission Investigation*, www.wada-ama.org/sites/default/files/resources/files/wada_independent_commission_report_1_en.pdf

Rumsby, B. (2015). Mo Farah 'asleep' for missed drugs test. *Telegraph*, 26 June, www.telegraph.co.uk/sport/othersports/athletics/mo-farah/11702508/Mo-Farah-asleep-for-missed-drugs-test.html, accessed 4 August 2018.

Stokes, S. (2018). UCI says no reasoned decision will be released for Froome case, elaborates on related topics. *Cycling Tips*, 7 July, https://cyclingtips.com/2018/07/uci-says-no-reasoned-decision-will-be-released-for-froome-case-elaborates-on-related-topics/, accessed 8 August 2018.

Sunday Times (2015). The Doping Scandal. http://features.thesundaytimes.co.uk/web/public/2015/the-doping-scandal/index.html#/, accessed 11 August 2018.

Thornley, A. (2012). The 2012 London Olympics. What legacy? *Journal of Policy Research in Tourism, Leisure and Events*, 4 (2), 206–210.

Weed, M., Coren, E., Fiore, J., Wellard, I., Chatziefstathiou, D., Mansfield, L., & Dowse, S. (2015). The Olympic Games and raising sport participation: a systematic review of evidence and an interrogation of policy for a demonstration effect. *European Sport Management Quarterly*, *15*(2), 195–226.

Wilkinson, M. (2016). Paula Radcliffe doping allegations: I was set up by MPs who damaged my reputation. *Telegraph*, 26 January, www.telegraph.co.uk/sport/othersports/athletics/12121783/Paula-Radcliffe-doping-allegations-I-was-set-up-by-MPs-who-damaged-my-reputation.html, accessed 10 August 2018.

Chapter 14

Is Froome's performance on the 2015 Tour de France credible?

A sociological analysis of the construction of the performance's authenticity in cycling

Flora Plassard and Lucie Schoch

Introduction

Imagine yourself in front of the television watching the Tour de France. Riders are climbing a crucial mountain pass and the leader of the race is giving a spectacular performance, completely outperforming the competition. How would you judge this performance? There is little doubt that only a few viewers would undoubtedly trust in this performance. Indeed, many doping scandals have disrupted the credibility and transformed the reputation of cycling in the past: the Festina (1998) and Armstrong (2012) affairs, the Puerto (2006) and Contador (2010) scandals. In addition, we have witnessed a loss of confidence in anti-doping institutions that have not always been able to fight against doping. Those elements contribute to a loss of confidence towards performance in cycling.

Yet, it seems essential that people trust in the natural character of the performance and the liability of the rankings. If people cannot be sure that the winner is clean, the race will be meaningless. Based on a meritocratic ideal, sports rankings imply a belief in the equality of the capacity and in the fact that performances reflect natural physical capacities. Thus, each competition transforms equal athletes at the start to an unequal classification at the end (Marchetti, Rasera, Schotté, & Souanef, 2015: 3). Therefore, sport has created categories to organise athletes based upon biological particularities (sex, weight, handicaps), which can create inequalities of opportunities to perform. And as doping compromises the equity between competitors, it is considered as a major threat to the credibility of rankings and sport.

In cycling, the international federation (UCI) tries to control the rankings and to impose itself as the main regulator (Aubel & Ohl, 2015: 4). To this end, it establishes annual ranking for riders and teams, based on the riders' results on a certain number of events (37 in 2018). Those rankings determine the 18 teams allowed to participate to the World Tour. Thus, they regulate the access to the competitions and the possibility of recruitment of the teams. Therefore, they determine the revenue and the 'value' of the riders (Aubel & Ohl, 2015: 10). Riders generally consider that, with the exception of doping, the rankings are fair. They share a 'doxa' (Bourdieu, 1994) that makes them adhere to a set of norms, codes, and values which are obvious to them and actually tend to naturalise sporting excellence and rankings. In reality, disparities between teams' resources produce inequalities and the precariousness has a direct impact on the choice to use doping (Aubel & Ohl, 2015).

Actors involved in cycling are well aware that doping scandals are harming the credibility of their sport. Some of them try to restore the reputation of cycling. Brian Cookson, the former UCI president, mentioned in his 2017 manifesto that 'maintain[ing] the restored credibility in sport and the UCI'[1] was on his priority list. In 2007, some professional cycling teams created the Movement for Credible Cycling (MPCC) to promote their credibility against doping by imposing stricter rules than the anti-doping code. For example, a rider who was suspended for doping for more than six months cannot be hired by the MPCC's teams for two years after its suspension ends. Some riders also try to improve the image of cycling by claiming within the media that they belong to a new generation of clean riders. It was the case of Thibaut Pinot, a French cyclist, who declared to *Le Monde*: 'We can be on a podium of a famous Tour and even win today and being clean. I am convinced' (*Le Monde*, 30 July 2016). Thus, the issue of credibility seems to be recurring in cycling and the following chapter proposes investigation of the mechanisms that shape people's confidence in cycling.

Confidence is a social relation between people constructed on the basis of a judgement. To judge whether a performance is trustworthy, people have to take into account (1) their knowledge of the situation or the context, (2) the reputation of the people whose performance is questioned (Origgi, 2015), and (3) the devices of confidence which give information to reduce the uncertainty of the credibility of the performance (Quéré, 2011). A controversy surrounding a performance is an interesting terrain to analyse those mechanisms of confidence, because several actors involved in the production of the performance express diverging opinions that highlight the power relations between those actors. That is why we have decided to analyse the controversy on Froome's performance during the 2015 Tour de France.

During the tenth stage, on 14 July, Froome began the day in first place on the General Classification. On the ascent of La Pierre-Saint-Martin, he attacked his rivals six kilometres before the finish line. He did a very impressive performance and he won the stage. Commentators on a France TV channel were very impressed but they also expressed their scepticism regarding the authenticity of Froome's performance:

> And here, we have the feeling that Christopher Froom's bicycle is cycling by itself, it moves alone. It's incredible! It's amazing to see that, but the road is 12% steep, thus we need to ask ourselves some questions.[2]

TV consultants are largely recognised as experts. Therefore, the scepticism they expressed has encouraged the expression of suspicions from other actors towards

Froome's performance. This created a favourable field for a debate, which we can consider as a controversy. Indeed, we observe interactions involving conflict by opposing actors that express different representations and wishes (Huet & Sarrouy, 2015). This conflicted process is characterised by a *triadic structure* that refers to a dispute between two parties staged in front of a public audience (Lemieux, 2007). In the case of Froome's performance, there are first those who express doubts or suspicion (media, experts, some sporting actors). Second, those who try to defend their work: cyclists and team staffs attacked (sport director, manager, head of performance, etc.). Third, the public observe the controversy and sometimes takes part in it by expressing its doubts or its support within the media and social networks. None of these actors is entirely right or wrong, and it contributes to create a situation of controversy (Pestre, 2015). When actors give a judgement on Froome's performance, they put their own professional credibility at stake. We will see in our analysis that it can be a way to gain legitimacy or recognition and to defend themselves, in reaction to the receipt of an attack on personal credibility. Thus, it seems that the actors' position statements are in tension, due to interdependency between them. All together, they try to define the authenticity of Froome's work. The authenticity refers to the traceability of a product, a document or an act (Heinich, 2009), which allows, in our case, to make the link between the performance and its intentionality: is Froome's performance on the 10th stage a 'natural' and genuine performance or is it doping?

During the controversy surrounding Froome's 2015 Tour de France, the media clearly played a key role in the construction of the debate and thus deserve focus for their contribution. Through their choices in terms of data, experts, interviewees, images, and their editorial treatment, they shaped the controversy. Their actions increased the suspicions or eased the tensions as they put forward more information or interpretations. Moreover, as observer and commentator of sporting events, they are highly interested in the credibility of performance and it seems fundamental for them to show that rankings reflect the real merit of athletes. But the media also construct their position depending on competitors' positions and are partially autonomous towards the social spaces they mediatise (Marchetti, 2005). Thus, we would like to analyse how they took part in the controversy and how it reveals the power relations they are engaged in and that they contribute to redefine within the debates.

Theoretical perspective

Language is not just communication, it can also be performative (Austin, 1962). And sportspeople have to produce a double performance. They have to perform on the field and also in their narrative to ensure that their performances are recognised as 'real'. In order to avoid any suspicions of doping or corruption, they need to give proof that their performances are legitimate. Their discourses interact with other actors' such as researchers, sports fans, and the media.

Controversies arise from many actors that contribute to the valorisation, critique, or belittling of the riders' performances. However, one of the key actors are the journalists because they have the power to provide visibility to the various actors, including themselves. So, they strongly influence the way controversies are expressed in the public arena.

Andrew Abbott's research on systems theory of professions (1988) is inspiring in our analysis of the interrelated relations between the groups of actors involved in the controversy. Although his work is mainly observing how actors interact to gain specific jurisdiction, which is not really an issue in our research, he also suggests the idea of an interdependence between the various ecologies. For the specific case of sport performance, the groups of actors interacting and the public constitute an 'audience', which can be both spectators of and actors in the controversy. Behaviours of actors are influenced and, in return, have some effects on the other actors of the audience. So, the interactions between people (Goffman, 1974) within the cycling audience operate according to an ecological system in which journalists, physicians, cyclists, coaches, fans, researchers interact (Abbott, 1988). However, the audiences are not homogeneous; there may be conflicts of interests between actors, diversity of judgements, and values. Because actors are not in the same situation, they do not necessarily share the same interests and have to face different constraints. As a consequence, the audience constitutes a complex structural interaction that can be understood as 'linked ecologies' (Abbott, 2003: 30).

Second, Bourdieu's theory on symbolic capital and symbolic power helps us to understand how the positions of the actors involved in the controversy are shaped and modified within this process. Symbolic capital refers to all the forms of capital (cultural, religious, artistic or in our case: sporting, journalistic, scientific, management, etc.) that are recognised within the society or specific fields (Bourdieu, 1994: 161). We can distinguish two forms of symbolic capital. First, a specific symbolic capital related to the occupation of actors. It is a particular status recognised by the other actors of the field (Bourdieu, 1994: 161) but not necessarily outside of them. For example, in cycling, a teammate's work is recognised by the riders and the team staff but most of the time is ignored by the public. Second, there is a more global and transversal symbolic capital that has a larger recognition. The status of a champion or famous journalist gives recognition in several areas, such as among other professional sports or entertainment icons. Footballer David Beckham modelling Calvin Klein underwear is a prime example of this process. Therefore, recognition can be sometimes converted for professional reconversion or economic capital. The symbolic power depends on the level of symbolic capital. It is a power 'which is achieved only with the complicity of those who don't want to know that they suffer from it or exercised it' (Bourdieu, 1977: 405). A high level of symbolic capital allows an actor to have a higher power position. Depending on the type of symbolic capital, symbolic power will apply in a specific area or within several fields. Consequently, the higher the symbolic status of an actor, the more legitimate it will be for them to intervene in the controversy recognised by the audience.

Methodology

To analyse the role of the media during the controversy that has surrounded Froome's performance during the 2015 Tour de France, we analysed a corpus of 320 press articles and 15 videos. The articles come from four French daily newspapers: *Le Figaro*, *Libération*, *L'Équipe*, and *Le Monde*. The videos were broadcasted on the French channel *France TV*'s *YouTube* platform. We have selected all the articles and videos where the name of « Froome » was mentioned. The period analysed (27 June 2015–2 August 2015) covers the Tour de France 2015, but also the week before and the week after the race. The newspapers were selected because of their representativeness of the diversity of the French press: *Le Figaro*, is a right-wing newspaper. It is the main political opponent of *Libération*, a leftist newspaper. *Le Monde* is a broadsheet newspaper that claims to have a neutral political position. *L'Équipe* is the only French sports newspaper. Finally, *France TV* is the French public broadcasting channel. It had the exclusive TV rights for the 2015 Tour de France. The corpus is only composed of French media, a choice we made because of the scale the controversy took in France, consequence of the symbolic value of the Tour de France in this country.

We used the software Nvivo to code the articles and videos and proceed to a discourse analysis. The aim was to highlight the way actors try to position themselves during the controversy. Moreover, through their public talk, actors try to legitimate themselves by performing a role. Thus, we have conducted an analysis of the performativity of the discourses (Austin, 1962) to see how actors create discourses in order to defend their professional interests.

Results

To understand how media participate within the controversy surrounding Froome's performance during the 2015 Tour de France, we analysed the way they interact with the other key actors of the ecosystem of the cycling performance: (1) the scientific experts who are at the beginning of the controversy, (2) the cyclists and the teams who defend themselves after the firsts attacks, and (3) the other media and journalists who take part in the controversy. We also studied how, by doing so, they contribute to change the power relations between other actors in the controversy and how they change the ecosystem.

Who tells the truth about Froome's performance? The relationship between media and experts

The audience of Froome's controversy has particular expectations concerning the interactions between actors involved in the debate. They expect credible discourses that can explain or question Froome's performance. Many members of the audience are also expecting some support to be able to assess the discourses and to know who lies and who tells the truth. To shape their opinion on the cyclists' discourses, relying on the analyses of some experts seems to be an important resource. The media may contribute to build the arguments of those experts as a 'credible story', by giving them legitimacy. They also use this process to gain credibility and position themselves in the controversy. For example, on 19 July, on the TV show 'Stade 2', a famous sports programme on France TV, Pierre Sallet is presented as follows:

> This evening in Stade 2, we offer you a scientific demonstration with foolproof numbers and markers. [...] Pierre Sallet has a Phd in physiology and his team of statisticians works for ASO, for the organiser. [...] Pierre Sallet was interested especially to the performance of Christopher Froome [...] in the ascent of La Pierre-Saint-Martin.[3]

Presenting Pierre Sallet as a PhD and emphasising the robustness of his analyses is a way for the channel to give him credit. The channel provides him a status of expertise which gives him a high level of prestige and strengthens the potential impact of his discourse. Indeed, it exists as a shared belief that experts' knowledge is 'true', giving them a high symbolical power and a certain legitimacy, on the contrary to laymen's knowledge (Blais, 2006, referring to Foucault). Thus, when the channel names Sallet as an expert, it is a performative speech act (Austin, 1962). This process is reinforced by the fact that during the report, Sallet stresses the high scientific reliability of his method, which allows estimation of the power developed by the riders from the time required to accomplish the ascent: 'It's a reliable mathematical model which gives us an average power for the whole ascension: 425 Watts. [...] Those things are validated by the scientific community. Those methods are used for several decades and are very reliable'.[4] This allows him to 'consolidate his power by establishing his authority on the truth' (Blais, 2006: 153) about Froome's performance. According to him, Froome's profile is suspect. France TV and Sallet transform the argument of the expert in a demonstration of truth by emphasising the scientific nature of the method. This process allows the channel to legitimise its report by showing that the arguments presented are formulated by an expert. It reinforces Sallet's and Stade 2's symbolic capital because their expert authority can be recognised widely, especially by the public.

Other media took position in the debate after the broadcast and Stade 2's attempt to impose a 'true' analysis. In order to strengthen their own position as sports news producers, they have invited 'their' expert to discuss Froome's power meter profile. The French Newspaper *Le Monde* interviewed Antoine Vayer, who uses the same watt estimation method as Pierre Sallet. He also expressed criticism towards Froome's performance. The newspaper presented Vayer as an expert by emphasising his level of skill in the analysis of the physical performance:

> Antoine Vayer, measures and analyses for Le Monde for several years the power produced by the riders of the Tour in mountains. [...] The specialist of the sporting performance has published the video and SRM (power sensor brand) data of Froome on social network.
>
> (*Le Monde*, 16 July 2015)

Two days later, another newspaper, *Le Figaro*, chose to give a voice to Frédéric Grappe. The newspaper credits him as an expert because of his scientific abilities: 'Frédéric Grappe, head of performance of FDJ (Française des Jeux) and Senior Lecturer at Besançon gives us an update'. Grappe expressed criticism towards the watt estimation method (that Sallet and Vayer presented respectively on France 2 TV and in *Le Monde*): 'Analyses about Froome are just a model. It doesn't measure the power directly on the bike. There are [...] different variables and we estimate a power output. But the error is more or less 5%'. Finally, he criticises the low level of expertise of some other experts that would only use the controversy to show up. He obviously refers to Pierre Sallet and Antoine Vayer, thus nourishing the controversy: 'But some people make too much buzz and I wanted to say they are intellectually dishonest. Moreover they are pseudo-scientists who aren't validated by the scientific community [...] It's a big trap.' (*Le Figaro*, 18 July 2015).

The experts can refer to distinct data, method and analysis. Therefore, we observe that they argue through the different media, which is a way to reinforce their own credibility. It gives rise to a controversy between experts within the controversy on Froome's performance in which they struggle to defend their specific capital. Indeed, actors are all interested in intervening in the controversy because their discourses on the performance allow them to legitimate their own position. To this end, they defend their professional skills, which give value to their specific symbolic capital. That contest is orchestrated but also instrumentalised by the media, which find here a way to take power in the controversy. By giving an important credit to the experts, the media redefine the ecological relation between the actors involved in the controversy.

The media are an ambivalent resource for sporting actors in terms of creating credibility

The media give space to sporting actors, who can take advantage of this media coverage to improve their image, present themselves positively, especially by arguing against the suspicion of doping. It can be an opportunity for them to defend their reputation, how they think they are seen (Origgi, 2015: 8), to face the attacks of some experts. Their discourses in the media have potentially a big impact. Sports champions are traditionally expected to be role models, representing the values of equity and morality that are associated to sport (Dorvillé, 2002: 26) and have a high transversal symbolic capital. This provides them and their public speeches a certain credibility (Blais, 2006: 152). This facet can be observed for example in *L'Équipe's* article entitled 'I will never flout the yellow jersey' (*L'Équipe*, 27 July 2015) which gives – it is obvious just from the title – the cyclist a public arena to defend the value of his performance. It is also the case in this article from *Le Figaro*:

> Chris Froome remains a strong yellow jersey. Impervious to the attacks and doubts: 'I stay focused on my race. After the Tour, I'm ready to pass physiological test, if some independent experts wish it. [...] That's normal questions, in view of the past, but at a moment, it's about a lack of respect to the job done. I'm training 9 months per year, often from 6 am to 10 pm, let people come see me and said that I'm not clean ...'
>
> (*Le Figaro*, 16 July 2015)

Le Figaro gives Chris Froome an opportunity to attest to the credibility of his performance. It is also an opportunity for him to defend the quality of his work (Karpik, 1989), by underlining that his performance is due to hard training and not doping, and thus to preserve as much as possible his symbolic capital. By doing so, the newspaper tempers the critics towards Froome's performance and the controversy. A place is also given to the staff members to defend themselves:

> A feeling which Nicolas Portal had also diffused. 'It's very frustrating', regrets French sport director of team Sky. 'Those former riders and managers are supposed to know the sport at their fingertips and they launch things freely'. A former manager on RMC[5] (Cyrille Guimard) says that there are couple of things wrong. But if it's wrong for him it's because he understands nothing at all, and it's too bad.
>
> (*L'Équipe*, 19 July 2015)

Interviews in this newspaper provide access to the public arena for Sky's staff to discredit the critics. However, the journalists can decide to support riders' explanations or to question and discredit the testimonies. It is the second case here, where the journalist shows that the yellow jersey avoids the principal topic of the discussion:

> Before the Tour, Froome has treated as 'clowns' those who interpret the power markers for expose the cheaters without positive controls. Interviewed last Tuesday about this video, he merely answered that 'Those are the data from 2013'. And added, failure to respond to this request: 'We are focused on the race, nothing going to distracted us from it'.
>
> (*Le Monde*, 16 July 2015)

Here, the journalist discredits Froome's discourse by deconstructing its authority argument. He shows that the yellow jersey avoids the principal topic of the discussion. The journalist's speech act not only discredits Froome's performance, but it is also performing his own professional value. He has to show that he is a 'good' critical journalist, relevant in his analysis and source, and not afraid of being critical towards the leader of the Tour de France. He feeds the controversy because as a broadsheet newspaper, he has a solid reputation, even if sports news is not its main domain of expertise.

Because Team Sky and Froome are part of the bigger ecology of professional cycling, the journalist's analysis and more broadly the controversies may change the perception of the whole corporation. Indeed, according to Aubel & Ohl (2015), the existence of the team depends on the loyalty and the confidence of the sponsors, which are attracted by credible positions in credible ranking. A lack of interest from the sponsors is a real threat for the teams and the riders. Thus, discrediting Froome's testimony can potentially have an impact on the position of its team, but also on the power positions in the field of cycling and it can modify its economy.

Sporting actors are the masters of their own speeches, notably during the press conferences that are the main way elite cyclists communicate. However, the way their discourses are mobilised afterwards by the media, is not under their control. The media are an ambivalent resource for them in the sense that they can use cyclists' testimonies to give credit or discredit them. Therefore, the media have the power to influence the beliefs about the authenticity of the performance.

Newspapers treat the controversy in order to confirm their position in the media field

This third part will focus on the structure of the press and will show that the role of the media within the controversy also depends on: their position within the French media field, the way the others take part in it, and the way they assert their authority. Thus, we will see that social conditions can explain the performativity of speech. Marchetti (2005: 65) has shown that the autonomy of a journalistic specialisation towards the social space it mediatises depends partly on 'the degree to which one or the other imposes its problematic and its principals of hierarchisation'. Therefore, being critical towards the authenticity of a performance, and denouncing a potential 'cheater' can be a way for a journalist and a newspaper to grow its status within the media field (Boltanski, Darré, & Schiltz, 1984: 40): 'try to reclaim, this tangible salvation which is only accessible by the granting of others'. Effectively, it allows the newspaper to enforce its point of view on the authenticity of the performance and to put the question of the 'truth' at the centre of the discussions. This kind of treatment can have a big impact on cycling ecology by affecting the reputation of the cyclists and teams. But, in the first place, it is a way for a journalist to increase his capacity to influence the social space more than his competitors, which in turn increases the journalist's power in the media field.

During the controversy, *Le Monde* was the newspaper which expressed the most virulent suspicions toward the rider's credibility:

> And if we speak about doping for Sky, I have heard that the data stole on their computers and that we can see on the video of Froome in the Ventoux in 2013 are … 'normal'. Oh so? Because is it 'normal' to win Quintana at the red flame with a heart beating at 157 beats. Like me when I put my bike out of the car at Longchamp …
>
> (*Le Monde*, 18 July 2015)

Le Monde emphasised the inconsistency of Froome's physiological data. It qualified the cyclist's performance as abnormal, therefore as artificial, and clearly threw doubts over its credibility. This treatment was recurring throughout all the controversy: 'While others riders don't hide it, Froome refuses, for example, to communicate his VO2max (maximal consumption of oxygen), a determining factor in endurance sports' (*Le Monde*, 16 July 2015).

The newspaper also showed its lack of confidence towards Froome and even compared him to Lance Armstrong at the end of the race:

> The Britain has preferred to stress the fact that the yellow jersey was 'deserved'. […] In 2005, Lance Armstrong, at the end of his 7th victorious Tour de France, had to say goodbye, used those famous words: 'I would like to send a message to people who don't believe in cycling, to the cynics, to the sceptics. I'm sorry that they don't believe in the miracles, in the dreams. Too bad for them'.
>
> (*Le Monde*, 28 July 2015)

This broadsheet newspaper is well known for its investigative journalism (Marchetti, 2002: 38), including on doping in cycling, as the paper revealed the Festina affair. Thus, it has to confirm this position within this controversy by being critical towards the yellow jersey.

Libération, a leftist newspaper that is historically in political opposition with *Le Figaro*, takes part in the controversy by questioning and expressing doubts about Froome's performances: 'Cycling is not healed', said to *Libération* an angry leader. 'There are some bandits who take advantage of this. We are back five or six years ago' (*Libération*, 16 July 2015). The newspaper, which has to respond to its critical editorial line adopts an argumentative and judgemental approach. He does it sometimes indirectly, by quoting the judgement of some other critical actors:

> Nicolas Portal, [Froome]'s sport director admits that he lived a stage that we see 'one every five or six years.' Then, he remembers the demonstration of his English turbo at the Ventoux in 2013. 'Well, it's true that this is the second time in three editions' […] But in the peloton, they remain discreet.

> Marc Sergeant, the Lotto-Soudal's manager: 'In the first six, there are three Sky. That means that they are very strong. Oh, and the second of the stage, who is he? A Sky too?' True: Richie Porte. 'It is not easy to draw conclusions', says Jérémy Roy (FDJ).
>
> (*Libération*, 15 July 2015)

However, *Libération* stays less critical than *Le Monde* and calls for caution regarding suspicions towards Froome. For example, it uses the testimony of Christophe Bassons, a former French cyclist but also a prominent figure of anti-doping, who tries to take into account all the parameters that can explain Froome's performance:

> But a part of the peloton was also disgusted by the demonstration of strength of the British and his team. [...] To his defence, his performance at La Pierre-Saint-Martin was done with back wind, at lower level than his performance at Mont Ventoux in 2013. [...] 'It is not because the French are in difficulties that we have to suspect them of doping' nuances the ex-professional Christophe Bassons.
>
> (*Libération*, 16 July 2015)

The paper also underlines that physiological data are very hard to interpret: 'The goal: prove the natural character of "Froomey" ascents. A fool's game. Nobody is in position to interpret the data (the famous watts), that are beside incomplete' (*Libération*, 25 July 2015). *Libération* stays more critical within the controversy than *Le Figaro*. Indeed, *Le Figaro* is laudatory towards Froome's performance, like here for example: 'The British, winner by K.O, at the top of La Pierre-Saint-Martin, gave to his yellow jersey the radiance of a predictable coronation' (*Le Figaro*, 15 July 2015). The right-wing newspaper uses gratifying adjectives to speak about Froome and gives him a place to justify himself, despite the controversy:

> Hard to believe it although Chris Froome seems able to tame the percentages and the elements, he appeared ruthless for truss his opponents according to his sensations, clever to rule the race with the support of a team with unique soundness and seems impervious to the suspicion that pursue his performances.
>
> (*Le Figaro*, 17 July 2015)

Le Figaro clearly implements the celebration of cycling and, more precisely here, the leader of the Tour de France. We can wonder if it is not a way for this conservative newspaper to please its readership. Indeed, road cycling in France is mainly practiced and followed in media by people closed to business, who share traditional values. It is exactly the heart of Figaro's readership. Thus, the newspaper has no interest in being specifically critical towards doping in cycling and in harming the reputation of this sport or the Tour de France.

Finally, *L'Équipe*'s position within the controversy could be situated almost at the same level of criticism than *Libération*:

> However, around Sky's bus, the movie of his fierce demonstration of the day before, at La Pierre-Saint-Martin, was in all the mind and was feeding the discussions. What should we think about that? [...] As in 2013, the Froome 'unease' crystallised itself around his ease to beat his rivals, moreover with a terrifying thinness and an unorthodox pedalling style – not to say one of the most ugly – which can visually reinforce a strange impression.
>
> (*L'Équipe*, 16 July 2015)

The sports daily asks Froome's team to provide some physiological data to certify the performance: 'And what about the Team Sky? If it has nothing to hide, why does it persist to refuse to publish the power profile of its leader, while others team agree to do it' (*L'Équipe*, 16 July 2015). *L'Équipe* has been criticised in the past for its lack of investigation on doping in cycling, particularly during the Festina affair in 1998 (Dorvillé, 2002: 28). Thus, we can assume that expressing some doubts toward Froome's performance on the 2015 Tour de France is a way for the paper to show its professionalism and avoid any doubt of complacency. It might also be a way to prove its independence towards its holder, ASO, which is also the organiser of the Tour de France. *L'Équipe*'s treatment of the Froome controversy depends on its position in two different ecologies. (1) The sport ecology, where the newspaper plays a major role in providing information on sport and has to maintain its relationship with sport field. (2) The media ecology in which *L'Équipe* tries to defend its position of leader in sport information and that it can also be critical towards sport.

Structural aspects of the media field have a big impact on the journalists and their journalistic productions. In the case of the controversy on Froome, the four newspapers that we analysed reaffirm their position and traditional editorial line, more or less critical and investigative, in order to satisfy their readership and preserve their specific symbolical capital in the media field (Souanef, 2015: 78). This treatment is also built in comparison with what the other newspapers do and therefore determined by a competitive process (Marchetti, 2002: 3).

Conclusion

The controversy surrounding Froome's performance during the 2015 Tour de France subsided after the end of the race. We can consider that it more or less ended with the publication of Froome's physiological data in December 2015. The yellow jersey passed some physiological tests at a GlaxoSmithKline (GSK) laboratory in London in autumn 2015 to try to attest that his capacities are normal even if some actors didn't trust those results.

During the main period of the controversy, which we have studied in this chapter, the media clearly played a key role. Those we analysed took part in the controversy and participated in the process of the production of the credibility of the performance. Each had a unique way to proceed. Some expressed strong criticism (*Le Monde*), others choose to be more careful and balanced (*Libération*, *L'Équipe*) or to stay more neutral (*Le Figaro*). The media construct their position by mobilising cyclists' testimonies that they can legitimise or discredit. Thus, media control for a large part the reputation of the sporting actors. They also use expert's analyses that they choose, contributing in this way to 'make' them expert and to give them a higher power position to speak in the controversy. All of this allows media to build their own legitimacy. Their journalistic treatments are determined by the necessity to satisfy their readership (and depend therefore on their position within the media field) and to preserve their symbolical power within with regard to their competitors (Marchetti, 2002). Thus, controversy appears to be one situation in which the actors question power positions in their future relations with each other (Lemieux, 2007: 3).

Consequently, media modify the cycling ecology during the controversy because they possess the power of the visibility. They are able to act on the confidence relationships between the 'audience' (Abbott, 1988) by building the reputation of actors. They give visibility to the 'devices of confidence' (Quéré, 2011) that are a basis of information on which people can rely to build their judgement. Moreover, to be legitimate in an ecologic system like cycling actors need some specific symbolic capital. In the same time, to be legitimate in the controversy, actors hate to find a global recognition of their symbolic capital to have a discourse with a high level of authority and to be considered as the most trustworthy. As Pierre Bourdieu said (1977: 408–409): 'The different classes and fractions of classes are engaged in a symbolical struggle to impose the definition of social world the most faithful to their interests'. To this end, actors need a stage of visibility that depends on the media which are crucial actors of the controversy.

Notes

1 'Union Cycliste Internationale Presidential Manifesto 2017' https://static1.squarespace.com/static/59031a839de4bb3c2b218f87/t/592fdedfe58c62421ed772db/1496309472752/Brian+Cookson+2017+Manifesto+-+English+-+FINAL.pdf
2 '10th[e] stage: Froome banish Contador and Quintana!', 14 July 2015, France TV Sport: www.youtube.com/watch?v=8e39EMkpTpc consulted on 30 September 2017.
3 Stade 2, France TV Sport, 19 July 2015: www.youtube.com/watch?v=lf2K6fT-4Y4
4 Ibidem.
5 A French radio channel.

References

Abbott, A. (1988). *The System of Professions. An Essay on the Division of Expert Labour*. Chicago: The Univsersity of Chicago Press.

Abbott, A. (2003). Ecologies liées à propos du système des professions. *Les professions et leurs sociologies: Modèles théoriques, catégorisations, évolutions*, 1–37.

Aubel, O., Brissonneau, C. & Ohl, F. (2013). Le dopage comme analyseur du drame social du travail cycliste. In M. Perrenoud (Eds), *Les mondes pluriels de Howard S. Becker* (pp. 9–28). Paris: La Découverte.

Aubel, O. & Ohl, F. (2015). De la précarité des coureurs cyclistes professionnels aux pratiques de dopage. L'économie des coproducteurs du WorldTour. *Actes de la recherche en sciences sociales*, 4, 28–41.

Austin, J.L. (1962). *How to do Things with Words*. Oxford: Clarendon Press.

Blais, L. (2006). Savoir expert, savoirs ordinaires: qui dit vrai ?: Vérité et pouvoir chez Foucault. *Sociologie et sociétés*, 38, 151–163.

Boltanski, L., Darré, Y., & Schiltz, M.-A. (1984). La dénonciation. *Actes de la recherche en sciences sociales*, 3–40.

Bourdieu, P. (1977). Sur le pouvoir symbolique. *Annales. Economies, Sociétés, Civilisations*, 3, 405–411.

Bourdieu, P. (1994). *Raisons Pratiques sur la Théorie de l'Action*. Paris: Seuil.

Dorvillé, C. (2002). Ethique sportive, éthique journalistique: une mise en questions. *Les Cahiers du journalisme*, 18–33.

Foucault, M. (2003). *Le Pouvoir Psychiatrique. Cours au Collège de France. 1973–1974*. Paris: Gallimard.

Goffman, E. (1974). *Les Rites d'Interactions*. Paris: Les Editions de Minuit.

Heinich, N. (2009). L'administration de l'authenticité. *Ethnologie française*, 39, 509–519.

Huet, R. & Sarrouy, O. (2015). Le fleuve et ses berges: la sociologie des controverses, ou la négation de l'existence. *Hermès, La Revue*, 3, 101–108.

Hughes, E.C. (1976). The social drama of work. *Mid-American Review of Sociology*, *1*, 1–7.

Karpik, L. (1989). L'économie de la qualité. *Revue française de sociologie*, 30, 187–210.

Lemieux, C. (2007). A quoi sert l'analyse des controverses? *Mil neuf cent. Revue d'histoire intellectuelle*, 191–212.

Marchetti, D. (2002). Les sous-champs spécialisés du journalisme. *Réseaux*, *1*, 22–55.

Marchetti, D. (2005). Sub-fields of specialized journalism. In R. Benson & E. Neveu (Eds), *Bourdieu and the Journalistic Field* (pp. 64–82). Cambridge: Polity Press.

Marchetti, D., Rasera, F., Schotté, M., & Souanef, K. (2015). Les enjeux sociaux des classements sportifs. *Actes de la recherche en sciences sociales*, 4, 4–9.

Origgi, G. (2015). *La réputation. Qui dit quoi de qui*. Paris: Presse Universitaires de France.

Pestre, D. (2015). Controverse. In E. Henry et al. (Eds), *Dictionnaire critique de l'expertise* (pp. 91–98). Paris: Presses de Science Po.

Quéré, L. (2011). Confiance et reconnaissance. *Social Science Information*, 375–390.

Souanef, K. (2015). Ecrire sur les footballeurs d'un club professionnel. Contribution à l'analyse des logiques de production de l'information sportive. *Actes de la recherche en sciences sociales*, 4, 72–85.

Chapter 15

The clean corrective

Can thinking about clean cyclists enhance anti-doping?

Matt Englar-Carlson

The growing empirical base on anti-doping largely focuses on the factors that produce doping behaviour or on athletes that are either already on the path to doping and the methods for changing their existing illicit behaviour. The emphasis on doping itself exists despite athletes' overwhelming desire to engage in their sport without performance-enhancing substances (Morente-Sanchez & Zabala, 2013). There is less known about why athletes *do not* use performance-enhancing substances (Chan, 2015), especially in sports such as cycling where substance use pervaded the sporting culture from its origins (Brewer, 2002; Connelly, 2015; Dimeo, 2014; Thompson, 2008; Waddington & Smith, 2009). The focus on doping is not surprising, since doping is the 'deviant' behaviour to be eradicated and thus draws the most attention. Though the term 'clean' referring to athletes that do not dope has emerged as one of the targets of anti-doping, and 'clean' features in the language of educational programmes (Backhouse, 2015), the existing knowledge base is overly problem-focused on doping, on athletes' deficits, and enforcement of existing anti-doping policies and rules (Backhouse, 2015; Englar-Carlson, Gleaves, Macedo, & Lee, 2016; Hoberman, 2002). Whereas it is important to understand doping behaviour, it is equally important to investigate the behaviour, cultures, and contexts that promote cyclists who train and compete without using prohibited methods of performance enhancement. This chapter focuses on the central question of 'What happens when promoting clean sport becomes the focus of anti-doping efforts?' Another way of looking at this is to reframe the common research question of 'Why do athletes dope and how can we stop it?' to 'Why do athletes complete cleanly and how can we encourage it?[1]

There are calls to broaden our understanding of doping through cross disciplinary research from the humanities (Christiansen & Gleaves, 2013). Heeding that call, the emerging field of positive psychology provides a corrective frame that shifts the focus from doping to clean behaviour (Englar-Carlson et al., 2016). Positive psychology studies conditions and processes that contribute to the flourishing or optimal functioning of people, groups, and institutions (Gable & Haidt 2005). In cycling, a positive psychology frame posits that anti-doping is best comprehended by a clear understanding of both doping and clean behaviour with a focus on the well-being of athletes and the conditions, strengths, and virtues that allow clean athletes to thrive (Englar-Carlson et al., 2016). Highlighting and elevating clean athletes and existing clean behaviour provides a counterpoint to the accepted norm that doping behaviour is a pervasive social norm in cycling. Whereas in previous eras one could confidently suggest that mostly 'everyone was doing it[2]', anecdotal reports from professional cyclists[3] indicate that professional cyclists are able to compete today at the highest levels without using prohibited substances or methods to enhance performance. Perception of social norms matter, as the perceptions of normative group behaviours tend to guide behaviour by providing information about 'normal' behaviour in social environments and 'deviant' behaviour that is deemed unacceptable (Bicchieri, 2006). If a goal of anti-doping is to create sporting spaces where clean athletes are protected and valued by athletes themselves – and not solely enforced by authorities – then clean sport behaviour and the mechanisms that support it must be elevated and depicted as normal. Awareness of clean behaviour and the associated structures that sustain clean athletes could help identify how clean individuals and communities thrive and become more successful.

The conundrum with the use of *clean*

Before going further, it is important to comment on the use of the term 'clean' in relation to anti-doping. Often when I mentioned to friends or colleagues that I focus my research on clean professional cyclists, there are often two responses: (1) What is that? or (2) Do they even exist? It is understandable that the casual observer might not understand anti-doping and cycling, and instead adopt the prevailing dominant narrative that equates cycling and doping as one of the same – for example, the recent mockumentary *Tour de Pharmacy* (Hughes, Samberg, Miller, Szymanski, & Bernad, 2017). For many, the notion of 'clean' cycling does not exist (Van Reeth & Lagae, 2012). It is also quite telling about the state of anti-doping and cycling that there is uncertainty and debate even within the scholarly community about what to name athletes and/or behaviour that ostensibly adheres to anti-doping rules and the spirit of the sport. Henning (2017) notes that it is important for scholars to be clear what they are referring to when they talk about anti-doping.

'Clean' is a short-hand term used to describe athletes not engaged in doping practice, yet it is a loaded and 'murky' term (Dimeo, 2016; Englar-Carlson et al., 2016; Henning, 2017). *Clean* can be contrasted with *dirty*, which could be equated with subverting anti-doping standards and being found in violation of those standards. There is also a moral connotation that goes with the terms clean and dirty, with the idea that clean is equated with purity. The simple fact exists that there are cyclists who have not tested positive for performance-enhancing drugs and thus appear to be *clean* but are in fact using performance-enhancing drugs that violate anti-doping standards without being detected, and thus are actually *dirty*. What is considered clean can get even shadier when therapeutic use exemptions (TUEs), tainted supplements, the use of legal but questionable substances (i.e. tramadol[4]), and inadvertent use[5] is added to the mix. Despite these complications and due to the lack of a more suitable option, I continue to use the term clean in my scholarship. As my colleagues and I noted previously (Englar-Carlson et al., 2016), clean is often the language of athletes themselves and reflects the internal discourse and language used in the cycling community to refer to athletes who follow anti-doping rules. Taking it a step further, however, the *intentionality* of the athlete in being clean is critical. In this chapter, clean is used to refer to athletes who do not intentionally violate any anti-doping rules during training or competition and are not gaming the system through TUEs or legal but questionable substances. For these athletes, clean is part of their ethos and identity and is an intentional act. The clarification and extension of clean for this chapter is necessary as it is focused on exploring and promoting healthy behaviours that are not due to chance.

Changing the frame of the doping landscape

Doping is considered to be a complex behaviour (Aubel & Ohl, 2014; Ntoumanis, Ng, Barkoukis, & Backhouse, 2014) embedded within the history of cycling (Dimeo, 2014). Following the 1998 Festina scandal, efforts in anti-doping stepped up in professional cycling because the sport had a reputation for tolerating doping and not punishing professional cyclists sufficiently who did test positive (Brissonneau, 2015; Waddington & Smith, 2013). The Festina scandal was a watershed moment for the sport due to the awareness that doping had for the health of the sport of cycling (but also in terms of the well-being of cyclists themselves). The attention on doping within cycling placed more emphasis on anti-doping enforcement with the notion that increased detection with longer punishment could act as an effective deterrent to doping within the sport.[6]

To be clear, the emphasis on detection and punishment has dramatically reduced doping in cycling, but it has not necessarily eradicated the problem. The desire to detect and punish doping violators appears to have taken anti-doping, including anti-doping research, about as far as it can go. Anti-doping research has typically centred on the act of 'doping' itself with the existing knowledge base being overly problem-focused on athletes' deficits (Backhouse et al., 2007; Hoberman, 2002). Such research provides ideas about the pathways (i.e. Sport Control Drug Model) to understand the roads leading athletes to doping, but it offers little insight into how athletes who do not intentionally use banned performance-enhancing substances continue avoiding performance-enhancing substance misuse.[7] The focus is primarily on doping, rather than *anti*-doping or prevention. This idea is captured by Singler (2015), who observed 'what is understood by prevention in [doping in sport] consists largely of control measures, emphasising the threat of punishment after positive doping tests and raising fears about the side-effects of doping' (p. 246). Whereas no one can dispute that for the security of the sport of cycling and competition and for deterrent effects for athletes the emphasis on detection and enforcement is needed. Yet from a practical perspective catching athletes *after* they have used potentially harmful substances is not ideal and relegates anti-doping as a reactionary effort of secondary and tertiary prevention. For the most part, athletes not competing clean have already decided to dope (an exemption to this would be inadvertent violations[8]), risked their health and contributed to an un-level playing field. Though not beyond remediation, the behaviour of these athletes can be considered more established and entrenched. While detection and punishment are vital to enforcing anti-doping regulations, ultimately the more sustainable and long-term effective anti-doping strategy is one of primary prevention because these efforts would prevent doping before it occurs. Efforts that address how anti-doping can prevent athletes from using or desiring performance-enhancing substances from the beginning will ultimately reduce the incidence of doping over time.

Another consideration is that much anti-doping research rests upon questionable assumptions of doping as an individual behaviour or moral fault that rests within the athlete (i.e. micro focus) rather than seeing the systemic nature of doping that is embedded in contextual and social relations (i.e. macro focus), especially in relation to team organisation, employment conditions (Aubel & Ohl, 2014), and sporting culture (Pappa & Kennedy, 2013). Athletes who dope exist in systems, contexts, and cultures that promote or encourage doping behaviour to reach particular outcomes (Johnson, 2012; Engelberg, Moston & Skinner, 2015), and this may be particularly true in cycling where doping has been normalised (Pappa & Kennedy, 2013). It is fair to say that some systems promote doping more than others, and it is likely that other systems are more conducive to clean behaviour.

Though ample research indicates athletes do not begin sport with a desire to dope (Morente-Sánchez & Zabala, 2013), a knowledge gap exists around empirically identifying the specific reasons or factors as to why some athletes continue to abstain from doping, even when they perceive detection and punishment as ineffective deterrents. Further, the focus on athletes who engage in doping practices eclipses the fact that elite athletes overwhelmingly support wellness, health, and ethical sporting behaviour (Gleaves & Christiansen, in press). Yet very little is known about clean athletes, why they choose to stay clean, and how they do it. Doping is complex, understood as more than single bad apples or one poor decision; yet the same must also be true for being a clean elite cyclist – they are likely more than just good apples or good people, but most likely the positioning of being clean is layered rather around individual differences, and but also the macro level situational, cultural, contextual factors, and systemic factors (Johnson, 2012; Petroczi & Aidman, 2008). Though an understanding of both micro and macro influences provides a more holistic understanding of doping (Blank, Kopp, Niedermeier, Schnitzer, & Schobersberger, 2016; Johnson, 2012), it does not offer a clearer picture of clean athletes and their behaviour. We encourage athletes to say no to doping, but what do we want them to say yes to?

What are we missing?

The normalisation of doping within cycling has created a situation where it is difficult to separate doping from cycling. As such, doping draws considerable attention from fans, critics, and scholars. The unmasking of the sport by athletes, scholars, and whistleblowers indicated that cycling's reputation for doping was well deserved. Cycling's history with doping and the public struggles the sport has endured means that coming to terms with that past casts a large shadow on those cyclists who are and want to train and compete cleanly.[9]

A shift in anti-doping strategies and research towards understanding clean cyclists could reverse the perceived normalisation of doping. The recognition of clean athletes elevates a counternarrative about doping in cycling, namely that there is more to the story. This could lead to understanding the adaptive and proactive behaviour that cyclists engage in to compete cleanly, reveal points of resistance/communities that support clean cyclists, uncover the local knowledge of how clean cyclists are able to be clean and compete within WADA guidelines and be able to promote and reproduce it, create opportunities for proactive partnerships with community and industry forces aligned with clean sport, and best understand how athletes themselves can be empowered to manage, maintain, and promote healthy social norms about clean cycling so that clean becomes the dominant norm (Macedo, Englar-Carlson, Lehrbach, & Gleaves, 2017). This is the potential of what could happen when the promotion of clean sport becomes the focus of anti-doping efforts.

Reaching that potential is of course the challenge that anyone involved in anti-doping faces. One might assume that cyclists who stay clean face many of the same pressures and pathways into the sport as cyclists that use performance-enhancing substances, but they go a different direction. Yet we do not know if this assumption is even correct. It might be that the reasons athletes choose good/clean behaviours are different than the reasons athletes choose bad/doping behaviours – and the existing evidence suggests that is most likely true (Blank et al., 2016). This chapter focuses on looking at how psychological processes and variables can be harnessed in the service of clean sport.

Research in psychology has pointed out that psychological traits and processes are not inherently positive or negative; instead, what matters is whether psychological characteristics promote or undermine well-being (or whether something is considered a strength), and this often depends on the context in which they operate. To understand a behaviour, one must understand the context. In that sense, clean cycling behaviour is closely tied to the context and culture in which it occurs – meaning there may be healthier environments to be cyclist. Athletes, coaches, teams, and sporting institutions therefore provide the contextual focus and the sporting cultures for understanding clean behaviour – and we should truly understand clean contexts.

What is positive psychology?

Positive psychology provides a corrective that shifts the focus from doping to clean behaviour. Positive psychology studies conditions and processes that contribute to the flourishing or optimal functioning of people, groups, and institutions (Seligman & Csikszentmihalyi, 2000), the goals of which are to better understand and apply those factors in a manner to help individuals and communities thrive and become more successful (Magyar-Moe, Owens, & Conoley, 2015). Positive psychology is philosophically strengths-based,[10] but also has defined theories, constructs, models, and interventions that can be utilised in the process of bringing that philosophical stance to the forefront (Lopez & Magyar-Moe, 2006).

Magyar-Moe, Owens, and Scheel (2015) noted a common misperception of positive psychology is that those who study and apply it are naïve, ignoring problems that exist by only focusing on the positives (McNulty & Fincham, 2012). That is incorrect as positive psychology calls for a perspective in which people are understood according to *both* their weaknesses and strengths (Ivtzan, Lomas, Hefferson, & Worth, 2016; Lopez, Snyder, & Rasmussen, 2003). Thus, understanding problems (e.g. why cyclists cheat) is important and those findings can be utilised in anti-doping, but so is studying and incorporating information about what works for cyclists who are clean and what factors buffer them in their professional sporting life from difficulties and problematic outcomes (Magyar-Moe, Owens, & Conley, 2015; McNulty & Fincham, 2012). Awareness of clean behaviour and the associated structures that sustain clean athletes helps identify how clean individuals and communities thrive and become more successful. Positive psychology and psychologists 'are as concerned with building strengths and the best things life has to offer as they are with managing weaknesses and repairing the worst things in life' (Magyar-Moe, Owens, & Scheel, 2015: 509). Positive psychology's theoretical approach to athletes doping would be holistic in vision, being as interested in helping those who engage in doping to overcome it as they are in helping those who are clean lead the most fulfilling lives possible (Seligman & Csikszentmihalyi, 2000).[11] A positive psychology frame posits that anti-doping is best comprehended by a clear understanding of both doping and clean behaviour with a focus on the well-being of athletes and the conditions, strengths, and virtues that allow clean athletes to thrive.

There are other disciplines that have benefitted from a positive psychology perspective from which cycling could learn. These include medicine and public health through the wellness movement, the emphasis on primary prevention, parenting education, substance use and addiction treatment, and drunk driving campaigns (Kobau et al., 2011; Sanders, 2008; Schueller, 2009). Law enforcement uses a positive psychology model through community policing efforts. Another example is the United States Army's Comprehensive Soldier Fitness (CSF) programme (Casey, Jr., 2011). The CSF is an integrated, proactive preventive programme that seeks to enhance psychological resilience among all members of the Army community by changing from 'a culture in which behavioural health was once stigmatised to a culture in which psychological fitness is recognised as every bit as important as physical fitness' (Casey, Jr., 2011: 2). Positive psychology was used to develop new tests and to assess psychosocial fitness in emotional, social, family, and spiritual domains in order to maximise resiliency and determine areas where members of the Army community could use additional support (Peterson, Park, & Castro, 2011). The CSF was a complete movement from a 'treatment-centric' approach to a prevention mode that enhanced psychological strengths already present in personal. Casey, Jr. (2011: 2) noted the goal of CSF was the idea that 'soldiers can "be" better before deploying to combat so they will not have to "get" better after they return'. These are just a few examples of how positive psychology theory, research, and interventions have been used as a prevention approach to address risks.

Positive psychology and cycling

Positive psychology emphasises the study of strengths, successful living, and virtue over disease, weakness, and damage. In that way, it is similar to athletes' normal mentality and behaviour where they identify strengths and focus on improvement in their performance. Therefore, examining what clean cyclists are doing well, how the range of their relationships support their clean sporting behaviour, and the cognitive orientation to remaining clean are overlooked tools in preventing doping that could emerge out of a positive psychology approach. Further, positive psychology is focused on building in people what is right rather than merely fixing what is wrong. Translated to prevention efforts, the tangible factors that support clean sporting practices – i.e. 'what is right' – become the cornerstone of anti-doping education. Anti-doping efforts then become more proactive by growing and supporting healthy and optimal behaviour rather than the status quo of being primarily reactive via detection and punishment of doping. This approach could also help all stakeholders (e.g. cyclists, team managers and coaches, sporting officials, WADA officials, etc.) get a clear sense of what clean cycling looks like at a developmental and organisational level.[12] An interesting caveat to consider is that it is often much easier to support and continue an existing behaviour than trying to extinguish one. Consider the notion that every athlete starts playing or competing clean, so the challenge is to continue that existing behaviour over the lifetime from early sports involvement into the professional level. The more that is known about how to maintain clean behaviour, the easier this task becomes.

Four areas of positive psychology research related to clean cycling

Assessment of strengths is a critical step in positive psychology (Lopez et al., 2003). Interventions can then harness these strengths to prosocial means. These interventions support both the focus population and the larger social welfare. Enhancing health also decreases psychological vulnerabilities to future distress and risk, meaning that healthy and happy people are less likely to engage in harmful and deviant behaviour (Rashid, 2008). Positive psychology applies a common language and empirical approach to research. Below are four target interactive areas that could be used to examine the experiences of clean cyclists:

1 Positive emotions (happiness, gratitude, fulfilment, thriving);
2 Positive individual traits (optimism, resiliency, hardiness, grit, character strengths);
3 Positive relationships among groups (teammates, coaches, family, community, social groups);
4 Enabling institutions (schools, teams, organisations, sporting federations) that foster positive outcomes.

It is interesting to imagine how research into these four areas could offer insight into the ways that cyclists find fulfilment in their lives and profession as a cyclist. All of these areas ponder, 'What is working, healthy, and functional in a cyclist's ecology that helps maintain a clean status?' Uncovering the answers to that question permits a true understanding what is going well in the lives of cyclists and if there are structures and supports within cycling that help promote positive emotions and clean experiences. Identification and insight could provide invaluable real-life models for other athletes about how operating and thrive within the rules. Even though athletes may not trust the doping testing systems (Overbye, 2016), they could learn to develop more trust in each other as athletes (Macedo et al., 2017). Further these positive psychology foci elevate health and wellness as possible among athletes. Though highlighting the negative health effects of doping has been unsuccessful in terms of curbing doping behaviour (Engelberg et al., 2015), it could be that knowledge about clean behaviour and its positive side effects could prove to be more beneficial as it is moving athletes towards wellness and health and it is consistent with the rules of conduct for the sport.

It is not enough to simply use positive psychology to investigate and intervene with athletes themselves. Social ecological theory considers the notion that attitudes and behaviours are not driven by personal intrinsic factors of the athlete, but also by environmental influences. This would also include proximal athletes' network and the significant role of coaches and team-mates, but also peers and other influential people (Momaya, Fawal, & Estes, 2015). Coaches and trainers have a great influence on athletes (Huybers & Mazanov, 2012), but often do not consider doping prevention as their task (Engelberg & Moston, 2016) and many are unaware of existing doping prevention approaches. Copeland and Potwarka (2016) note that effective anti-doping preventive approaches should ensure the improvement of ethical team culture by including leadership elements. Thus, a positive psychology investigation would extend in the sporting culture and networks to focus on what is working well, what networks are supportive of clean athletes and environments, and how coaches and trainers can be part of resisting the theme of doping as usual within the sport.

Targeting social norms

Knowledge gained from research using a positive psychology approach could have important ramification for targeting social norms within cycling at all developmental levels. From a social psychological framework, perceptions of normative group behaviours guide behaviour by providing information about 'normal' behaviour in social environments and 'deviant' behaviour that is off limits (Bicchieri, 2006). In professional cycling, the idea of what is 'normal' behaviour is a bit unknown. It can be observed that doping behaviour is perceived as normative due to its strong association with the sport's history (Ohl, Fincoeur, Lentillon-Kaestner, Defrance, & Brissonneau, 2015; Connolly, 2015), and because there is constant uncertainly and questioning from within and outside the sport about cyclists and their performances. An example of this is the furor surrounding British cyclist Chris Froome and his overall victory in the 2018 Giro d'Italia. After a stage 1 crash and subsequent subpar performances in the early stages, Froome stormed back in the final stages – including a dramatic long-range solo victory on stage 19 – to take the overall victory. Not only were many questioning his ability to 'ride into shape' over the grueling three-week race, but his entire entrance in the race was clouded by a pending doping sanction due to elevated salbutamol levels from stage 18 of the 2017 Vuelta a España.

People are often influenced by their observations of others because the 'social proof' these descriptive norms provide saves time and cognitive effort while giving guidance about behaviour that is likely to be effective (Cialdini, 2013). Applied to cycling, perceptions of other cyclists' practices may provide information about how individual cyclists should act – or not act – in terms of the health behaviours they adopt. For clean cyclists to wield some influence on social norms, and thus actually change the social proof that clean cycling is possible and common, their clean behaviour must be elevated and depicted as normal.

Social norms are unwritten rules about how to behave (Cialdini, 2013). They provide an expected idea of how to behave in a particular social group or culture. The presence of others seems to set up expectations for how we should be. We do not expect people to behave randomly, but rather to behave in certain ways in particular situations. Each social situation entails its own particular set of expectations about the 'proper' way to behave. Such expectations can vary from group to group and exist on the group and societal level (Bicchieri, 2006). Social norms are learned through social interaction, not alone, thus social norms theory focuses on peers because they have been found to have the greatest influence in shaping individual behaviour (Walton, 2014; Yeager & Walton, 2011). According to social norms theory (Berkowitz, 2003), unhealthy (and healthy) behaviour is fostered by perceptions (often incorrect) of how one's peers behave. These misperceptions often occur in relation to problem or risk behaviours (which are usually overestimated) and in relation to healthy or protective behaviours (which are usually underestimated) and may cause individuals to change their own behaviour to approximate the misperceived norm. Social norms can be understood as either injunctive or descriptive (Cialdini, Reno, & Kallgren, 1990).

Injunctive norms involve *perceptions* of which behaviours are typically approved or disapproved by others – how someone should behave, and therefore assist in determining what is acceptable social behaviour. Injunctive norms could be considered the morals of a community. For example, in cycling, the injunctive norm is that doping is wrong or that you should not dope. Descriptive norms involve the perceptions of the behaviours of others that are typically performed, perceptions about how most people in a community *actually* behave. Descriptive norms motivate action by informing insiders about what is considered to be effective or adaptive in a particular context and provide a decisional short cut when choosing how to behave in a particular situation. Within cycling and in the absence of a clear baseline information about incidence rates around doping, the descriptive norm within some context might be, 'If others are doping, then it must be a sensible thing to do to be successful'. Due to the normalisation of doping culture within cycling (Smith, 2017) it is easy to make that assumption. Copeland and Potwarka (2016) note the importance of informing athletes about the actual prevalence of doping, thus challenging the descriptive norm around doping, yet this is easier said than done since the actual prevalence of doping within the professional peloton is unknown.

In regards to sports, injunctive or descriptive social norms can overlap (doping is wrong, and nobody does it), or conflict (doping is wrong, but many athletes are doing it; Englar-Carlson et al., 2016). For example, a cyclist might overestimate peers' involvement in doping, which would foster one's own involvement in using performance-enhancing substances. Such misperceptions (e.g. everyone is doping) may be used by a cyclist, trainer, manager, or others to justify doping. Of course, a cyclist might underestimate peers' adoption of healthy habits (e.g. clean behaviour), which would discourage the athlete from adopting healthy behaviour. Social norms, also, are context dependent. This is important, too, as cyclists are embedded in community cultures and practices (Wagner, 2010). Being part of a certain sporting culture might also mean adopting certain norms and beliefs the individual might not have had prior to entering this specific culture (Copeland & Potwarka, 2016).

Interventions that emphasise descriptive norms tend to be more successful in influencing behaviour and social change (Aronson, Wilson, Akert, & Sommers, 2015). In regards to health behaviour, while both types of norms are associated with health behaviour intentions, associations are stronger for descriptive norms than for injunctive norms (Rivis & Sheeran, 2003). Further, descriptive norms are more influential when they are focal and salient for an individual at the time of the behaviour (Cialdini et al., 1990). Therefore, the descriptive norms must originate from the appropriate social group (e.g. athletes or cyclists themselves) and accurately reflect that social group's experiences. A positive psychology approach would directly target descriptive norms that would illuminate actual clean behaviour and norms as practiced by other cyclists within their cycling. This is also in line with what Backhouse (2015: 236) referred to as a 'community responsive approach to doping prevention' and engages athletes as active and influential partners for change (Macedo et al., 2017). The connection between using positive psychology to understand actual anti-doping behaviour (e.g. clean behaviour) and the application of a social norms approach to promoting clean cyclists and their behaviour holds promise for the future of anti-doping efforts in cycling and beyond. For a clean athlete to wield some influence on social norms, and thus actually change the social proof that clean sport is possible and common, their clean behaviour must be known, shared, elevated, and depicted as normal.

Where this could lead cycling

This chapter has focused on the clean cyclist and the sport of cycling by putting forth the notion that a goal of anti-doping is to create spaces where clean athletes are protected and valued, but at first clean athletes and the networks around them need to be understood. The question is how can this change occur in professional cycling? It seems apparent that true change within cycling can only occur when there is a cultural change/shift that emphasises clean athletes and sport, meaning that the context itself has to shift. That shift occurs when anti-doping is less reactive to violations and more focused on the bigger issue of doping prevention. This chapter suggests one place to start is to shift from thinking about primarily doping and deviance to broadening the anti-doping focus to include elevating clean athletes, behaviours, and sporting cultures. Anti-doping cannot primarily be about deterrence and testing, rather it could be expanded to include more prevention efforts. One tool to help better understand clean sport is offered by the field of positive psychology. Positive psychology research is broad in scope, but incorporates concepts such as resiliency, self-efficacy, wellness, optimal and peak performance with an emphasis on health and adaptability as opposed to dysfunction and illness (Lopez et al.,

2015). A positive psychology perspective posits that anti-doping is best comprehended by a clear understanding of both doping and clean behaviour with a focus on the well-being of athletes and the conditions, strengths, and virtues that allow clean athletes to thrive.

For anti-doping, the definition of success has to be both relevant and achievable. Ultimately, success is not measured on whether anti-doping efforts stop all cheaters or eradicate doping completely. Rather success is achieved when professional spaces exist where clean athletes are protected and valued and feel that hard work and talent and luck will be enough to compete and train successfully. If anti-doping accomplishes that goal, it does not have to stop every doper. The cheaters will exist, but they'll be the anomaly, the outlier and not the norm. Sports culture will prize not just great competition, but great, clean, competition.

Notes

1 The reader may notice a bit of a contrarian tone throughout this chapter, namely that one way to think about the potential of clean cycling is to reverse most questions about doping by replacing 'clean' where the word dope or doping would usually be used.
2 See Gleaves' chapter in this book with the same title.
3 For example, in *Cycling Weekly*, 2018 Tour de France winner Geraint Thomas commented 'I can't say 100% for the peloton, but I'm 99% cent sure that everyone's doing it the right way, working hard'.
4 While legal, tramadol's use is somewhat frowned upon due to its strength as a painkiller. Many think it should be banned – the MPCC (Movement for Credible Cycling), a voluntary organisation that has stricter anti-doping rules, does not allow its members to use the substance. The World Anti-Doping Agency (WADA, 2018) found that 4.3% of all cycling tests conducted in-competition in 2017 were positive for tramadol, far more frequently than any other sport.
5 This is uncommon. Numerous studies (Backhouse, Whitaker, & Petróczi, 2013; Morente-Sánchez & Zabala, 2013) indicate athletes show moderate to high levels of awareness when a substance's use constitutes a doping violation. Most athletes are conscious and aware of their use of banned substances.
6 An interesting parallel can be derived from the field of public health and how it would approach a health outbreak or risk. In the case of a threat to the health of a population, detection and treatment are front line efforts to reduce risk and stop an outbreak, but the long-term approach to eradicating the harm is through health promotion and prevention. This has not been the approach within professional cycling or WADA.
7 A compelling analog to the impact of studies that investigate why investigating athletes who dope can be found in studies that examined adults and physical activity. Early research on this topic focused solely on adults that did not get the minimum required physical activity. These people cited busy schedules, time commitment, enjoyment, and lack of energy as reasons they did not exercise. However, interventions focused on these reasons did not improve exercise rates for sedentary people or create any change. Once researchers studied characteristics of people who successfully exercised and developed interventions to strengthen these characteristics in sedentary adults, the research team was able to increase sedentary peoples' physical activity. The focus of this chapter

suspects the same might prove true in anti-doping. The previous focus on athletes who violate anti-doping rules means that most studies focus on places where athletes went wrong. But this says little about why other athletes went right.

8 Inadvertent or unintentional doping refers to positive anti-doping tests due to the use of any supplement containing unlisted substances banned by anti-doping regulations and organisations (Martínez-Sanz et al., 2017).

9 American cyclist Andrew Talansky in 2015 noted how the doping is always hanging over riders who try to compete cleanly, noting

> We feel a responsibility to one another to do our jobs clean, to race clean, to be outspoken proponents of anti-doping, and to achieve the best results we can and then use that as a platform to show how far the movement for clean cycling has come.

10 Smith (2006) notes that the strength-based approach emphasises people's assets rather than their deficits or problems. It is a shift from a medical model focusing on pathology to a model that stresses developing assets. It asks 'what strengths has one used to effectively address life's challenges?' Importantly, the strength-based approach operates using the language of strengths and positive human qualities that are often unrecognised, unnamed, and unacknowledged.

11 This is an important point for cycling as anti-doping should be about maintaining clean sport, but also helping athletes make a healthy return to compete cleanly even if they violate doping standards. Among many others, the Scottish cyclist David Millar in his memoir *Racing Through the Dark* chronicled his descent into depression and addiction following his 2004 doping sanction. Rather than offer support of sanctioned riders in need, WADA code limits direct support of sanctioned riders, cutting them off from their sport and professional relationships. It is not surprising that many riders experience distress during this time.

12 Imagine the difference between peeling back the layers on a doping scandal compared to peeling back the layers on how cyclists train and compete cleanly. The former can potentially extinguish doping through sanctioning of riders, coaches, and medical personnel so that that avenue of doping and that particular rider is eliminated, but the latter could provide rich knowledge that clean professional cycling is possible and knowable, and that there are some structural supports that can be duplicated to help spread this local clean knowledge to others. One of those examples is more proactive and hopeful than the other.

References

Aronson, E., Wilson, T.D., Akert, R.M., & Sommers, S.R. (2015). *Social Psychology* (9th ed.). Upper Saddle River: Prentice Hall.

Aubel, O. & Ohl, F. (2014). An alternative approach to the prevention of doping in cycling. *International Journal of Drug Policy*, *25*(6), 1094–1102.

Backhouse, S., McKenna, J., Robinson, S., & Atkin, A. (2007). *International literature review: Attitudes, behaviours, knowledge and education–drugs in sport: past, present and future*. Retrieved from www.wada-ama.org/en/resources/social-science/international-literature-review-attitudes-behaviours-knowledge-and

Backhouse, S., Whitaker, L., & Petróczi, A. (2013). Gateway to doping? Supplement use in the context of preferred competitive situations, doping attitude, beliefs, and norms. *Scandinavian Journal of Medicine & Science in Sports*, *23*, 244–252.

Backhouse, S. (2015). Anti-doping education for athletes. In V. Moller, I. Waddington, & J. Hoberman (Eds), *Routledge Handbook of Drugs in Sport* (pp. 229-238). New York: Routledge.

Berkowitz, A.D. (2003). Applications of social norms theory to other health and social justice issues. In H.W. Perkins (Eds), *The Social Norms Approach to Preventing School and College-Age Substance Abuse* (pp. 258–279). San Francisco: Jossey-Bass

Bicchieri, C. (2006). *The Grammar of Society: The Nature and Dynamics of Social Norms*. New York: Cambridge University Press.

Blank, C., Kopp, M., Niedermeier, M., Schnitzer, M., & Schobersberger, W. (2016). Predictors of doping intentions, susceptibility, and behaviour of elite athletes: a meta-analytic review. *SpringerPlus*, 5(1), 1333.

Brewer, B. (2002) Commercialization in professional cycling 1950–2001: Institutional transformations and the rationalization of 'doping'. *Sociology of Sport Journal, 19*, 276–301.

Brissonneau, C. (2015). The 1998 Tour de France: Festina, from scandal to an affair in cycling. In V. Moller, I. Waddington, & J. Hoberman (Eds) *Routledge Handbook of Drugs and Sport* (pp. 181–192). Abingdon: Routledge.

Casey, G.W., Jr. (2011). Comprehensive soldier fitness: A vision for psychological resilience in the U.S. Army. *American Psychologist*, 66(1), 1–3.

Chan, D.K.C., Hardcastle, S., Dimmock, J.A., Lentillon-Kaestner, V., Donovan, R.J., Burgin, M., & Hagger, M.S. (2015). Modal salient belief and social cognitive variables of anti-doping behaviors in sport: Examining an extended model of the theory of planned behaviour. *Psychology of Sport and Exercise, 16*, 164–174.

Christiansen, A.V. & Gleaves, J. (2013). What do the humanities (really) know about doping? Questions, answers and cross-disciplinary strategies. *Performance Enhancement & Health, 2*, 216–223.Cialdini, R.B., Reno, R.R., & Kallgren, C.A. (1990). A focus theory of normative conduct: Recycling the concept of norms to reduce littering in public places. *Journal of Personality and Social Psychology*, 58, 1015–1026.

Cialdini, R.B. (2013). *Influence: Science and Practice* (5th ed. Rev.). Boston: Pearson.

Connolly, J. (2015). Civilising processes and doping in professional cycling. *Current Sociology*, 63(7), 1037–1057.

Copeland, R. & Potwarka, L.R. (2016). Individual and contextual factors in ethical decision making: A case study of the most significant doping scandal in Canadian university sports history. *Sports Management Review, 19*, 61–68.

Dimeo, P. (2014). Why Lance Armstrong? Historical context and key turning points in the 'cleaning up' of professional cycling. *The International Journal of the History of Sport, 31*, 951–988.

Dimeo, P. (2016). The myth of clean sport and its unintended consequences. *Performance Enhancement & Health*, 4(3), 103–110.

Engelberg, T. & Moston, S. (2016). Inside the locker room: A qualitative study of coaches' anti-doping knowledge, beliefs and attitudes. *Sports in Society, 19*, 942–956.

Engelberg, E., Moston, S., & Skinner, J. (2015). The final frontier of anti-doping: A study of athletes who have committed doping violations. *Sport Management Review, 18*(2), 268–279.

Englar-Carlson, M., Gleaves, J., Macedo, E., & Lee, H. (2016). What about the clean athletes? The need for positive psychology in anti-doping research. *Performance Enhancement & Health*, 4, 116–122.

Gable, S.L. & Haidt, J. (2005). What (and why) is positive psychology? *Review of General Psychology*, 9, 103–110.

Gleaves, J. & Christiansen, A.V. (in press). Athletes' perspective on the WADA code. *International Journal of Sport Policy and Politics*.

Henning, A. (2017, October). Seeking an alternative to clean. *INHR Newsletter*. Retrieved from http://ph.au.dk/en/research/research-areas/humanistic-sport-research/research-unit-for-sports-and-physical-culture/international-network-of-doping-research/newsletters/october-2017/indr-commentary-april-henning/

Henning, A. & Dimeo, P. (2015). Questions of fairness and anti-doping in US cycling: The contrasting experiences of professionals and amateurs. *Drugs: Education, Prevention and Policy*, *22*(5), 400–409.

Hoberman, J. (2002). Sports physicians and the doping crisis in elite sport. *Clinical Journal of Sport Medicine*, *12*, 203–208.

Hughes, M.E., Samberg, A., Miller, M., Szymanski., J., & Bernad., D. (Producers) (2017). *Tour de Pharmacy* [Motion Picture]. Home Box Office.

Huybers, T. & Mazanov, J. (2012). What would Kim do: A choice study of projected athlete doping considerations. *Journal of Sport Management*, *26*, 322–334.

Ivtzan, I., Lomas, T., Hefferson, K., & Worth, P. (2016). *Second Wave Positive Psychology: Embracing the Dark Side of Life*. New York: Routledge.

Johnson, M. (2012). A systemic social-cognitive perspective on doping. *Psychology of Sport & Exercise*, *13*(3), 317–323.

Kobau, R., Seligman, M., Peterson, C., Diener, E., Zack, M., Chapman, D., & Thompson, W. (2011). Mental health promotion in public health: Perspectives and strategies from positive psychology. *American Journal of Public Health*, *101*(8), e1–e9.

Lopez, S.J. & Magyar-Moe, J.L. (2006). A positive psychology that matters. *The Counselling Psychologist*, *34*, 323–330.

Lopez, S.J., Pedrotti, J.T., and Snyder, C.R. (2015). *Positive Psychology: The Scientific and Practical Explorations of Human Strengths*. Thousand Oaks: Sage Publications.

Lopez, S.J., Snyder, C.R., & Rasmussen, H.N. (2003). Striking a vital balance: Developing a complementary focus on human weakness and strength through positive psychological assessment. In S.J. Lopez, & C.R. Snyder (Eds), *Positive Psychological Assessment: A Handbook of Models and Measures* (pp. 3–20). Washington: American Psychological Association.

Macedo, E., Englar-Carlson, M., Lehrbach, T., & Gleaves, J. (2017). Moral communities in anti-doping policy: A response to Bowers and Paternoster. *Sports, Ethics and Philosophy*. doi: 10.1080/17511321.2017.1371791

Magyar-Moe, J.L., Owens, R.L., & Conoley, C.W. (2015). Positive psychological interventions in counseling: What every counseling psychologist should know. *The Counselling Psychologist*, *43*(4), 508–557.

Magyar-Moe, J.L., Owens, R.L., & Scheel, M.J. (2015). Applications of positive psychology in counseling psychology: Current status and future directions. *The Counseling Psychologist*, *43*(3), 494–507.

Martínez-Sanz, J.M., Sospedra, I., Mañas Ortiz, C., Baladía, E., Gil-Izquierdo, A., & Ortiz-Moncada, R. (2017). Intended or unintended doping? A review of the presence of doping substances in dietary supplements used in sports. *Nutrients*, 9(10), 1093.

McNulty J.K. & Fincham F.D. (2012). Beyond positive psychology? Toward a contextual view of psychological processes and well-being. *American Psychologist*, *67*, 101–110.

Momaya, A., Fawal, M., & Estes R. (2015). Performance-enhancing substances in sports: A review of the literature. *Sports Medicine*, *45*, 517–531.

Morente-Sánchez, J., & Zabala, M. (2013). Doping in sport: A review of elite athletes' attitudes, beliefs, and knowledge. *Sports Medicine*, *43*, 395–411.

Ntoumanis, N., Ng, J., Barkoukis, V., & Backhouse, S. (2014). Personal and psychosocial predictors of doping use in physical activity settings: A meta-analysis. *Sports Medicine*, *44*, 1603–1624.

Ohl, F., Fincoeur, B., Lentillon-Kaestner, V., Defrance, J., & Brissonneau, C. (2015). The socialization of young cyclists and the culture of doping. *International Review for the Sociology of Sport*, *50*(7), 865–882.

Overbye, M. (2016). Doping control in sport: an investigation of how elite athletes perceive and trust the functioning of the doping testing system in their sport. *Sports Management Review*, *19*(1), 6–22.

Pappa, E. & Kennedy, E. (2013). 'It was my thought … he made it a reality': Normalization and responsibility in athletes' accounts of performance-enhancing drug use. *International Review for the Sociology of Sport*, *48*(3), 277–294.

Peterson, C., Park, N., & Castro, C.A. (2011). Assessment for the U.S. Army Comprehensive Soldier Fitness Program: The Global Assessment Tool. *American Psychologist*, 66(1), 10–18

Petroczi, A. & Aidman, E.V. (2008). Psychological drivers in doping: the life-cycle model of performance enhancement. *Substance Abuse Treatment, Prevention, & Policy*, 3, 1–12.

Rashid, T. (2008). Positive psychotherapy. In S.J. Lopez (Eds), *Positive Psychology: Exploring the Best in People* (Vol. 4, pp. 187–217). Westport: Praeger.

Rivis, A. & Sheeran, P. (2003). Descriptive norms as an additional predictor in the theory of planned behaviour: A meta-analysis. *Current Psychology: Developmental, Learning, Personality, Social*, *22*, 218–233.

Sanders, M. (2008). Triple p-positive parenting program as a public health approach to strengthening parenting. *Journal of Family Psychology*, *22*(4), 506–517.

Schueller, S. (2009). Promoting wellness: Integrating community and positive psychology. *Journal of Community Psychology*, *37*(7), 922–937.

Seligman, M.E.P. & Csikszentmihalyi, M. (2000). Positive psychology: An introduction. *American Psychologist*, *55*, 5–14.

Seligman, M., Steen, T., Park, N., & Peterson, C. (2005). Positive psychology progress: Empirical validation of interventions. *American Psychologist*, *60*(5), 410–421.

Singler, A. (2015). Doping prevention–demands and reality: Why education of athletes is not enough. In V. Moller, I. Waddington, & J. Hoberman (Eds), *Routledge Handbook of Drugs in Sport* (pp. 239–248). New York: Routledge

Smith, E. (2006). The strength-based counseling model. *The Counseling Psychologist*, *34*(1), 13–79.

Smith, C. (2017). Tour du dopage: Confessions of doping professional cyclists in a modern work environment. *International Review for the Sociology of Sport*, *52*(1), 97–111.

Thompson, C. (2008) *The Tour De France*. Berkeley: University of California Press.

Van Reeth, D. & Lagae, W. (2012, May). *Public opinion on doping in cycling: How cycling interest, cycling activity and doping knowledge matter*. Presentation given at the Annual Congress of the Arbeitskreis Sportökonomie, Magglingen, Switzerland.

Waddington, I. & Smith, A. (2009) *An Introduction to Drugs in Sport: Addicted to Winning*. Abingdon: Routledge.

Waddington, I. & Smith, A. (2013). *Sport, Health and Drugs: A Critical Sociological Perspective*. London: Routledge.

Wagner, U. (2010). The International Cycling Union under siege- Anti-doping and the biological passport as a mission impossible? *European Sports Management Quarterly*, *10*, 321–342.

Walton, G.M. (2014). The new science of wise psychological interventions. *Current Directions in Psychological Science, 23*(1), 73–82.
World Anti-Doping Agency. (2018). *2017 Monitoring Program Figures.* Retrieved from www.wada-ama.org/en/media/news/2018-06/wada-publishes-2017-monitoring-program-figures
Yeager, D.S. & Walton, G.M. (2011). Social-psychological interventions in education They're not magic. *Review of Educational Research, 81*(2), 67–301.

Chapter 16

What to do with the TUE process? Bradley Wiggins, therapeutic use, and data sharing

A critical analysis

Andrew Bloodworth, Luke Cox, and Michael McNamee

Introduction: the therapeutic use exemption process in anti-doping policy

The majority of anti-doping scholarship has focused on the rationale for such a policy itself, and the problems arising from the consideration of substances and methods for the Prohibited List (PL). More recently, the therapeutic use exemption process (commonly referred to as the TUE process) is an aspect of anti-doping policy that has come under scrutiny. This scrutiny was heightened after Russian hackers 'Fancy Bears' managed to hack and disclose some of the World Anti-Doping Agency's (WADA's) records of top athletes and the therapeutic use exemptions they had been granted (Fancy Bears, 2016). The data published by the Russian hacking organisation, Fancy Bears, and in particular the details of Bradley Wiggins' therapeutic use exemptions also formed part of a UK Parliamentary Inquiry into Combatting Doping in Sport (Digital, Culture, Media and Sport Committee, 2018). This chapter will offer an ethical analysis of the problems arising from the application of the TUE process. This includes a discussion of proposals to (i) abolish the TUE process altogether; (ii) and make details of athletes' TUE applications and awards more widely (even publicly) available, as a way of discouraging exploitation or dishonest use of the process.

The WADA TUE policy allows an athlete with a medical condition (that meets the criteria outlined below) to receive controlled access to a substance on the Prohibited List (see WADA, 2018). Based on WADA's criteria (stated below) a substance may only be permitted for an athlete's use on the basis that it will merely restore normal function for that athlete, rather than offer an enhancement to performance. Below are WADA's criteria for obtaining a TUE:

> An Athlete may be granted a TUE if (and only if) he/she can show, by a balance of probability, that each of the following conditions is met:
>
> a The Prohibited Substance or Prohibited Method in question is needed to treat an acute or chronic medical condition, such that the Athlete

would experience a significant impairment to health if the Prohibited Substance or Prohibited Method were to be withheld;

b The Therapeutic Use of the Prohibited Substance or Prohibited Method is highly unlikely to produce any additional enhancement of performance beyond what might be anticipated by a return to the Athlete's normal state of health following the treatment of the acute or chronic medical condition;

c There is no reasonable Therapeutic alternative to the Use of the Prohibited Substance or Prohibited Method;

d The necessity for the Use of the Prohibited Substance or Prohibited Method is not a consequence, wholly or in part, of the prior Use (without a TUE) of a substance or method which was prohibited at the time of such Use.

(WADA, 2016: 10)

Athletes are in principle entitled to the appropriate treatment of acute or chronic medical conditions, even if such a treatment requires the use of a substance on the Prohibited List. Use of such a substance, however, must be 'highly unlikely' to result in an additional enhancement beyond restoration of the athlete's normal function.

A complex anti-doping policy instrument such as this raises a number of questions. At the root, the policy offers a distinction between therapy (or treatment) and enhancement. Challenges to this distinction bring into question not only the TUE policy, but also the entire anti-doping effort.[1] The literature within the philosophy of medicine attests to the fact that it is also notoriously difficult to define health, and what constitutes a significant impairment to health (Boorse, 2011; Nordenfelt, 2001; Schramme, 2007) in an indisputable way. Certainly, the TUE policy inherits some of these difficulties and differences that may prove harmonising the policy a challenge. Moreover, the qualification that the drug be 'highly unlikely' to produce additional enhancement has raised questions in the literature pertaining to vagueness (Pike, 2018). Previous versions of the policy (WADA, 2011) more straightforwardly stipulated that no additional enhancement to the athlete receiving a TUE was permissible. The introduction of the term 'highly unlikely', however, can be understood as a recognition that the practice of medicine and medical science cannot grant assurance that therapies would be categorically non-enhancing. The clause 'highly unlikely' might therefore create a space where athletes have proper access to medications while preventing reasonably foreseeable exploitation and avoiding an anti-doping rule violation.

One possible line of argument is to focus not on the policy itself, as the origin of ethical and practical difficulties, but on the exploitation of the process by dishonest athletes and athlete support personnel. The full extent of TUE exploitation is unclear. The scholarly and journalistic literature suggests athletes perceive that the system is being exploited (Overbye & Wagner, 2013) and presents some first-person confessions of such practices (Coyle & Hamilton, 2012). Analogous to the problem of ascertaining valid estimates of the prevalence of doping itself,[2] the actual extent to which TUE exploitation is a widespread problem is unclear. By 'exploitation of the policy' we refer to the approved access to otherwise prohibited medications via the TUE process in an attempt to gain an advantage over competitors, rather than merely to restore their normal function. It is thought that athletes could, by manipulating the extent of an existing condition, or even fabricating such a condition altogether, gain access to medication (or an enhanced dosage) in an undeserved manner that may prove beneficial to them in performance terms. Such abuse should, it could be argued, be prevented or detected by a stringent administration of the process itself (for further details of the process, and how it is handled, see The International Standard for Therapeutic Use Exemptions (WADA, 2016: b)). The practice of medicine, however, relies not only on scientific data, but on the reporting of symptoms by the patient, and treatment will of course follow in part on the basis of this reporting of conditions whose causes are uncertain or disputed (as in the case of all 'syndromes'). This inescapable feature of medical practice may well offer scope for exploitation.

A tale of (Triamcinolone acetonide and) two Sirs

The accusation of TUE exploitation has been levelled at cyclist Sir Bradley Wiggins in recent UK Parliamentary committee hearings. It should be noted that Sir Bradley is Britain's most decorated Olympian. The details of Wiggins' TUE use, which he later commented upon publicly (Gibson, 2016), were illegally revealed as part of the Fancy Bears hack of WADA's database. There, and in subsequent discussions and media reports, it became clear that Wiggins was granted a therapeutic use exemption certificate for the administration of glucocorticoids prior to three major races. Wiggins did not commit any anti-doping rule violation in obtaining controlled access to these drugs, which he used for the prevention of hay-fever induced asthma (Armstrong, 1996). The anti-doping authorities were aware of this condition and had approved its use. Controversy, however, followed the disclosure. Some cyclists and indeed some scientific evidence suggested that the substance for which Wiggins was treated had an enhancing effect (Raul, Cirimele, Ludes, & Kintz, 2004; Duclos, 2010). It should be noted that the validity of these claims is not without challenge. If evidence were indeed compelling for an effect of this nature, the TUE for the drug should not have been granted. Granting the TUE suggests that the enhancing question is at the very least contested, and that due process has not been challenged by commentators, we may conclude that those granting the TUE thought additional enhancement was 'highly unlikely'.

Nevertheless, the timing of the TUEs, and the nature of the drug, has led some to suggest that this has contributed to the very significant reputational loss for both Wiggins' and Team Sky's much vaunted reputation for 'clean' success.

The situation for Team Sky, and for its head Sir David Brailsford worsened during a Digital, Culture, Media and Sport Committee (UK Government) review into doping in sport (DCMS, 2016), including the use of the TUE process. During the inquiry a number of those involved failed to identify precisely the contents of a so-called 'mystery package', delivered to Wiggins for another race in 2011. This package was the subject of a subsequently dropped UK Anti-Doping inquiry. Subsequently, Team Sky disclosed that the package contained the decongestant Flumicil, which is not on the Prohibited List. This disclosure became the subject of considerable debate not least because of the delay in identifying the medication, but the inadequacy or incompleteness of medical records pertaining to the Fumicil disclosure and other treatments to Team Sky riders. Members of the Committee queried why Brailsford was unaware of the details of his athlete's medical records given the historical cynicism around doping in elite cycling and the much-publicised clean approach of Team Sky. Nevertheless, Brailsford maintained that he was not privy to the details of Wiggins' medical treatment (DCMS, 2016). Members of the committee seemed unhappy with this response. Quite whether Brailsford's defence concerning medical confidentiality is as weak as suggested by some will be the subject of discussion below.

The Parliamentary Enquiry reported its findings in the early part of 2018. Practices at Team Sky came under significant criticism for a number of issues (i) the apparent exploitation of apparent grey areas, for example the use of medications not on WADA's Prohibited List (such as tramadol or out-of-competition corticoid use) for their alleged enhancing effects; (ii) the poor keeping of medical records; and (iii) their lack of support for a subsequent UK Anti-Doping enquiry. Somewhat surprisingly, the Enquiry also inferred that Wiggins did seek to exploit the TUE process for performance gain. For this conclusion to be properly founded, however, it would depend on access to Wiggins' medical records and an understanding of his intention neither of which is presented in their report. Wiggins continues to deny vehemently that he sought to exploit the TUE process in this fashion.

Should we abandon the TUE process altogether?

The foundational question concerning the TUE process is whether it should exist at all. In light of the significant risk of exploitation does its presence compromise anti-doping efforts? Dimeo and Møller (2017) argue that it is time to scrap the TUE system altogether. It is notable, however, that despite their strong line, the very last few sentences of their article suggest room for a slightly softer stance, suggesting that WADA explore ways to soften this blow for those in genuine need. Their argument in favour of scrapping the TUE process comes in three parts: (1) the potential for exploitation of the system; (2) the lack of consistency in administration of the process; and (3) that scrapping the system would be both in the short-term and long-term interests of athletes' welfare.

Our view aligns to some extent with the reasons offered here, and the need to address them. But, we argue, these reasons do not sufficiently support the abolishment of the TUE policy: effectively, their cure is worse than the condition it seeks to ameliorate.

First, we consider their account of the potential exploitation of the TUE policy. Dimeo and Møller offer some evidence of either perceived exploitation of the process, or suggest that the culture of elite sport is such that unscrupulous athletes will use it to try and obtain some form of advantage. There ought to be no denying this possibility. Inventing a condition to obtain a prohibited substance would be following neither the spirit nor letter of the law so to speak. Rather, it would be merely a deception in order to dope. But Dimeo and Møller might refer here to an example of an athlete seeking the most powerful drug that might reasonably be thought of as a treatment for a condition, and the highest dose of it, to try and gain some benefit that extends beyond the restorative. This is obviously problematic, were it to occur, and the suggestions are that this is occurring, and athletes are gaining an unfair advantage over their competitors. The process is being used as a way of making further marginal performance gains. Dimeo and Møller suggest that cycling coach Shane Sutton has said as much in a recent television programme. The *Guardian* newspaper reports the dialogue from the BBC programme:

> If you've got an athlete that's 95% ready and that little 5% niggle or injury that's troubling them, if you can get the TUE to get them to 100%, of course you would in them days.
>
> The business you're in is to give you the edge on your opponent and ultimately it's about killing them off but you definitely don't cross the line and that's something we've never done.
>
> [Asked if] finding the gains might mean getting the TUE, [Sutton repeated the question, before adding:]
>
> Yes, because the rules allow you to do that.
>
> (Fotheringham, 2017)

First, we should note a relevant ambiguity in Sutton's comments. Sutton may be interpreted as referring to marginal gains supported by a restoration of health rather than using the TUE process to extend performance beyond normal function (enhancement). Indeed, this is the more generous interpretation. The potential for the TUE process to lead to enhancement is a serious issue. Pike (2017) argues persuasively, that healthcare professionals are unable to foresee all the effects of taking a medication on the PL, intended and unintended, and make concrete conclusions regarding the potential for enhancement. This would require the professional to be confident that in each individual, who may well react in different ways to a substance (as we have seen in the discussion of Chris Froome's recent Adverse Analytical Finding), the effects of the drug can be more or less precisely predicted in terms of ensuring restoration only, and any secondary effects prevented. Expecting this degree of precision from current medical knowledge seems unreasonable. Indeed Pike (2018) suggests that WADA should loosen their criteria to allow for moderate enhancement, a move that he argues is more reflective of the current state of play. Importantly though, Pike does not suggest that this loosening is a threat to the TUE process altogether.

Pike offers an original application of the doctrine (or Principle) of double effect to anti-doping. Reserved commonly for discussions of healthcare professionals, the distinction is often used to support or decry the hastening of a dying patient's death or indeed abortive practices. Its justification splits philosophers and bioethicists equally (Kamm, 1999; McMahan, 1994). Roughly put, defenders focus on the original intention in pursuit of ethically valuable ends, while detractors focus on the negative foreseeable consequences. In the context of the present discussion the salient difference between athletes using medications should not be understood in terms of the complex effects of the medications themselves, but in terms of the intentions behind the use of such medications (Pike, 2018). This negates the assumption that the abuse of the TUE process is the primary goal of the athlete (or their support system). Dimeo and Møller are nevertheless concerned with those who intend to cheat, and the possibility of the TUE process to provide a useful vehicle for achieving this without detection, or indeed with the approval of the anti-doping authorities. Pike's work is ultimately critical of WADA's current lack of interest in the intentionality of athletes, at least in this process, to determine whether an anti-doping rule has been committed. We do not engage with the difficult issue as to how best to incorporate intention into anti-doping policy here. We do note, however, that the use of strict liability elsewhere in the prosecution of ADRVs means at least that their approach is consistent. Moreover, it would add a layer of complexity and finance to attempt to revise the regulatory framework and processes to a degree where a panel could be 'comfortably satisfied' of the athlete or their doctors intentions, or even come to such a decision on the 'balance of probabilities' – a stronger jurisprudential conclusion.

Our recommendations with regard to the TUE policy, and in particular with regard to concerns as to its exploitation raised above, echo Pike's own defence of the process. We should retain the policy, although we would not object to an adjustment of the language employed to more adequately reflect the ambiguities at play here. In short, we shall argue for the importance of the TUE policy as a just policy that protects athletes' welfare and livelihoods where they might suffer from a genuine, potentially chronic medical condition. We argue for the policy despite the potential for enhancement and indeed exploitation that might exist. It is the lesser of two evils so to speak.

First, in support of this argument, grant a basic point. From the fact that a rule can be exploited we cannot conclude automatically that there is something wrong with the rule itself. Diving ('simulation' in FIFA-speak) in football has a number of similarities to the exploitation of the TUE process. It involves deception, in order to seem as if one is playing by the rules, while in fact the attempt is for an illegitimate advantage. We might argue over whether the foul in football is a rule more central to the sport than the anti-doping rules and TUE process. But we might also suggest that the response to diving should be the same as the response to the TUE process. Target more directly those in the wrong who are trying to cheat, rather than change rules or policy.

Second, we acknowledge that there is potential for enhancement inherent in the TUE process. This is not the place (neither are we the people!) to conduct a review of the science. Medicine may not currently possess the precision required to limit the effects of the medication to the purely restorative, or to limit the secondary effects that impact upon performance. We still argue that fairness dictates athletes, where necessary, have access to substances on the Prohibited List for medical treatment. Loland develops an idea of fairness in sport based upon 'Equality of opportunity to perform' or the Fair Opportunity Principle (FOP). The crux of Loland's Fair Opportunity Principle is as follows:

> we should eliminate or compensate for essential inequalities between persons that cannot be controlled or influenced by individuals in any significant way and for which individuals cannot be deemed responsible.
>
> (Loland, 2010: 118)

Essential inequalities are understood as inequalities with a significant influence on sporting performance. Assuring athletes fair opportunities to perform does not just require adequate classification to moderate the effects of differences like size, weight, or financial inequalities. It requires that athletes unlucky enough to suffer from a medical condition have an opportunity for compensation in the form of appropriate medical treatment. Athletes with medical conditions cannot simply, via training, compensate for the effects of these conditions. Where the condition is unlikely to impact upon training or performance the TUE should not be granted. But where there is likely significant impact upon performance, this also concerns the potential for significant disruption to athletes' careers and livelihoods, or indeed prevention of some individuals from taking up the sport at an elite level altogether. Justice may in some instances not require equality, but the differing treatment of those in differing need. Some athletes are unequal in respect of suffering from a medical condition that impacts upon their sporting participation, justice requires that anti-doping policy may be applied *mutatis mutandis*. Where an athlete genuinely requires access to medications, even those on the PL, they ought to have access to them to the degree relevant to their medically relevant circumstances.

A further point, raised by implication should be considered. One can only wonder what implications there might be for Paralympic sport were Dimeo and Møller's proposals taken on board more generally. What, for example, would a consistent position be on those who require various treatments and devices in order to compete in the first place? Any policy based, at least in part, on compensatory justice is likely to create problems of line drawing. Our position is a principled one: we uphold the primacy of athletes' right to healthcare and medical treatment over their prohibition from competition on the grounds of unmerited medical conditions.

Attempts to classify athletes in this fairness-promoting way in sport cannot rely upon exact sciences. Good and wise judgement is the best we may hope for, and that is likely to generate exceptions and even some unpalatable conclusions. Likewise, the TUE process, limited as it is by the application of current medical knowledge, cannot guarantee an entirely level playing field. This issue of perceived unfairness that the TUE can give rise to, however, is not as significant as that which would result in preventing the competing of those on the grounds of a medical condition, or at least preventing them receiving standard medical treatment for the condition and competing.

A defence of the process in terms of justice does not of course remove the potential for exploitation. Indeed, our analysis, in acknowledging potential indirect enhancing effects, leaves this as a distinct possibility. Our suggestion here would be to challenge the ethics of those involved, athletes, and indeed athlete support personnel, rather than seek to remove a process that can support those with a genuine medical condition to continue in their occupation. If problematic norms exist that would normalise exploitation then it is the norms be addressed, rather than policy further shift to reflect these ethically problematic behaviours. This is of course easier said than done. One solution should be the development of auditing to deter abuses, either by athletes or 'rogue' doctors. Athlete profiles could be monitored in a manner analogous to the current use of Athletes' Biological Passports or the so-called steroid profile. This view would be consistent with the medically conservative one that exploitation of the TUE process involves the *misuse* of medical means, properly understood as aimed at the relief of suffering and restoration of function (Edwards & McNamee, 2006). A separation of performance and medical functions, organisationally and in terms of their respective aims, might discourage those otherwise inclined to pressure or utilise medical professionals in the pursuit of competitive advantage. This separation might be further strengthened where the fate of coaching staff, if results are poor for example, is not in anyway tied to the fate or job security of medical teams or departments.

Second, Dimeo and Møller cite an inconsistency in application and indeed understanding of the process. Again, we are in agreement with many of the points here. The first appears to suggest that the process creates an injustice, whereby those with certain injuries must rest, but those with conditions that might respond to certain treatment do not, and can seek rectification via the TUE process. This, we hold, is an inescapable inequality in sport, some injuries respond better to different forms of treatment. The key part of the process is to ensure approval of the appropriate treatment, even if this involves a banned substance. The following points, however, raise some concerns central to the practice of elite sport in general. First, it is argued that those with privileged knowledge and access will be more likely to use the process, and thus compete, while others without such knowledge may be unable to perform or return to play. Indeed, Loland (2010) has indicated his own concerns with uneven access to sports science systems support in general. Here we might say, in agreement with Dimeo and Møller, that there is plenty of work to be done in educating relevant athletic (and media) populations concerning anti-doping policy, namely the TUE policy, and its challenges. But the aim here should be to democratise access to sports science support and sports medicine support more generally. That way sport can test the athletes' hard work and natural ability, not their access to sports science support or knowledge of the intricacies of anti-doping policy. This might of course sound a somewhat idealistic line. Essentially, we reject policy changes that promote or strengthen the currently inequitable distribution of sports science and sports medicine support. Instead we support Loland's view of sport that seeks to democratise such access, while retaining a policy that is essentially in the interests of sick athletes. Our argument would be to continue with a rigorous anti-doping education, in order to better inform athletes of the appropriate processes should they be ill or injured, and possibly require prohibited substances.

Dimeo and Møller also express concern that some athletes, hindered by their own ethical sensibility, will be less likely to use the process, and thus place themselves at a disadvantage. This seems a pertinent concern. We might think of students in a university, and the reticence of some to use the extenuating circumstances system to gain a deadline extension, despite good reason, as a comparator. Again, we might question whether the solution should be the abolition of the process. Instead, as we suggest above, perhaps through increased education, we could facilitate proper use of the process. It is, after all, there for those that *need* it. They *need* medical treatment in order to compete at normal function, and the appropriate medical treatment is a banned substance. Students and athletes might choose not to use the process, either autonomously electing to suffer the disadvantage, or because they are not sure that their condition really affects their performance so significantly.

Dimeo and Møller's final abolitionist argument is a paternalistic one concerning the potentially damaging effects on athletes' long-term and short-term health. Athletes would, they suggest, be better off resting than competing having received the treatments that the TUE process allows. Are some interventions concerned with the restoring of the health of athletes, or have they extended to be more concerned with getting the athlete back competing regardless as to whether this in the athlete's longer term or shorter term best interests? The latter is a conceptual inflation of medicine beyond its traditional aims of restoration, and into the realm enhancement, sporting, goals (Edwards & McNamee, 2006). The aim should be to attain the *treatment* that best reflects the autonomous desires of the athletes themselves. They might be willing to accept some risk in order to compete, or, in adopting a more holistic less physical conception of health, claim that competing would actually be in their best interests both in terms of health and more broadly. Ensuring the athlete's decision is a free one, without coercion, requires careful consideration of the elite sport environment, and the context in which such decisions are made.

Sociologists Malcolm and Waddington (Waddington & Roderick 2002; Malcolm & Scott, 2013: Malcolm 2016; Waddington, Scott-Bell, & Malcolm, 2017) have produced extensive literature depicting elite sport environments in which medical confidentiality is not protected, can be affected by the conflicts of interests that medical professionals in these contexts face, and have questioned the nature and quality of the consent players might offer for the sharing of medical data. While our concerns here do not concern confidentiality and medical data directly they are relevant. To what extent is athlete autonomy being respected with regard to the TUE process? Are athletes able to offer their informed consent to treatments without interference perceived or otherwise from performance focused staff? The research of Malcolm and Waddington in this depicts an environment less attentive to these important issues of consent and autonomy, and more concerned with the ease of sharing information in the interests of the team or club as a whole.

Athletes seeking medical advice must be assured that their medical data will only be shared with their informed and considered permission. This should assure that their confidentiality is respected. This is an important step in ensuring that the decision to race, or to use medical treatment including a TUE in order to do so, is the athlete's own, made after careful contemplation of the risks involved. Organisations such as governing bodies and teams must be cognisant of the way in which team goals, and the longer term best interests of the athlete in terms of health may differ. Structures and functions, such as separation of medicine and performance functions, would help to ensure that where risks to health, or some impact upon longer term health is accepted, as is fairly commonplace in elite sport, this is a result of the informed judgement of the athlete, not the pressures of the environment within which they work. As an aside it should also be stated that the aim of the process is to rectify significant impairments to health, and also allows athletes suffering from chronic conditions to continue to compete, not just the often discussed response to an acute ailment.

In short, our defence of the TUE process in response to the criticisms of Dimeo and Møller concerns the relationship between the arguments offered and the conclusion. We acknowledge a problematic ethos within some sections of elite sport, and the implications of this for a process such as the TUE policy. We argue that while many of the reasons hold, a more optimistic view of the possible culture of elite sport, rather than an acceptance of current norms, makes room for changes that address these practices, rather than rule changes. In the following sections, we seek to explore one possible way of addressing and reducing the possible exploitation of the TUE process.

Enhancing the therapeutic use exemption process: confidentiality, transparency, and medical data sharing

Having tentatively defended WADA's TUE process as it stands we move to consider ways of enhancing it via exploitation-reducing measures. The controversy over Bradley Wiggins' TUEs are a useful start point with which to consider potential solutions. Our concern, however, is a more general one. As we have noted Team Sky's Sir David Brailsford has been criticised for not being fully aware of the medications or treatments that his riders were receiving. Having endured such criticism it is perhaps unsurprising that Brailsford has proposed an entirely transparent TUE process (Butler, 2016), in which data concerning medications are shared not only within teams and performance staff, but also to the public. This may have some sort of advantage in terms of restoring trust in the process itself. Elsewhere, however, we have argued against an essentially public TUE process, suggesting that this is an indefensible invasion of athlete's privacy (Cox, Bloodworth, & McNamee, 2017). Waddington, Scott-Bell, and Malcolm (2017) demonstrate that a weaker version of transparency is already in existence in some form. In this form data is shared freely within teams, between medical and performance staff. This should not be necessarily seen as a transgression of patient confidentiality, where effective medical treatment is indeed a team affair (McNamee, 2014). This might help ensure proper oversight and adherence to anti-doping policy. The advantages are clear. Those in a position such as Brailsford's, ultimately accountable we might argue, will be able to retain oversight over medications, and ensure due process.

Before raising some concerns some conceptual ground needs charting. In using the concept of 'privacy' we are referring to a state or condition of limited access to a specified thing (Beauchamp & Childress, 2013) under the discretion of the individual seeking to protect that access (Solove, 2005). In medical interactions, we might expect certain information to remain completely private (not to be disclosed further) and some only to be disclosed in a manner in line with the professional relationship with which both the doctor and patient are engaged. A breach of confidentiality would concern information being disclosed in a fashion that deviates from this typical interaction, in a manner in which I, the patient, have not consented to.

Pike (2018) has argued in favour of a public TUE policy, and indeed one in which the athletic community are involved in the decision-making process over whether they are granted. Here we have been predominantly focused on a defence of the policy itself. An ethical analysis of a transparent TUE policy is the topic for another paper. At this stage though we note two important reservations. First, objections might be made purely in terms of the importance of respecting autonomy of athletes' decision, and related to this, respecting of their privacy. In the current anti-doping climate, it might be difficult for athletes to decline to release their data in this way, without looking like they are trying to hide something. A process that itself requires the release of data, rather than being an athlete choice, raises serious questions as to the balance between supporting anti-doping efforts and pressures on athletes to accept privacy invasions not expected in other occupations. The hacking of WADA's databases should serve as a warning here.

Second, even if advocates of a transparent TUE process are not persuaded by appeals to autonomy and privacy of this nature, the overall consequences of such an approach may compromise the justice that the policy seeks to promote. Pete Sampras was said to guard his medical conditions exceptionally closely so that his opponents could not exploit them. A similar point may be made of any athlete whose injury status might be exploited – quite legitimately – by opponents. Under some conceptions of transparent therapeutic data process to access otherwise prohibited medications, athletes may be coerced into disclosing conditions that unfairly render them at a competitive disadvantage.

Conclusion

Our primary focus has been the defence of the TUE process as it stands. We acknowledge potential for exploitation and enhancement inherent in the process but offer some tentative proposals for addressing an ethos that accepts exploitation, rather than doing away with a valuable policy. Fairness, as we have argued, is an important goal in sport. Following Loland (2002), we have argued that enabling access to medical treatments under conditions of necessity and with highly unlikely enhancing effects, seems the least worst policy on offer. It affords athletes rights to healthcare while retaining (some) oversight of zealous or permissive athletes, sports medicine, and science support team. These rights extend to those concerning the proper access to what are considered private medical data. We have expressed concern that the proper goals of sports medicine appear to be under pressures of conceptual inflation (Edwards & McNamee, 2006), from the therapeutic to enhancement goals. Conflicts of interest arise at the close intersection of sports medicine goals and those concerned with performance. The exploitation of the TUE process is an example of these distorted ways in which some view sports medicine.[3] Separating the functions of medicine and performance within teams and organisations, rather than increasing the transparency of the TUE process, may in the longer term be a better way of demonstrating the separateness of the process from performance and enhancement aims.

Notes

1 A discussion of this is beyond the scope of this chapter. See Morgan (2009); Daniels (2000).

2 For a recent review on the prevalence of doping, and some of the problems in conducting research of this nature, see de Hon, Kuipers, and van Bottenburg (2015).

3 We should note here that recent empirical interviews and questionnaires with sports medicine professionals have suggested a group wholly attentive to their responsibilities to patients first and foremost. So our comment is not intended as a report on the values of the profession generally.

References

Armstrong, D. (1996). Sympathomimetic amines and their antagonists. In D. Mottram (Eds), *Drugs in Sport* (pp. 56–85). London: Chapman & Hall.

Beauchamp, T. & Childress, J. (2013). *Principles of Biomedical Ethics*. New York: Oxford University Press.

Boorse, C. (2011). Concepts of health and disease. *Philosophy of medicine*, 13–64.

Brailsford, D. (2016). Team Sky considering making all TUEs public in order to boost transparency. Retrieved from www.insidethegames.biz/articles/1042071/team-sky-considering-making-all-tues-public-in-order-to-boost-transparency Accessed 13 January 2018.

Butler, N. (2016) 'Team Sky considering making all TUEs public in order to boost transparency' Inside the Games: Available Online www.insidethegames.biz/articles/1042071/team-sky-considering-making-all-tues-public-in-order-to-boost-transparency Accessed 5 February 2018

Cox, L., Bloodworth, A., & McNamee, M. (2017). Olympic doping, transparency & the therapeutic use exemption process. *International Academic Journal on Olympic Studies*, *1*, 55–74.

Coyle, D. & Hamilton, T. (2012). *The Secret Race: Inside the Hidden World of the Tour de France: Doping, Cover-ups, and Winning at All Costs*. UK: Transworld Publishers.

Daniels, N. (2000). Normal functioning and the treatment-enhancement distinction. *Cambridge Quarterly of Healthcare Ethics*, 9(3), 309–322.

de Hon, O., Kuipers, H., & van Bottenburg, M. (2015). Prevalence of doping use in elite sports: A review of numbers and methods. *Sports Medicine*, 45(1), 57–69.

Digital Culture Media Sport. (2016). Combatting doping in sport. Retrieved from www.parliamentlive.tv/Event/Indexfe5a6178-448d-44cc-835d-7ee6cd91b6e4 Accessed 20 January 2018.

Dimeo, P & Møller, V. (2017). Elite sport: time to scrap the therapeutic exemption system of banned medicines. Retrieved from https://theconversation.com/elite-sport-time-to-scrap-the-therapeutic-exemption-system-of-banned-medicines-89252 Accessed 20 December 2017.

Duclos, M. (2010). Glucocorticoids: a doping agent? *Endocrinology and Metabolism Clinics of North America*, 39(1), 107–126.

Edwards, S. & McNamee, M. (2006). Why sports medicine is not medicine. *Health Care Analysis*, *14*(2), 103–109.

Fancy Bears. (2016). Hack Team. Retrieved from https://fancybear.net Accessed 20 January 2018.

Fotheringham, W. (2017) Shane Sutton defends Bradley Wiggins's use of TUEs for 'marginal gains' *Guardian*, www.theguardian.com/sport/2017/nov/18/shane-sutton-bradley-wiggins-tues Accessed 17 May 2018.

Gibson, O. (2016) Bradley Wiggins tells Andrew Marr 'I did not seek an unfair advantage' in the *Guardian*. Accessed Online www.theguardian.com/sport/2016/sep/24/bradley-wiggins-andrew-marr-unfair-advantage 5 February 2018.

Kamm, F.M. (1999). Physician-assisted suicide, the doctrine of double effect, and the ground of value. *Ethics*, *109*(3), 586–605.

Loland, S. (2010). 'Fairness in sport: An ideal and its consequences'. In M.J. McNamee (Eds), *The Ethics of Sports: A Reader*. London: Routledge.

Loland, S. & McNamee, M. (2000). Fair play and the ethos of sports: an eclectic philosophical framework. *Journal of the Philosophy of Sport*, *27*(1), 63–80.

Malcolm, D. & Scott, A. (2013). Practical responses to confidentiality dilemmas in elite sport medicine. *British Journal of Sports Medicine*, 0, 1–4.

Malcolm, D. (2016). Confidentiality in sports medicine. *Clinics in sports medicine*, *35*(2), 205–215.

McMahan, J. (1994). Revising the doctrine of double effect. *Journal of Applied Philosophy*, *11*(2), 201–212.

McNamee, M. (2014) *Sport, Medicine, Ethics*. Abingdon: Routledge

McNamee, M., Bloodworth, A., Backhouse, S., & Cox, L. (2017). *Sports Medicine Professionals and Anti-Doping: Knowledge, Attitudes, Behaviours and Ethical Stance*. (Unpublished research).

McNamee, M. & Phillips, N. (2009). Confidentiality, disclosure and doping in sports medicine. *British Journal of Sports Medicine*, *45*, *174–177*.

Morgan, W.J. (2009). Athletic perfection, performance-enhancing drugs, and the treatment-enhancement distinction. *Journal of the Philosophy of Sport*, *36*(2), 162–181.

Nordenfelt, L. (2001). On the goals of medicine, health enhancement and social welfare. *Health Care Analysis*, 9(1), 15–23.

Overbye, M. & Wagner, U. (2013). Between medical treatment and performance enhancement: An investigation of how elite athletes experience therapeutic use exemptions. *International Journal of Drug Policy*, *24*(6), 579–588.

Pike, J. (2018). Therapeutic use exemptions and the doctrine of double effect. *Journal of the Philosophy of Sport*, *45*(1), 68–82.

Raul, J., Cirimele, V., Ludes, B., & Kintz, P. (2004). Detection of physiological concentrations of cortisol and cortisone in human hair. *Clinical Biochemistry*, *37*(12), 1105–1111.

Schramme, T. (2007). A qualified defence of a naturalist theory of health. *Medicine, Health Care and Philosophy*, *10*(1), 11.

Solove, D.J. (2005). A taxonomy of privacy. *U. Pa. L. Rev.*, *154*, 477.

Thompson, T. (2017). 'Duty of Care in Sport Review'. Retrieved from www.gov.uk/government/publications/duty-of-care-in-sport-review Accessed 13 September 2017.

WADA. (2011). International Standard for Therapeutic Use Exemptions (ISTUE). Available Online www.wada-ama.org/en/resources/therapeutic-use-exemption-tue/international-standard-for-therapeutic-use-exemptions-istue Accessed 5 October 2018.

WADA. (2016). International Standard for Therapeutic Use Exemptions (ISTUE). Available Online www.wada-ama.org/en/resources/therapeutic-use-exemption-tue/international-standard-for-therapeutic-use-exemptions-istue Accessed 5 October 2018.

WADA. (2018). Prohibited List. Available Online www.wada-ama.org/en/resources/science-medicine/prohibited-list-documents Accessed 5 October 2018.

Waddington, I. & Roderick, M. (2002). Management of medical confidentiality in English professional football clubs: some ethical problems and issues. *British Journal of Sports Medicine*, *36*(2), 118–123.

Waddington, I., Scott-Bell, A., & Malcolm, D. (2017). The social management of medical ethics in sport: confidentiality in English professional football. *International Review for the Sociology of Sport*, *20*(12), 1053–1056.

Chapter 17

Doping relevance and the World Anti-Doping Code

Marjolaine Viret

In August 2017, multiple World Champion and Olympic medallist in cross-country skiing Therese Johaug was sanctioned by the Court of Arbitration for Sport (CAS) with an 18-month ban for using a balm to treat a sunburn on her lips. The balm turned out to contain the prohibited substance 'Clostebol', as she discovered when her urine sample was reported positive upon an out-of-competition test. The balm had been procured by her team doctor, and it was common ground that its application could not possibly have influenced her performances. The ban, which caused Johaug to miss the 2018 Pyeongchang Winter Olympic Games, was issued by the CAS based on a reasoning perfectly congruent with the rules imposed by the World Anti-Doping Code (WADC) (Rigozzi, Viret, & Wisnosky, 2017).[1]

In 2013, Lance Armstrong famously made his public confession to practising doping throughout his cycling career on an interview with US TV show host Oprah Winfrey. At that time, he had already been stripped of his victories and banned by the US Anti-Doping Agency (USADA) after a large-scale investigation. But he had never tested positive. Fast forward a few years and investigations into widespread doping practices in Russian sport revealed that doping conducted at institutional level had not disappeared, allowing athletes to cover up suspicious analytical findings, potentially robbing hundreds of competitors of a world champion or Olympic title. Even a few days before the start of the Olympics, participants and sport fans were left feeling perplexed as proceedings pending before the CAS lingered and uncertainty as to the legitimacy of the Russian athletes admitted to compete under neutral banner remained.

In these circumstances, it is understandable that the public would question the credibility of a system that tolerates such apparent discrepancies in its outcomes. It has become fashionable indeed to describe anti-doping programmes implemented under the WADC as both unfair on innocents and ineffective on cheats. Former WADA Director General David Howman, reportedly stated on various occasions that only the 'dopey doper' gets caught by routine testing protocols.[2] Similarly, former WADA President Dick Pound has been cited as supporting the position that those who fail a doping test fail two tests: an IQ test and a doping test.[3] Legitimate questions arise therefrom: are anti-doping programmes striking the targets they are shooting for? Should the goals of the anti-doping community to protect the 'clean athlete' from cheaters be restated to encompass more clearly protecting that same athlete from inadvertently becoming a 'dirty' one?[4] Finally, what can longitudinal monitoring of biological athlete values, in which cycling has been a pioneer, contribute to that effect?

This contribution aims to take a look at these questions. It is less concerned with cheaters that slip through the cracks, than with those athletes who, like Johaug, have their sample reported positive for relatively banal deeds. Before condemning the doping control system as a whole, it is important to acquire some essentials of the rationales underlying the WADC and the regulation set forth therein, specifically those underlying its evidentiary mechanics. This is necessary if we wish to have a productive, cross-disciplinary debate and suggest paths to improvement. To this aim, the contribution presents the evidentiary approach chosen by the WADC and analyses to what extent a 'failed doping test' can be considered indication of 'doping relevant' behaviour.

After clarifying the concept of 'doping relevance' and setting out the fundamentals of the WADC's evidentiary framework, the contribution compares violations based on traditional 'adverse analytical findings' (AAF) and those based on the 'Athlete Biological Passport' (ABP) for their doping relevance. With the increasing sophistication of detection tools, the historical evidentiary assumptions underlying the WADC may not always lead to satisfactory results for maintaining doping relevance of analytical findings, which makes certain adaptations to the system necessary. While some of those adaptations are already in place, the contribution concludes with suggestions to further enhance the doping relevance of analytical findings.

How to circumscribe 'doping relevance'

This contribution aims to assess the evidentiary approach of the WADC from the perspective of doping relevance. The term 'doping relevance' as used here is meant to identify the type of conduct that the fight against doping seeks to deter and punish under the WADC.

In social sciences, determining how the relevant athlete population understands 'doping' is a critical factor for the interpretation of studies aimed at assessing the prevalence of doping. Studies conducted through questionnaires reveal that athletes who use prohibited substances may not consider themselves to be 'doping', because they associate doping with an illegitimate way of improving sports performances, whereas their use occurred for recreational or medical purposes. Assessment of doping prevalence is thus complicated by possible discrepancies between what is prohibited by the WADC and what athletes believe to be prohibited (Lentillon-Kaestner & Ohl, 2011). From personal experience, asking 'what is doping?' when lecturing, or speaking to lay audiences, will invariably trigger answers involving a connotation of 'lack of fair play', 'illegitimate aim to improve performances', and a certain 'morally reprehensible' component.

These answers fit in well with the values behind the 'spirit of sport' as described in the Introduction of the WADC, which aims to protect what is intrinsically valuable about sport, or '*how we play true*'. In fact, it was one of the stated goals of the 2015 WADC revision to be harsher on the real cheats, and provide a more flexible framework for inadvertent violations (Rigozzi, Viret, & Wisnosky, 2013: 18).

During the workshop, Dr Pierre-Edouard Sottas, scientific advisor to WADA, presented a pragmatic approach to anti-doping, in the sense that the goal of the World Anti-Doping Program, namely '*to protect the Athletes' fundamental right to participate in doping-free sport*' (see section Purpose, Scope, and Organization in the WADC), could be achieved not through an elusive eradication of doping, but through a decrease of its 'effect-size', i.e. a reduction of doping practices (substances used and dosage) to an extent that 'clean' athletes retain a realistic prospect of winning. Dr Sottas identified the 'big 3' as EPO (blood doping), testosterone (steroid doping), and growth hormones. The introduction of the Athlete Biological Passport programme in cycling undoubtedly had an impact on the use of EPO. Dr Sottas showed how the number of cases successfully prosecuted for blood doping in all sports has increased by 300% since the introduction of the ABP. The ABP thus has a strong deterrence effect in terms of prevalence of violations, but also in terms of potential effect of these violations: 'game-changing' EPO and blood doping practices in general have considerably decreased, leaving space at most for more limited, sophisticated, protocols involving micro-dosing, with much lower impact on competition and the athlete's health.

From a policy perspective, then, focus on the 'effect-size' implies that the fight against doping is directed at behaviours that reach a level of significance sufficient to threaten the 'clean' athlete and jeopardise the latter's prospects of winning by playing fair. From a legal perspective, a similar, but more formal, test is to ask whether situations caught through doping control fall within the realm of the criteria set up by the WADC for defining the scope of the prohibition, i.e. for including a substance or method on the Prohibited List. These criteria are: potential for performance-enhancement, health risk, and violation of the spirit of sport (Article 4.3 WADC). Two criteria out of these three must be fulfilled in order for a substance or method to be contemplated for inclusion.[5] Therefore, an analytical finding arising from circumstances meeting none of the criteria deemed to warrant a prohibition cannot easily be considered doping relevant and ought not to lead to punishment.[6]

An initial finding is thus that circumscribing 'doping relevance' is not a straightforward task; perceptions seem to vary between the addressees of the rules, the policy-maker and the actual contents of the regulations. Indeed, what is regarded (or ought to be regarded) as doping could well form the subject of a separate analysis. For purposes of this contribution, we can work from the smallest common denominator and simply ask what is clearly not doping relevant in anyone's view. This would include any situation in which: (i) the athlete's performance could not possibly have been impacted in a way that would distort competition, nor was the athlete trying to enhance performances; and (ii) the athlete could not possibly be aware that a prohibited substance was entering his or her body, or was at most inadvertent (e.g. was negligent in context unrelated to his or her sports activities).

Fundamentals of the regulatory framework

The WADC defines 'doping' through a catalogue of 'anti-doping rule violations' set forth in its Articles 2.1–2.10 (Article 1 WADC). This contribution only considers the two standard violations that together account for the core of the doping prohibition. Those are: presence of a prohibited substance (or its metabolites or markers) in an athlete's sample (Article 2.1), and use of a prohibited substance or method (Article 2.2).

Per Article 2.1.1, a violation of 'presence' can only be established through a so-called 'adverse analytical finding', i.e. a report from a WADA-accredited laboratory that identifies in a sample the presence of a prohibited substance (or its metabolites or markers).[7] Unless the athlete is able to invalidate the AAF by demonstrating the existence of flaws in the testing or analytical process that could reasonably have caused the findings,[8] such a report is sufficient evidence to establish a violation of 'presence'. A violation of 'use', by contrast, can be established through 'any reliable means', per the general rule of the WADC (Article 3.1).

In spite of their different wording, both provisions ultimately aim at prohibiting the same circumstances: Article 2.1 is, in its roots, no more than a special means of evidence – detection of a prohibited substance in a doping control sample – that has been elevated to the rank of a violation *sui generis* to ease the evidentiary burden on anti-doping organisations (see below). In situations of suspected doping in which it is not possible to produce an AAF, anti-doping organisations are forced to fall back on Article 2.2 and prosecute the violation as one of 'use' through other evidence.

ABP cases are the most publicised category of 'use' violations,[9] and the one that has been most extensively formalised in WADA regulations.[10] From the very outset, cycling has been at the forefront of the development and implementation of the ABP as an effective tool of reducing so-called 'blood doping' (Zorzoli & Rossi, 2010). Beyond the demonstrated effectiveness of the approach in cycling (see above), the experience accumulated in this sport also eased the learning curve for other sports and for national anti-doping organisations to implement their own programmes. Unlike the AAF which is based on a single sample collection session, the ABP monitors biological parameters over time, to establish a longitudinal profile in which abnormalities can be detected when values excessively depart from the athlete's expected values and baseline. An AAF is frequently referred to in jurisprudence and literature as 'direct' evidence or 'direct' detection of doping. Cases based on abnormal ABP values (so-called adverse passport findings, APF), by contrast, are referred to as 'indirect'.[11]

The strict liability principle applies to both Article 2.1 and Article 2.2 violations. There is often confusion around the scope and meaning of this principle. A definition of strict liability was introduced during the 2015 WADC revision, whereby: '*it is not necessary that intent, Fault, negligence, or knowing Use on the Athlete's part be demonstrated by the Anti-Doping Organization in order to establish an anti-doping rule violation*' (Appendix 1 WADC). In other words, the prerequisites for establishing a strict liability violation are purely 'objective' (objective presence or occurrence of use)[12]; 'subjective' components related to the athlete's mind set (intention, negligence) are irrelevant. Unlike what is believed at times, strict liability does not mean that consequences necessarily entail for the athlete found to have committed a violation. The only automatic consequence is disqualification of results obtained in the competition in connection with which the testing took place (i.e. in-competition testing only; Article 9 WADC). The mandatory public disclosure of the violation (save for minor athletes; Article 10.13) could also be characterised as an automatic consequence.

Importantly, the strict liability principle does not extend to disciplinary sanctions *stricto sensu*, specifically the ineligibility provided for in the WADC. Even within the context of sports matters, it is accepted that no disciplinary sanction can be imposed in the absence of any fault.[13] Producing an AAF or establishing use of a prohibited substance or method only constitutes a *prima facie* case that the standard sanctions contemplated in Article 10 WADC (for a first offence: four or two years) are warranted. However, the burden of proof then shifts to the athlete to establish such an absence of fault, including the factual background behind the AAF, i.e. produce an explanation as to how the substance entered his or her body. The default sanction for a first offence depends on the type of analytical finding at stake, namely whether a so-called 'specified substance' is involved or not. The categories that are to be considered as non-specified are defined through Article 4.2.2 WADC and the Prohibited List. Specified substances are, per the WADC drafters, not to be '*considered less important or less dangerous than other doping substances*', but simply '*more likely to have been consumed by an Athlete for a purpose other than the enhancement of sport performance*' (Comment to Article 4.2.2). For non-specified substances, the presumption is one of intentional violation and the default sanction is four years; the burden is in full on the athlete to show grounds for reduction or elimination of that sanction. For specified substances, the default sanction is two years, and the burden of proof is on the anti-doping organisation to establish intentional doping (Article 10.2.1 WADC). This is the only exception in which the anti-doping organisation bears the burden of proof with respect to fault. In all other situations, the burden is on the athlete to convince the panel to depart from the default full sanction, which in practice proves one of the main hardships of the system (see below)

The standard of proof is one aspect through which the WADC seeks to take into account the athlete's position for greater fairness. For establishing a violation, the standard of proof on the anti-doping organisation is '*comfortable satisfaction*'. There has been much debate before CAS panels as to the exact bearing of this standard, but it is generally accepted that the standard lies somewhere between the 'beyond reasonable doubt' standard used in criminal law, and the 'balance of probability' standard used in common law civil proceedings.[14] In practice, this standard leaves a lot of flexibility for panels to adapt their assessment to the seriousness of the violation and the cogency of the evidence. Wherever the burden of proof is on the athlete, by contrast, the standard is by a mere '*balance of probability*' (Article 3.1 WADC). In short, this standard means that the fact alleged must be more likely than not to have occurred (i.e. the probability exceeds 50%; Viret, 2016: 86–88).

In its design, the WADC thus rests on the assumption that the presence of a prohibited substance typically results from intentional or at least significantly negligent use of the substance by the athlete. Every athlete who falls outside the realm of this assumption but is unable to convince the disciplinary panel of an 'innocent' explanation for the finding is, so to say, 'collateral damage' of the system.

Comparing doping relevance of adverse analytical versus adverse passport findings

Direct versus indirect evidence – a deceptive distinction?

As explained above, disciplinary panels adjudicating doping disputes often identify the AAF as 'direct' evidence or detection, as opposed to findings based on the ABP characterised as 'indirect'. The opposition 'direct' versus 'indirect' typically implies a closer versus more remote connection with a pre-defined reference standard, a certain degree of 'immediacy'. The term 'direct' conveys a sense of superiority, of higher legitimacy and reliability of the evidentiary findings made via such direct means. It also implies that the risk of erroneous findings of fact is lower, since the panel has the benefit of evidence that does not require further assumptions, known as 'inferences' in the evaluation of the evidence. Or, as the National Anti-Doping Panel in the cycling matter *Tiernan-Locke v UKAD* stated: '*An adverse analytical finding is, in general, an objective fact, whereas the conclusions to be drawn from deviations from a longitudinal profile require scientific judgement as to the significance of observed abnormalities*'.[15]

The question, then, is: what is the reference standard in this particular usage of the opposites, and is it true that an AAF does not require any inferences as to its significance?

This is certainly not the case if we consider doping relevance (as defined above) as a reference standard. For example, the report of an AAF for cocaine may give extremely reliable evidence of the presence of cocaine in the sample, but it does not tell us anything per se about the circumstances that led to this presence, nor about their doping relevance: the AAF may have arisen from actual 'intentional' doping (use for performance enhancement),[16] just as much as from recreational use, contamination through food or beverage (mate coca tea), sabotage,[17] or environmental contamination outside the athlete's control (banknotes, 'French kiss').[18] Finding which of the above scenarios occurred will require further evidence and inferential reasoning on the part of the disciplinary panel; the determination cannot be made directly based on the AAF alone.

Viewed from this angle, AAFs and ABP findings are both equally valid evidentiary methods, each targeting a different marker of a potential act with doping relevance. The first detects the presence of a substance in athlete fluids – which may (or may not) have impacted their physiology and may (or may not) result from a deliberate act of cheating. The second detects modifications in physiological values that could be due to such cheating, or to another cause. One marker is not a priori 'more direct' than the other. Instead, every piece of evidence requires the panel to draw inferences and assess whether the evidence presented is sufficient to establish the facts in dispute and the parties' respective scenarios (Viret, 2016: 102).

A more plausible interpretation is that the implicit reference standard when comparing the 'directness' of the AAF and the ABP is whether they allow for the finding of an anti-doping rule violation as defined in the catalogue of the WADC. Here, one can indeed argue that the AAF is immediate proof of 'presence' under Article 2.1, while ABP findings require experts to evaluate whether the values are sufficiently indicative of use of a prohibited substance or method under 2.2. This, however, is only because Article 2.1 erects 'presence' of a prohibited substance in a sample into a violation *sui generis* (see above). This does not automatically entail that doping-relevant inferences can be drawn from such a presence.

Here again, the WADC addresses this issue by standardising the assessment that the disciplinary panel is to conduct. The WADC considerably restrains panels when it comes to AAFs, by dictating the inferences to be drawn therefrom:

- AAF(s) = finding of doping, i.e. an anti-doping rule violation under Article 2.1;
- For specified substances = presumption of doping with significant fault;
- For non-specified substances = presumption of intentional doping.

In sum, labelling an AAF as direct evidence is only accurate in a very narrow sense, rooted in the regulatory technique of the WADC. The label is technically correct only if one takes as a reference the wording of the rule. But does this bring us any further? As explained, Article 2.1 and Article 2.2 have the same rationale: they sanction athletes who use (in the strict liability sense, i.e. as a purely objective fact) a prohibited substance or method (see above). The opposition 'direct' versus 'indirect' evidence thus obscures rather than clarifies the role and value of analytical evidence used in anti-doping (Viret, 2016:

694–700). It wraps the AAF into an aura of infallibility, and casts unwarranted doubts on the value of ABP data. The terminology may be appropriate for lawyers who are aware of the symbolic character behind the distinction, and of its limits. To the anti-doping community at large, to athletes and the general public, describing the AAF as direct evidence of doping implies that presence of a prohibited substance in a sample mandates an automatic inference that the athlete 'doped'.

Safeguards for guaranteeing doping relevance

Since the distinction 'direct' versus 'indirect' evidence proves of little value to characterise the significance of the AAF and ABP findings, it seems more to the point to ask how the system ensures the doping relevance of the two categories.

In the ABP system, when the profile values fall out of a reference range that is constantly refined based on the individual athlete's prior tests, the system will issue a flag (an atypical passport finding). The flag means no more than a warning that there is (too) little likelihood to observe these values assuming the athlete is 'normal', i.e. clean and not suffering from a pathology. It does not say anything, in and by itself, about the causes behind these abnormalities, in particular the likelihood of doping. The task of evaluating possible causes and weighing them against each other is assigned to an expert panel. The expert review compares three hypotheses: the athlete is doping; the athlete has a normal physiology (and is a statistical outlier); the athlete has a medical condition. As part of the process, the athlete is provided with the file and asked to explain the abnormalities. If the athlete has no explanations to present, or if the explanations are unanimously not considered sufficiently plausible compared to the hypothesis of doping, the experts decide to forward the case to the anti-doping organisation and recommend that an adverse passport finding (APF) be issued and disciplinary proceedings initiated.[19]

The essential point to retain from this summary overview is that doping relevance is an integral part of the expert review. Of equal importance, the burden of proof is in full on the anti-doping organisation to show that the hypothesis of doping (use of a prohibited substance or method) is established to comfortable satisfaction.[20] The maximum rate of false positive of the initial flag (atypical passport finding) is known, and the reference values are based on an estimation of the prevalence of doping in the athlete population. We have analysed elsewhere how the evaluation of ABP findings would benefit from a greater proficiency of experts and hearing panels in forensic standards and dealing with probabilities (Viret, 2016: 727–777). Nevertheless, if properly applied, the ABP is a tool that allows for taking into consideration the doping relevance of its findings; in fact, makes such consideration mandatory before an APF can be issued, and, *a fortiori*, before a finding of an anti-doping rule violation can be made.

This stands in stark contrast to the situation in which an AAF is reported. In the previous example of an AAF for cocaine (see above), scenarios involving consumption of ordinary foodstuff or contamination at trace level clearly do not fall within the realm of the criteria that justify the prohibition of cocaine under the WADC (i.e. they are not 'doping relevant' as we defined above), yet the AAF is identical and must be reported. From a viewpoint of doping relevance, an AAF thus ought to represent a starting point rather than the end of the story. Not so under the WADC: provided the AAF is 'valid' (i.e. not undermined by procedural flaws, see above), the AAF is declared 'absolute' evidence of an anti-doping rule violation. If an AAF is present, the disciplinary panel has hence no choice but to render a finding of an anti-doping rule violation There is no room for a case-specific assessment of doping relevance at this stage. In particular, the rate of false positive is not considered, and generally not accessible to the athlete. The assumption is probably that the rate of false positive inherent to the analytical method itself is too low to impact the evaluation of the evidence. However, this does not solve the issue of possible true (in the sense of analytically correct) positives arising from contamination of the sample or the athlete, which is important data to assess doping relevance. There is no information either as to how the prevalence of doping, especially with the substance detected and in the athlete's population, is taken into account, an important factor in weighing the a priori likelihood of a doping-relevant finding.

At the level of the disciplinary sanction, where the WADC allows for consideration of the evidentiary value of the AAF, it does so in an extremely generic way. Thus, AAFs for specified substances enjoy a more lenient treatment, since these only trigger a presumption of doping with significant fault or negligence (rather than intentional), and thus a default two-year period of ineligibility (which can be further reduced to a reprimand if no significant fault or negligence is established). Another type of situation on which the 2015 revision of the WADC sought to enhance fairness for athletes is for contaminated products. If the athlete can establish that the AAF came from a contaminated product (defined as a product that did not label the Prohibited Substance, nor was the presence of the Prohibited Substance identifiable through a '*reasonable internet search*', WADA Definitions, Appendix 1) then they can reduce their sanction down to a reprimand, provided also that they establish no significant fault or negligence.

In sum, while the AAF is generally referred to as 'direct' evidence, ABP findings are subjected to an expert evaluation with respect to their significance that presents a much better guarantee of doping relevance (see above) if properly applied, and in this sense a better protection of the athlete. Though, in theory, an anti-doping rule violation for an AAF should not automatically lead to disciplinary sanctions, in practice the system that shifts the burden of proof onto the athlete to explain the AAF (see above) results in sanctioning the athlete based on the AAF alone whenever the athlete is not in a position to provide such explanation. Because the AAF is, in principle, reported without regard to its possible causes, two categories of athletes are most at risk for the maximum four-year ban available for a first offence: the athlete who intentionally doped, but also the athlete who genuinely has no idea what the cause of the AAF could be.[21] In addition, the automatic disqualification of results may be the athlete's main or only concern (e.g. if an Olympic medal is at stake), and public disclosure of the violation may be career-ending and ruin the athlete's reputation. Both these consequences arise directly out of the AAF (see above); there is no defence against them and absolutely no room for an assessment of doping relevance.

Gradual erosion of assumptions underlying the regulation

The conundrum of enhanced analytical capacities

We have seen previously that the AAF dictates various assumptions to the disciplinary panel, in particular that the presence of a non-specified substance originates from intentional doping, whereas a specified substance originates at least from significant fault (see above). It is for the athlete to prove otherwise. It is worth exploring whether these assumptions can still claim general validity: is the athlete truly in a better position to explain the AAF than the anti-doping organisation?

In order to answer this question, it is worth recalling that the WADC was designed with 'zero tolerance' as a default setting (Article 2.1.3 WADC), and with the assumption that the challenge would be to develop analytical methods sufficiently sensitive to catch dopers. The WADA system thus supports an approach in which anti-doping laboratories are encouraged to constantly improve their capabilities in this respect. In order to be accredited, laboratories must be able to guarantee certain minimal capacities (so-called Minimal Required Performance Levels, MRPL); by contrast, the idea was that there should be no limits to laboratories striving for additional sensitivity (Viret, 2016: 344–349). As exemplified by the Johaug matter and other cases described in this contribution, a new challenge may now confront anti-doping organisations: how to restrict analytical findings to truly relevant ones.

The solution of choice, of course, is to enhance the significance behind the report of an AAF in and by itself, by making the analysis more sophisticated rather than improving its sensitivity. For example, Glucocorticoids (class S.9) are only prohibited via certain paths of administration per the WADA Prohibited List. Detection of a specific metabolite for the Glucocorticoid 'Budesonide' now allows anti-doping laboratories to determine whether a prohibited oral, or an authorised inhaled mode of administration has been used.[22] More generally, extracting as much additional analytical data as possible from the sample can greatly enhance the significance of the AAF. For example, the ratio between the parent drug and its metabolite(s), and the type of metabolite detected, can be useful information in determining the causes behind the AAF.

The presence of metabolites also rules out the hypothesis of a sample contamination during testing.

Whenever the science does not (yet) allow for enhancing the significance of the AAF, the rules can be adapted to account for the limited doping relevance in certain concentrations or circumstances:

- First, this can be done by imposing boundaries on the prohibition itself, i.e. introducing a threshold or other type of 'decision limit' to delimit the prohibited from the authorised findings (Saugy, Viret, & Giraud, 2016: 21–25). Below the threshold, there is no case to answer. The WADC system uses thresholds primarily for substances that can also be produced endogenously (naturally) by the human body. In isolated cases, thresholds have been used to limit other non-relevant findings (e.g. for the cannabis metabolite Carboxy-THC) or to identify permitted therapeutic usage.[23]
- Second, limitations (so-called reporting levels) can be set on the reporting duties of the laboratories. Here, the limit is a purely technical one: laboratories are invited not to report an AAF below the reporting level. The wording of the WADA Technical Document on MRPL is ambiguous ('*should*' not), so that there is no clarity regarding actions to take should an AAF be reported below the reporting level (Saugy, Viret, & Giraud, 2016: 20). More importantly, reporting levels are introduced on a generic basis – e.g. for all substances prohibited in-competition only, the reporting level is set at 50% of the MRPL. It is not clear how such a single fixed percentage can accurately correlate with doping relevance and potential effects at the reporting level, given the individual pharmacokinetics of each substance and its unique excretion curve.[24]

In other situations, the violation itself is not questioned, but the path for athletes to eliminate or reduce their sanction is facilitated. So-called 'recreational' drugs, for example, benefit from a few options for a privileged assessment. The prohibition of cannabis, in particular, has been disputed for some time among stakeholders in anti-doping. As a result, a Comment was introduced to the 2015 WADC in the Definition section (Appendix 1 WADC), whereby an athlete may establish no significant fault or negligence by '*clearly demonstrating that the context of the Use was unrelated to sport performance*'. This assessment has been extended, by analogy to cases of cocaine consumption, both by the UCI Tribunal (*UCI v. Paolini*) and a CAS panel (*FIFA v. Fernandez*).[25]

There are also cases in which the system simply does not offer satisfactory solutions. The substance 'Clenbuterol' is a good illustration of a situation in which accumulation of AAFs arising from common foodstuff makes their lack of doping relevance undeniable, forcing anti-doping organisations to seek solutions outside the regulatory framework. To this day, there is no threshold and no reporting level for Clenbuterol. Clenbuterol may also be used as a potent anabolic agent (class S1.2) and there are no analytical means to differentiate intake for doping purposes from meat contamination. The position adopted by WADA, however, is for Clenbuterol AAFs to be treated on a case-by-case basis: depending on the estimated concentration and the context, it is considered that the case should not go forward, which relieves the athlete from having to prove absence of fault.[26] Clenbuterol is thus currently dealt with in contradiction with the WADC rules, under which any AAF for a non-threshold substance must result in a finding of an anti-doping rule violation, shifting to the athlete the burden of proof with respect to the origin of the substance.

Outlook: an increase in non-doping relevant findings?

Beyond situations such as the mass occurrence of AAF for a specific substance that compel anti-doping authorities to react with extraordinary measures, there are those individual cases in which disciplinary panels struggle to justify the lenient treatment they feel would be appropriate for the athlete, while still remaining within the boundaries of the WADC. Cases in which athletes are sanctioned for unfortunate circumstances in spite of the panel's sympathy have always existed,[27] but athletes may get increased exposure to this risk as the sensitivity of analysis continues to improve.

What might increasingly prove a key problem of legal technique is that the test of 'No (Significant) Fault or Negligence' (Appendix 1 WADC) does not incorporate a component of doping relevance, or at least leaves relatively little space for taking into account this component. Athletes can be terribly dumb or even reckless in their everyday behaviour, but in a way that is totally unrelated to their performance and sports activity, which may place panels into a true dilemma. This dilemma was perceivable in the UCI Tribunal *UCI v Paolini* decision cited above, where the single judge drew a line between what would commonly be considered 'unreasonable' (i.e. consume cocaine for recreational purposes),[28] versus what the fight against doping aims to combat (i.e. athletes may consume whatever they wish as long as they do not return to competition with the drug still present).[29] Thanks to this reasoning, both Paolini and Fernandez (before CAS) obtained the benefit of a reduced sanction. Not every athlete is as lucky: during the same period, a football player who smoked out of a 'shisha' pipe during a birthday party the weekend before a match, unaware that the pipe also contained cocaine, was found to have been significantly at fault and received a two-year ban from CAS for not inquiring about the contents of the pipe.[30]

In our view, the thinking behind the *Paolini* and *Fernandez* cases could be transposed to any assessment of no (significant) fault or negligence, when the conduct: '*clearly can be dissociated from the sporting sphere*'.[31] Unless the anti-doping movement is to evolve into a morality police, dubious lifestyle choices should not automatically be equated with doping relevance, when there was neither impact on the sport performance nor violation of the spirit of sport, and the athlete's health was arguably not put at risk. Similarly, it should not be a prime objective of anti-doping programmes to punish stupidity. Therese Johaug paid, at most, for a certain degree of carelessness. She certainly did not pay for something that would remotely qualify as 'doping' as most would understand it.

An even more concerning prospect is the idea of AAFs arising from circumstances entirely out of the athletes' control and without their awareness. In these cases, athletes are dependent on chance, as much as on the readiness of their anti-doping organisation to get to the roots of the AAF. In 2016, a case study reported in Forensic Sciences International describes a Swiss athlete testing positive to Hydrochlorothiazide (HCTZ), a diuretic prohibited at all times. The origin was established to be the ingestion of a common non-prohibited NSAIDs drug (ibuprofen), purchased from a German pharmacy. Further analysis revealed that HCTZ was present in the drug at levels below the carry-over amounts allowed under pharmaceutical Good Manufacturing Practices (GMP), so that they could not be detected by the manufacturer of the drug. The athlete was only rescued by coincidence (he had one coated tablet of the ibuprofen left) and the anti-doping organisation's willingness to get to the bottom of the matter, in particular to order controlled administration studies that confirmed the levels recovered from urine after administering the tablets to volunteers were consistent with the levels detected in the doping control sample. The authors, among them WADA-accredited laboratory scientists and representatives of the Swiss national anti-doping agency, conclude: '*such a contamination represents a serious issue for elite athletes as doping control analytical assays are designed and tailored to utmost sensitivity for compounds prohibited according to the regulations of* WADA' (Helmlin et al., 2016: 171). The authors further recommended to consider introducing reporting levels for all specified substances and to systematically report an estimated concentration as a support for results management.

It is not clear what steps have been taken as a result of the case. The new Technical Document on MPRL 2018 does not introduce reporting levels for HCTZ, and in fact there is no reason to suspect that HCTZ would be the only potential contaminant in the pharmaceutical industry. More importantly, however, to our awareness, no warnings have been issued by anti-doping organisations to inform athletes that even licenced pharmaceuticals – probably the most tightly regulated products on earth – may be contaminated by prohibited substances in amounts that can lead to an AAF. Given the known widespread use of NSAIDS in elite sport, especially in close proximity to competitions (Fournier, 2012; Tscholl, Vaso, Weber, & Dvorak, 2015) it would not be surprising for other cases to arise. And in fact, a similar case seems to have been dealt with by the US Anti-Doping Agency (USADA) in late 2017. Though little information is accessible about the background, USADA reported that volleyball player Alexandra Klineman accepted a finding of no fault or negligence for a double AAF of both HCTZ and triamterene. During the investigations, the athlete provided to USADA records of intake of an authorised prescription medication (not named in the press release), but '*detailed laboratory analyses subsequently conducted on the medication tablets*' revealed contamination by the two prohibited substances, which were not named on the label.[32]

Of note, similar issues may arise with respect to ubiquitous medications (of which HCTZ is a prime example) ending up in ground water. Several cases have been reported over the past years in which such a possibility was evoked, sometimes successfully,[33] sometimes in vain.[34]

Suggestions for more relevant approaches, or how to minimise collateral damage

Today, every athlete runs the risk of testing positive to a prohibited substance for futile mistakes or circumstances entirely outside his or her control. The exact risk level is difficult to assess, but gaining a better understanding of such a risk would help determine whether the level is still acceptable to the 'clean' athlete that the World Anti-Doping Program aims to protect, especially given the strong indications that doping control still fails to nail large-scale doping schemes, and thus does not guarantee them a fair competition as a compensation. Having more accurate data on the current risk-level for each substance could also be vital to relativise the impact of an AAF on the athlete's reputation and awaken public perception to the (potential) lack of doping relevance of certain publicly reported findings.

The proportionality of the consequences to which athletes are liable in case of a positive test is crucial to the fairness of the system. One limb of the proportionality test is whether the sanction incurred is capable of meeting its justifiable aims. In our view, this requirement is not met if athletes are sanctioned for circumstances that could not influence their performance nor impact their health, especially if these circumstances are due to mere general inadvertence or could not be avoided at all. If the goal of WADA is to decrease the 'size-effect' in terms of types of substances used and their dosage so that 'clean' athletes retain a realistic prospect of winning (see above), this goal is thus primarily one of deterrence from 'genuine' doping practices. A deterrence effect, however, can only be created if athletes are capable of adjusting their conducts to avoid an anti-doping rule violation. Insofar as it proves impossible to avoid a violation, the deterrence effect becomes questionable and the system is not capable of achieving its stated goals, and thus arguably disproportionate.

Many of the suboptimal features described above can be explained through the limitations inherent in the very nature of an AAF. Since the AAF only provides a single-point value in the excretion curve, there is no straightforward way to tell where the sample collection lies in the detection window, thus whether the detected 'low' value is truly a trace level from environmental contamination or the remainder of an intake for doping purposes. Operating with zero tolerance, in these cases, leads to placing the risk of contamination unilaterally on the athlete tested, where the risk should be shared equally between the tested and the tester (and fellow competitors). Case-by-case management in crisis situations such as Clenbuterol allows to by-pass this problem, but shakes the credibility of the regulatory framework by operating ostensibly outside its boundaries.

In this respect, the ABP proves an interesting tool to strengthen doping relevance, especially in the sport of cycling that played a pioneer role in implementing the Athlete Biological Passport. The comparative views proposed in this contribution should hopefully reinstate the ABP into stronger evidentiary legitimacy: while the ABP is often seen as producing less 'straightforward' (and thus less solid) results than the AAF, it proves a tool superior to traditional doping control in terms of doping relevance if properly applied, in that ABP findings are subjected to a mandatory expert evaluation to determine their significance.[35]

Combined approaches could thus represent a 'quality label' for doping relevance. Sports which, like cycling and the Cycling Anti-Doping Foundation (CADF, in charge of doping control for the Union Cycliste Internationale), invest into developing a test distribution plan and use the data gathered from the ABP for intelligent testing are more likely to catch genuine doping cases, and therefore also less likely to catch the odd inadvertence case than random testing methods. A meaningful use of the ABP is to analyse ABP values to direct target testing or order additional analyses on samples in accordance with an underlying suspected doping pattern and thus produce AAFs which can then be prosecuted under Article 2.1 (Zorzoli & Rossi, 2010). Recent cases in cycling show the effectiveness of this approach.[36] These are not only a more efficient use of the anti-doping organisation's resources, but they also guarantee more relevant findings, since the AAF is backed up by biological parameters showing an effective impact of the substance on the athlete's physiology and frequently the possibility to construct a 'doping scenario'.

Where combined approaches are not available, much will depend on the nature of the substance at stake. For certain substances, the plausibility of a non-doping relevant explanation is rather remote (e.g. EPO). By contrast, for others, especially in low concentrations, doubts may arise as to whether the assumptions that led to the burden of proof being shifted onto the athlete when designing the WADC are still valid. These assumptions were that the likelihood of a truly 'innocent' – i.e. neither faulty nor even significantly negligent athlete – becoming a victim of the system was extremely unlikely and that such cases would remain marginal. In other words, it was considered close to impossible to be beyond reproach and nevertheless test positive, and one could suspect that this view is probably still widespread in the public. At the very least, it was expected that the athlete was the better party to explain the positive findings, which justified shifting the burden of proof to them. As various cases described above show, even this assumption may not always hold true.

Currently, unless reporting can be halted through a threshold or reporting level, doping relevance is only considered generically, and to a certain extent, for specified substances and contaminated products. Even then, the athlete still has to be capable of identifying the cause behind the AAF as a prerequisite for showing an absence of fault. Ironically, those athletes who are totally at loss for explaining the finding are those who enjoy the weakest protection under the WADC. The system offers no solution where the cause is so much out of the control of the athlete that it cannot be uncovered, or where the athlete acts stupidly but in a way that is completely irrelevant to anti-doping purposes.

Cases of trace-level contamination in licenced drugs are of particular concern here. It is somewhat surprising that the two cases described have not been more publicised (see above), and it is unclear what actions have been taken to prevent further cases from occurring. It may be that those carry-overs are actually exceptional; their frequency is probably difficult to assess since they are below GMP standards and would therefore not lead to any kind of action on the part of the manufacturers, nor possibly even be detectable by them. Another, gloomier, hypothesis is that athletes who test positive as a result are simply unable to explain their AAFs, being unaware that such contamination is even possible, so that the association with an authorised pharmaceutical drug is never made in the first place.

One way forward here, as recommended by the authors of the Swiss case study (see above), could be to generalise the use of reporting levels. Unless and until this is done, the role of communication by anti-doping organisations appears essential. In particular, athletes ought to be advised to systematically retain some sealed blisters of any licenced medication they use (as they should do for nutritional supplements). While there may be an understandable reluctance for anti-doping organisations to communicate about this risk, for fear of opening new lines of defence for cheats, in our view the concern of protecting the 'clean' athlete should prevail here. Where doping relevance cannot be achieved through analytical means alone, athletes should at the very least be empowered to avoid an anti-doping rule violation, or to maximise their prospects of showing that their circumstances warrant elimination or strong reduction of the sanction.

Notes

1 CAS 2017/A/5015, *FIS v. Johaug & NIF* & CAS 2017/A/5110, *Johaug v. NIF*, 21 August 2017.
2 WADA Website, speech in Melbourne, October 2015, www.wada-ama.org/en/media/news/2015-10/speech-by-wada-director-general-david-howman-challenges-to-the-integrity-of-sport; speech to the UNESCO Convention assembly in Paris, November 2011 (www.smh.com.au/sport/only-dopey-dopers-get-caught-20111115-1nh7x.html)
3 See e.g. https://uk.reuters.com/article/uk-sport-doping-wada/new-doping-allegations-hard-to-prove-says-former-wada-chief-idUKKCN0Y22UK
4 WADA press release of 24 March 2015, www.wada-ama.org/en/media/news/2015-03/wada-ado-symposium-prioritizes-protecting-clean-athletes
5 An additional, separate category encompasses substances that can mask use of another, prohibited, substance or method (Article 4.3.2 WADC).

6 We are truly questioning here the 'doping relevance' from a policy standpoint, not whether an anti-doping rule violation is formally committed under the WADC in an individual matter. The WADC explicitly precludes athletes from challenging the rationales for including a substance or method on the Prohibited List (Article 4.3.3).
7 More precisely, a combination of AAFs in A and B samples if the B sample is analysed, as described in Article 2.1.2 WADC.
8 For the exact mechanics, see Article 3.2.1 to 3.2.3 WADC.
9 'Use' violations may include purely non-analytical cases, such as the high-profile Australian 'Essendon' matter, in which players of an Australian football team were sanctioned on the basis of investigations only (see CAS 2015/A/4059, *WADA v. Bellchambers et al.*, 11 January 2016).
10 WADA APB Operating Guidelines (v.6.0), www.wada-ama.org/en/resources/athlete-biological-passport/athlete-biological-passport-abp-operating-guidelines
11 For recent examples: CAS 2017/A/4949, *Chernova v. IAAF*, 18 July 2017, para. 7; CAS 2016/O/4883, *IAAF v. ARAF & Trofimov*, 17 May 2017, para. 55; CAS 2015/A/4008, *IAAF v. ARAF, Kaniskina & RUSADA*, 25 April 2016, paras 8 & 81; UCI Anti-Doping Tribunal, 13 September 2017, *UCI v Diniz*, paras 6 & 53; UCI Anti-Doping Tribunal, 17 August 2017, *UCI v Moreira Lacerda*, para. 59. This distinction seems to have been introduced from the early days of ABP cases: CAS 2010/A/2235, *UCI v. Valjavec & OC Slovenia*, 21 April 2011, para. 7; UK Anti-Doping Panel, *British Cycling v. Tiernan-Locke*, 15 July 2014, paras 2/3.
12 Use as defined in the WADC refers to any objective form of administration: '*utilization, application, ingestion, injection or consumption by any means whatsoever*' (Appendix 1 WADC).
13 Explicitly in Comment to Article 2.1.1 WADC.
14 CAS 2015/A/4059, *WADA v. Bellchambers et al., AFL & ASADA*, 11 January 2016, paras 104–106.
15 UK Anti-Doping Panel, *British Cycling v. Tiernan-Locke*, 15 July 2014, para 12.
16 CAS 2014/A/3475, *Van Snick v. FIJ*, 4 July 2014.
17 CAS 2014/A/3475, *Van Snick v. FIJ*, 4 July 2014.
18 CAS 2009/A/1926 & 1930, *ITF v. Gasquet*, 17 December 2009.
19 The process is detailed in the WADA APB Operating Guidelines.
20 However, the UCI Tribunal in a recent case considered that the athlete bears a certain duty to cooperate and put forward plausible explanations other than doping ('*Beweisnotstand*'); UCI Anti-Doping Tribunal, 13 September 2017, *UCI v Diniz*, para. 69.
21 And who was unlucky enough to test positive to a non-specified substance.
22 WADA Technical Document on MRPL, note j, www.wada-ama.org/en/resources/science-medicine/td2018mrpl-0. According to the WADA HMR Committee Meeting of 29–30 August 2017, similar research is ongoing for certain Beta 2-agonists (Minutes, p. 3). www.wada-ama.org/sites/default/files/resources/files/minutes_hmr_committee_august_29-30_2017_final.pdf
23 WADA Technical Document on Decision Limits . Beta-2 agonists are a hybrid category: e.g. Salbutamol has a threshold, but athletes are still entitled to prove that the values resulted from a permissible consumption, through a controlled administration study on themselves.
24 Only in special situations have reporting levels been introduced specifically for one substance: e.g. Meldonium, after the crisis that ensued when the substance was placed on the Prohibited List in 2016 without awareness of its extremely long excretion pattern.
25 UCI Anti-Doping Tribunal, *UCI v Paolini*, 13 April 2016, para. 48; CAS 2016/A/4416, *FIFA v. CONMEBOL & Fernández*, 7 November 2016, paras 68 *et seq.*
26 WADA Statement, 2 April 2017: www.wada-ama.org/en/media/news/2017-04/wada-statement-on-ard-documentary

27 See e.g. in 2004 the case of Torry Edwards sanctioned with a two-year ban for a glucose tablet containing nikethamide (CAS OG 04/003).
28 UCI Anti-Doping Tribunal, *UCI v Paolini*, 13 April 2016, para. 43: *'Obviously, a "reasonable person" would never have consumed drugs to begin with, in particular drugs like cocaine the addictive character of which is well known'.*
29 UCI Anti-Doping Tribunal, ADT n°02/2015, *UCI v Paolini*, 13 April 2016, para. 43: *'However, from the standpoint of the fight against doping there is, in principle, no issue if these drugs are ingested in a recreational context unrelated to competition as long as the athlete does not return to competition with the drug still present in his or her system'.*
30 CAS 2016/A/4452, *Belaili v.* CAF, 4 November 2016, para. 69.
31 UCI Anti-Doping Tribunal, *UCI v Paolini*, 13 April 2016, para. 43.
32 USADA Press Release of 6 November 2017, www.usada.org/alexandra-klineman-accepts-finding-no-fault/
33 CAS 2014/A/3487, *Campbell-Brown v. JAAA & IAAF*, 24 February 2014; Sports Dispute Resolution Centre of Canada, *Burke v. Cycling Canada*, 2 October 2013.
34 CAS 2015/A/3925, *Smikle v. JADCO*, 10 August 2015.
35 Even though the expert review does not directly extend to evaluation of the athlete's fault, it is hardly imaginable how athletes could inadvertently commit a violation involving the blood passport, e.g. administer EPO or blood transfusions without at least some considerable degree of negligence. More difficulties may ensue if cases were to be prosecuted based on abnormal steroidal passports, in which one could more easily imagine scenarios arising from mere inadvertence. See the discussion in CAS 2016/A/4707, *Schwazer v. IAAF & NADO Italia & FIDAL & WADA*, 30 January 2017.
36 AAFs produced through intelligence-led testing: www.uci.ch/pressreleases/uci-statement-the-vuelta-ciclista-internacional-costa-rica/

References

Fournier, P.E. (2012). Prise d'anti-inflammatoires chez le sportif: limitons les abus. *Schweizerische Zeitschrift für Sportmedizin und Sporttraumatologie*, 60(4), 147–149.

Helmlin, H.J., Mürner, A., Steiner, S., Kamber, M., Weber, C., Geyer, H., Guddat, S., Schänzer, W., & Thevis, M. (2016). Detection of the diuretic hydrochlorothiazide in a doping control urine sample as the result of a non-steroidal anti-inflammatory drug (NSAID) tablet contamination. *Forensic Science International*, 267, 166–172.

Lentillon-Kaestner, V. & Ohl, F. (2011). Can we measure accurately the prevalence of doping? *Scandinavian Journal of Medicine & Science in Sports*, 21(6), 132–142.

Rigozzi, A., Viret, M., & Wisnosky, E. (2013). *Does the World Anti-Doping Code Revision Live up to its Promises?* Jusletter. Available at SSRN: https://ssrn.com/abstract=2411990

Rigozzi, A., Viret, M., & Wisnosky, E. (2017). *Johaug CAS award – Too harsh?*, Available at http://wadc-commentary.com/johaug/

Saugy, M., Viret, M., & Giraud, S. (2016). The View of the Laboratory and the Scientist (The WADA Code 2015 – most relevant changes). In M. Bernasconi (Eds), *Arbitrating disputes in a modern sports world.* Bern: 5th Conference CAS & SAV/FSA.

Tscholl, P., Vaso, M., Weber, A., & Dvorak, J. (2015). High prevalence of medication use in professional football tournaments including the World Cups between 2002 and 2014: a narrative review with a focus on NSAIDs. *British Journal of Sports Medicine*, 49, 580–582.

Viret, M. (2016). *Evidence in Anti-Doping at the Intersection of Science and Law.* The Hague: T.MC Asser Press/Springer.

Zorzoli, M. & Rossi, F. (2010). Implementation of the biological passport: the experience of the International Cycling Union, *Drug Testing and Analysis*, 2(11–12), 542–547.

Index

Milton Keynes UK
Ingram Content Group UK Ltd.
UKHW020314111024
449327UK00040B/937